W9-BEP-607

Health Policy and Politics

A Nurse's Guide

Health Policy and Politics

A Nurse's Guide

SECOND EDITION

JERI A. MILSTEAD, PhD, RN, FAAN

DEAN AND PROFESSOR
SCHOOL OF NURSING
MEDICAL COLLEGE OF OHIO
TOLEDO, OHIO

JONES AND BARTLETT PUBLISHERS
Sudbury, Massachusetts
BOSTON   TORONTO   LONDON   SINGAPORE

World Headquarters

Jones and Bartlett Publishers
40 Tall Pine Drive
Sudbury, MA 01776
978-443-5000
info@jbpub.com
www.jbpub.com

Jones and Bartlett Publishers
Canada
6339 Ormindale Way
Mississauga, ON L5V 1J2
CANADA

Jones and Bartlett Publishers
International
Barb House, Barb Mews
London W6 7PA
UK

Jones and Bartlett's books and products are available through most bookstores and online booksellers. To contact Jones and Bartlett Publishers directly, call 800-832-0034, fax 978-443-8000, or visit our website at www.jbpub.com.

Substantial discounts on bulk quantities of Jones and Bartlett's publications are available to corporations, professional associations, and other qualified organizations. For details and specific discount information, contact the special sales department at Jones and Bartlett via the above contact information or send an email to specialsales@jbpub.com.

The authors, editor, and publisher have made every effort to provide accurate information. However, they are not responsible for errors, omissions, or for any outcomes related to the use of the contents of this book and take no responsibility for the use of the products and procedures described. Treatments and side effects described in this book may not be applicable to all people; likewise, some people may require a dose or experience a side effect that is not described herein. Drugs and medical devices are discussed that may have limited availability controlled by the Food and Drug Administration (FDA) for use only in a research study or clinical trial. Research, clinical practice, and government regulations often change the accepted standard in this field. When consideration is being given to use of any drug in the clinical setting, the health care provider or reader is responsible for determining FDA status of the drug, reading the package insert, and reviewing prescribing information for the most up-to-date recommendations on dose, precautions, and contraindications, and determining the appropriate usage for the product. This is especially important in the case of drugs that are new or seldom used.

Copyright © 2004 by Jones and Bartlett Publishers, Inc.

All rights reserved. No part of the material protected by this copyright may be reproduced or utilized in any form, electronic or mechanical, including photocopying, recording, or by any information storage and retrieval system, without written permission from the copyright owner.

ISBN-13: 978-0-7637-3158-8
ISBN-10: 0-7637-3158-7

Library of Congress Cataloging-in-Publication Data
Health policy and politics: a nurse's guide/edited by Jeri A. Milstead.—2nd ed.
    p. ; cm.
Includes bibliographical references and index.
  ISBN 0-7637-3158-7
1. Nurses—United States—Political activity. 2. Nursing—Political aspects—United States. 3. Medical policy—United States. 4. Medical care—Political aspects—United States.
  [DNLM: 1. Legislation, Nursing—United States. 2. Health Policy—United States. 3. Politics—United States. WY 33 AA1 H399 2004] I. Milstead, Jeri A.
  RT86.5.M54 2004
  362.17'3'0973—dc22   2003021208
6048

Production Credits

Acquisitions Editor: Kevin Sullivan
Production Manager: Amy Rose
Associate Production Editor: Renée Sekerak
Editorial Assistant: Amy Sibley
Marketing Manager: Joy Stark-Vancs

Manufacturing Buyer: Amy Bacus
Composition: Shepherd Incorporated
Cover Design: Kristin E. Ohlin
Printing and Binding: Malloy, Inc.
Cover Printing: Malloy, Inc.

Printed in the United States of America
10 09 08 07 06   10 9 8 7 6 5 4 3

Contents

Contributors

Elizabeth Ann Furlong, PhD, RN, JD
Associate Professor
School of Nursing
Creighton University
Omaha, Nebraska

Renatta S. Loquist, RN, FAAN, MN
Director of Congregational Care
Northeast Presbyterian Church
Columbia, South Carolina

Jeri A. Milstead, PhD, RN, FAAN
Professor and Dean
School of Nursing
Medical College of Ohio
Toledo, Ohio

Ramona Nelson, PhD, RN
Professor and Co-Director of Health Care
 Informatics Program
College of Health and Human Services
Slippery Rock University of Pennsylvania
Slippery Rock, Pennsylvania

Patricia Smart, PhD, RN, FNP
Professor and Faculty Assistant to the
 Provost and Assistant to the President
Clemson University
Clemson, South Carolina

Ardith L. Sudduth, PhD, RN, FNP
Assistant Professor
School of Nursing
University of Louisiana at Lafayette
Lafayette, Louisiana

Mary K. Wakefield, PhD, RN, FAAN
Director, Center for Rural Health
University of North Dakota
Grand Forks, North Dakota

Marlene Wilken, PhD, RN
Assistant Professor
School of Nursing
Creighton University
Omaha, Nebraska

Preface

This book is a research-based, contributed text for advanced practice nurses (APNs). The scope of the content covers the whole process of making public policy. Components of the process are addressed within broad categories of agenda setting; government response; and program design, implementation, and evaluation. The primary focus is at the federal and state levels, although the reader can adapt concepts to the world or local level. Some nurses are sophisticated in their political activity. They have served as Senate or congressional district coordinators for the American Nurses Association, volunteered as campaign managers or workers for elected officials, or presented testimony at congressional or state hearings. However, even these nurses often think legislation when they hear policy. Few know the reality of how a bill becomes a law, where ideas for those bills are derived, or how the decisions to create one program rather than another are made. This book addresses the policy process as a broad range of decision points, strategies, activities, and outcomes that involve elected and appointed government officials and their staffs, bureaucratic agencies, private citizens, and interest groups. The process is dynamic, convoluted, and ongoing; not static, linear, or concise. Knowledgeable nurses in advanced practice must demonstrate their commitment to action by being a part of relevant decisions that will ensure the delivery of quality health care by appropriate providers in a cost-effective manner.

Nursing as a profession is based on practice. For many years that practice has been interpreted as direct, hands-on care of individuals. Although this still is true, the profession has matured to the point where the provision of expert, direct care is not enough. Nurses of the third millennium can stand tall in their multiple roles of provider of care, educator, administrator, consultant, researcher, political activist, and policy maker (Milstead, 1997). The question of how much a nurse in advanced practice can or should take on may be raised. The information explosion continues to present new knowledge exponentially. Nurses have added more and more tasks that seem important to the professional nurse and essential for the provision of quality care to the client. Is political activism necessary? All health professionals are expected to do more with fewer resources. Realistically, how much can a specialist do?

Drucker (1995), in addressing the need for more general-practitioner physicians rather than specialists, redefines the generalist of today as one who puts multiple specialties together rapidly. Nursing can benefit from that thought. In Drucker's definition, the APN must be a multidimensional generalist/specialist. This means that the APN combines knowledge and skills from a variety of fields or subspecialties in order to function effectively in the new paradigm of health care or, more importantly, to actually design the new paradigm. This also means that the APN must demonstrate competence in the multiple roles in which he or she functions. To function effectively in the role of political activist, the APN must realize the scope of the whole policy process, and the process is much broader than how a bill becomes a law.

It is natural for nurses to talk with bureaucrats, agency staff, legislators, and others in public service about what nurses do, what nurses need, and the extent of their cost-effectiveness and long-term impact on health care in this country. For too long, nurses talked to each other. *Each* knew their value; each told great stories; they "preached to the choir" of other nurses instead of sharing their wisdom with those who could help change the health care system for the better. Today's nurses, especially those in advanced practice who have a solid foundation of focused education and competent experience, know how to market themselves and their talents and know how to harness their irritations and direct them toward positive resolution. As nurses, each must embrace the whole range of options available in the various parts of the policy process. The opportunity to sustain an ongoing, meaningful dialogue with those who represent the districts and states and those who administer public programs is theirs to initiate. Nurses must become indispensable to elected and appointed officials. APNs must demonstrate leadership by becoming those officials and by participating with others in planning and decision making.

Why a Second Edition?

The first book was well-received and has been used by nurses in at least five countries. When the original publisher changed focus from health, education, and criminal justice to law and business, Jones and Bartlett picked up the option for this book and encouraged us to write a second edition. The contributors were enthusiastic and agreed that it was time. The Information Age is upon us and everyone struggles to stay current. The political agenda changes quickly, in spite of incremental changes in political systems. So, what's new?

Each chapter has been updated with current thought and references. Beth Furlong, in Chapter 2, includes new agenda-setting research. Additionally there is a wonderful story about how an army nurse, Diane Carlson Evans, created the Vietnam Women's Memorial. Dr. Furlong also updated how the National Institute of Nursing Research (NINR) contributes to the profession of nursing and added more practice implications for APNs. In Chapter 4, Renatta Loquist discusses the impact of the nursing shortage on regulations and licensure. Her insightful thought provides a policy dimension to the problem. Pat Smart includes in Chapter 5 more information about economics, noting that this topic is becoming integrated in policy courses. Dr. Smart also expanded and updated relevant Web sites. Marty Wilken, in Chapter 6, writes about the umbrella legislation that has occurred in many states. This legislation will be introduced in Nebraska as a bill to require all four types of APNs to have the same title, APRN. Dr. Wilken also discusses direct reimbursement, prescriptive authority, and physician supervision, especially as these issues may spawn problems in finding work sites for nurse practitioners. Ardie Sudduth re-titled Chapter 7 as Program Evaluation rather than Policy Evaluation. Although the two topics are similar, there is a difference in scope. Dr. Sudduth argues that APNs should become involved in the process of evaluating programs and offers practical and helpful suggestions in weaving through the process. She also broadens the discussion of outcome-based evaluation and the ethics of program evaluation. In Chapter 8, Ramona Nelson updated and revised all Internet sources and links—a formidable task in the fast-changing world of information technology. Dr. Nelson discusses the impact of the Internet on all steps of health policy development. Chapter 9 presents the Milstead Model, a comprehensive framework for studying nursing and health policy across countries and cultures. The model integrates policy components and the role of the advanced practice nurse. We think you will appreciate and like the changes.

Target Audience

This book is intended for several audiences:

1. Nurses who work in advanced practice in clinical, education, administrative, research, or consultative settings can use this book as a guide for understanding the full range of the policy components that they did not learn in graduate school. Components are presented with theoretical foundations and are brought to life through actual nursing research and nurses' experiences. This book will help the nurse who is searching for knowledge of how leaders of today influence public policy toward better health care for the future. Nurses in leadership positions clearly articulate nursing's societal mission. Nurses, as the largest group of health care workers in the country, realize that the way to make a permanent impact on the delivery of health care is to be a part of the decision making that occurs at every step of the health care policy process.

2. Graduate and doctoral students in nursing can use this text for in-depth study of the full policy process. Works of scholars in each segment provide a solid foundation for examining each component. This book goes beyond the narrow elementary explanation of legislation and bridges the gap toward understanding of a broader policy process in which multiple opportunities for involvement exist.

3. Faculty in graduate programs and other current nursing leaders can use this book as a reference for their own policy activity. Faculty and other

leaders should be mentors for those they teach and for other nurses throughout the profession. Because the whole policy process is so broad, these leaders can track their own experiences through the policy process by referring to the components described in this book.

4. Other health care professionals who are interested in the area of health care policy will find this book useful in directing their thoughts and actions toward the complex issues of both health care policy and public policy. Physicians, pharmacists, psychologists, occupational and physical therapists, physician's assistants, and others will discover parallels with their own practices as they examine case studies and other research. Nurses cannot change huge systems alone. APNs can use this book as a vehicle to educate other professionals so that, together, everyone in the health care profession can influence policy makers.

5. Those professionals who do not provide health care directly but who are involved in areas of the environment that produce actual and potential threats to personal and community health and safety will find this book a valuable resource regarding how a problem becomes known, who decides what to do about it, and what type of governmental response might result. Environmental scientists, public health official sociologists, political scientists, and other professionals involved with health problems in the public interest will benefit from the ideas generated in this book.

6. Interest groups can use this book as a tool to consider opportunities to become involved in public policy making. Interest groups can be extremely helpful in changing systems because the passion for their causes energizes them to act. Knowing how and when to use their influence to assist APNs at junctures in the policy process, interest groups can become partners in the political activity of nurses.

7. Corporate leaders can use this book to gain an understanding of the broad roles within which nurses function. Chief executive officers (CEOs) and other top business administrators must learn that nurses are articulate, assertive, and intelligent experts in health care who have a solid knowledge base and a political agenda. The wise CEO and colleagues will seek out APNs for counsel and collaboration when moving policy ideas forward.

Using This Book

Each chapter is freestanding; that is, chapters do not rely, or necessarily build, on one another. The sequence of the chapters is presented in a linear fashion, but readers will note immediately that the policy process is not linear. For example, readers of the Policy Implementation chapter will find reference to scholars and concepts featured in the Agenda Setting and Policy Design chapters. Such is the nature of the public process of making decisions. The material covered is a small portion of the existing research, argument, and considered thought about policy making and the broader political, economic, and social concepts and issues. Therefore, readers should use this book as a starting point for their own scholarly inquiry.

This book can be used to initiate discussions about issues of policy and nurses' opportunities and responsibilities throughout the process. The research studies that are presented should raise some questions about what should have happened or why something else did not happen. In this way, the book can serve as a guide through what some think of as a maze of activity with no direction but actually is a rational, albeit chaotic, system.

The Instructor's Manual is ideal for planning a class or addressing an audience. There are many activities presented, and I hope that they will serve as a stimulus to the readers' own creative thoughts about how to engage others. Gone are the days of the "sage on stage"—the teacher who had all the answers and lectured to students who had no questions. Good teachers always have learned from students and vice versa. Today's teachers/learners are interactive, technically savvy, curious and questioning, and capable of integrating large amounts of data and information. The manual can serve as a guide and a beginning.

References

Drucker, P. F. (1995). The age of social transformation. *Quality Digest,* February, pp. 36, 39.

Milstead, J. A. (1997). Using advanced practice to shape public policy: Agenda setting. *Nursing Administration Quarterly 21*(94), 12, 18.

Acknowledgments

Only a few nurses in the United States with master's degrees in nursing also hold earned doctorates in political science. Each such contributor to this book has researched a different component of the policy process and, therefore, a book immediately came to mind. The authors realize that there is much more to public decision making than the process of writing laws and that this knowledge affords them the opportunity and responsibility for contributing seriously to public policy. When I approached these nurses about contributing to this book, each agreed enthusiastically. Therefore, special thanks must go to Dr. Beth Furlong, Dr. Patricia Smart, Dr. Ardith Sudduth, and Dr. Marlene Wilken for their scholarly endowment. The two chapters on government response are a welcome addition due the importance of the content. Dr. Mary Wakefield served as chief of staff for North Dakota senators Quentin Burdick and Pete Conrad for several years. She has "been there, done that" and can explain just how a bill really does become a law. She adds the strong dimension of informal communication and negotiation that occurs as ideas are formalized into laws. Renatta Loquist, former executive director of the State Board of Nursing for South Carolina and past president of the National Council of State Boards of Nursing, is the most knowledgeable person I know to write about the regulatory process. In many ways a parallel process to legislation, the process of devising and approving regulations often is not recognized by nurses as important or as an opportunity for nursing input. Both Mary and Renatta were essential to the completion of this book. Dr. Ramona Nelson's contribution brings the nurse in advanced practice into the third millennium by identifying electronic resources that can assist the advanced practice nurse in preparing material, studying issues, and locating assets. There is a plethora of data that nurses can share with colleagues and officials. Dr. Nelson is one of the leaders in nursing informatics, and her investment in this book is substantial.

I must thank Jones and Bartlett Publishers for their encouragement and guidance in writing this second edition. I also thank the readers of this book for their interest in the policy process. For those of you who have integrated these components and concepts into your nursing careers, I applaud you. You already have contributed to the profession and to the broader society. For those readers who are struggling with how to incorporate one more piece into your role as an advanced practice nurse, remember that you are advancing the cause of nursing and health care delivery in this country and throughout the world every time you use this book. Nurses are a powerful force and can exercise their many talents to further good public policy, which, ultimately, must improve health care for patients, consumers, and their families.

Finally, I acknowledge with lots of love my four children, their spouses and significant others, and three grandchildren. They are always there for me and provide continuous support, encouragement, and unconditional optimism. I love you, Kerrin, George, Sunny, and George Biddle; Joan Milstead, Kevin Milstead, and Gregg Peace; Sara, Steve, and Matthew Lott. You make me smile.

Advanced Practice Nurses and Public Policy, Naturally

1

Jeri A. Milstead, PhD, RN, FAAN

Key Terms

Advanced practice nurse (APN)   A registered nurse with a master's degree in nursing, who demonstrates expert knowledge, skills, and attitudes in the practice of nursing.

New organizational paradigm   Conceptual approach to the arrangement of work from the traditional hierarchical bureaucracy to systems appropriate to the current information age.

Nursing's agenda for health   Policy expectations of a vision for nursing practice that includes prevention of illness, promotion of health, empowerment of individuals to assume responsibility for the state of their own health, expertise in the provision of direct nursing care, delegation and supervision of selected care to appropriate individuals, and the political influence to accomplish these goals.

Policy process   The course of bringing problems to government and obtaining a reply. The process includes agenda setting, design, government response, implementation, and evaluation.

Public policy   Actual directives that document government decisions; also, the process of taking problems to government agents and obtaining a decision or reply in the form of a program, law, or regulation.

Introduction

The advanced practice nurse of the third millennium must be technically competent, use critical thinking and decision models, possess vision that is shared with colleagues and consumers, and function in a vast array of roles. One of these roles is policy expert. In spite of the influence of Florence Nightingale in the 19th century, nurses in the 20th century nearly lost the role of the nurse in the political arena. Only at the end of the 1990s was this aspect of the role becoming integrated into the scope of practice of the advanced practice nurse. Policy and politics is a natural domain for nurses, and the full integration into practice chronicles nursing's heritage and the evolution of the profession and the health care system. Major changes in the profession and society mirror the evolution: changes in the practice of nursing, the emerging political role of nurses, finding a foundation in theory, and a new organizational paradigm.

Changes in the Practice of Nursing

The changing paradigm in the delivery of health care of the late 20th century is reflected in changes in the practice of nursing. In the early 1900s when nurses traditionally worked in homes or did home visits through an organized nursing service, nurses focused on personal care of individuals who were sick. As hospitals took on the function of workshops for physicians, nurses were employed to provide care to many individuals in one site. Just as organizational theorists were trying to establish the structure and function of institutional arrangements that developed with the industrial age, nurses were trying to establish the roles and functions of organizational employees in a system that was becoming very complex. Nurses categorized patients as those with primarily medical or primarily surgical problems, which led to the early differentiation of types of "floors" or areas in which nurses worked and which also differentiated nursing expertise in specific areas. Some nurses became organizational experts as they managed nursing units and whole hospitals.

As early as the 1940s, nurses were creating typographies of areas of nursing. Psychiatric, pediatric, obstetrical, medical, and surgical nursing were considered distinct clinical areas that were required for basic practice and, as such, were tested in early examinations for licensure. By the 1950s, nursing programs long had recognized the teaching of nursing as an area that required knowledge beyond the traditional baccalaureate degree. Bachelor of science degrees in nursing education (BSNE) had been offered at the undergraduate level to prepare nurses to teach in diploma schools of nursing. BSNE programs were phased out as specialization in all areas of nursing education, and clinical practice was ascribed to the master's level.

After World War II, veterans (including nurses) pursued college degrees through the GI bill. With the dearth of advanced nursing education programs, many nurses enrolled in education majors. Students and faculty in many areas were struggling with the impact of an explosion of knowledge and questioned whether their fields were "science" and whether the discipline fit the definition and expectations of a profession. For example, the discipline of political economy changed its name to political science and many nursing programs became "nursing science" programs. Practitioners of nursing adopted the scientific process and embraced the scientific theory of assessing, planning, implementing, and evaluating what nurses do. Nursing education programs sought courses in the natural sciences (chemistry and physiology) and social sciences (sociology and psychology) to provide a foundation for the nursing courses that were evolving with theories and models. Research became important to confirm nursing's position as a profession, but many of the studies examined the behavior of the nurse or the system of nursing education rather than clinical practice. The endorsement of the scientific approach as a logical, linear, and sequential process concomitantly rejected any indication of intuition or discernment of knowledge in any way other than what could be calculated by quantitative measures. The wisdom that was transferred through generations of nurses almost was lost by the insistence in academic programs of a focus on "hard" science.

By the 1960s, special care areas were surfacing in hospitals. As machines were invented for diagnostic testing and monitoring of patients, as early computers were developed, and as statistics evolved into a special branch of mathematics, physicians and nurses were placing patients into geographic and medically focused units where care could be concentrated. The emergence of coronary care units was quickly followed by the creation of intensive care units that soon became differentiated as surgical, trauma, neonatal, and other narrow domains. Nurses and physicians needed more knowledge and clinical skills to understand the medical, nursing, and technological advances that were occurring, and specialization became formalized into programs.

As nurses came to understand more about what constituted the practice of nursing, the boundaries of nursing expanded. Breaking free of the old-fashioned perspective of the nurse as handmaiden to the physician, nurses in the 1970s and 1980s sought autonomy as independent practitioners of *nursing*. Nurse practitioner programs were created to relieve a shortage of physicians. However, rather than becoming "junior doctors," nurse practitioners pushed out the margins of the discipline of nursing. Physical examinations, formerly limited to the scope of practice of physicians, were incorporated into nursing education programs, and physical examinations became essential to clinical nursing practice. Assertiveness training was taught in schools of nursing, which produced articulate registered nurses who could speak up. The nursing process became the watchword of the profession, and national standards were adopted based on assessment, diagnosis, planning, implementation, and evaluation criteria. Nursing theories were developed and research was conducted to test the theories. Certification in specialty areas acknowledged the clinical competence of nurses in distinct practice areas. Intensive care nurses became certain of and comfortable with their clinical knowledge and used it to provide physicians with indispensable data and to suggest treatment options. The rise in the number of baccalaureate-prepared nurses triggered a move toward graduate education. The number of doctoral programs in nursing was increasing. Although the improving image of nursing still did not command the respect from physicians, nurses gained respect and trust with the public.

By the 1990s, nurses were found in many settings. In addition to staff nurses, hospitals employed nurses as unit managers, educators in staff-development departments, coordinators of outpatient services, senior administrators, and creators of data-and-information systems. Nurses also served as infection-control officers, materials coordinators, patient-relations officials, and heads of quality improvement. Outside the hospital, nurses provided direct care in hospices and homes, in occupational health departments of business and industry, in prisons and correctional facilities, in schools, in interdisciplinary teams concerned with the health of astronauts, and in a host of military situations. Nonhospital, nondirect care opportunities found nurses directing their own continuing education companies, staffing professional and specialty associations, and combining nursing knowledge and skill with law and business degrees, in marketing and product sales, in pharmaceutical companies (as salespersons, researchers, and lobbyists), and in computer sales. Professional nurses also were contributing their expertise through positions as executive directors or members of boards of directors of social and health-related associations such as Planned Parenthood, Inc. Nurses were appointed to state boards of nursing; a few ran for public office; and some nurses directed or staffed offices of federal and state legislators, legislative committees and commissions, and bureaucratic agencies. The scope of nursing practice had expanded, and most state nurse practice acts reflected the changes in their legal definitions of nursing.

Laws that govern nursing define the practice of nursing and set the scope of practice of professional nurses. Early definitions of practice focused on the provision of direct care; later definitions added functions and roles such as "teaching, counseling, administration, research, consultation, supervision, delegation and evaluation of practice" and "observation, care, and counsel of the ill, injured, infirm, the promotion and maintenance of health" (*Laws Governing Nursing,* 1994, p. 3). Clearly, the role of the nurse had been expanded beyond caring for the sick patient. Laws governing advanced practice have emerged to offer title protection and legal guidance. Because all laws are the result of compromise, nurse practice acts reflect what is acceptable at the time, not the ideal.

The Emerging Political Role of Nurses

As early as the 1960s, social scientists from a broad array of disciplines had investigated the concept of occupational and professional roles. Concepts such as role ambiguity, role congruence, role conflict, and role taking were frequently cited in the literature (Argyris, 1962). Haas's (1964) early study of nurses clarified that role had four dimensions: task, authority or power, deference or prestige, and affect or feelings. In spite of Haas's study, however, the term *role* still is synonymous with *task* in most of the literature, and readers miss, therefore, a full understanding of the concept. There has been a major shift in the roles that nurses assume. In addition to clinical experts, nurses have become entrepreneurs, decision makers, and political activists. Many nurses realized that in order to control practice and move the profession of nursing forward as a major player in the health care arena, nursing and nurses had to be involved in the legal decisions about the health and welfare of the public, decisions that often were made in the governmental arena.

For many nurses, political activism meant letting someone else get involved. For some nurses, political activism meant dusting off the page in the high school or college *Problems in Government* textbook that presented an algorithm about how a bill becomes a law. A focus on the legislative process in which bills are drafted and passed by the Senate and the House of Representatives stimulated some grassroots connections between nurses and their legislative members. Nurses began to "tune in" to bills that affected a specific disease entity (e.g., diabetes), a population (e.g., the elderly), an issue (e.g., drunk driving), or a personal passion. Nurses learned to write letters to congresspersons and to visit them in their offices on occasion.

Organized nursing, especially the American Nurses Association (ANA), realized early that decisions that affected nurses and their patients often were made in Washington, DC. ANA moved its national headquarters to that city in 1992 (Kelly and Joel, 1995) to establish visibility and make a statement about the seriousness of purpose of the organization. ANA created political action committees (PACs) that developed processes for endorsing public officials through statements or with financial contributions to their campaigns. ANA also created a department of governmental affairs that employed full-time registered lobbyists who developed ongoing relationships with elected and appointed officials and their staffs. The development of staff relationships was especially critical as nurses learned that the way to access governmental decision makers was through their staff. By developing credibility with those active in the political process and demonstrating integrity and moral purpose as client advocates, nurses slowly became players in the complex process of policy making.

The ANA and its state and district levels educated nurses about the political process through continuing education programs, legislation committee structures, and the creation of Senate and congressional district coordinators. The latter were nurses who volunteered to create ongoing relationships with their U.S. senators and representatives in order to serve as liaisons between legislators and organized nursing. The creation of the Nurses Strategic Action Team (N-STAT) and state nurses association Legislative Liaison programs provided a grassroots network of nurses throughout the country who are informed when immediate action is needed and who respond quickly to their legislative representatives.

Political appointments of nurses were sporadic but strong appointments. Kristine Gebbie, RN, served as the "AIDS Czar" in the 1990s. Sheila Burke, RN, was chief of staff to Senate Majority Leader Bob Dole, and Dr. Mary Wakefield, RN, was chief of staff for Senators Quentin Burdick and Pete Conrad. Carolyne Davis, RN, served as head of the Health Care Financing Administration, the agency responsible for the third-largest federal budget and for shaping

Medicare and Medicaid policy. Virginia Trotter Betts, RN, a former president of ANA, was appointed senior health policy advisor of the U.S. Department of Health and Human Services during the Clinton administration. Also during that administration, Dr. Beverly Malone, RN, another former ANA president, served as deputy assistant secretary for Health and Human Services. Dr. Malone went on to become the general secretary of the Royal College of Nursing in England, Scotland, and Northern Ireland. These prestigious and powerful appointments came after many years of involvement in politics and with policy makers.

Nurses learned that by using nursing knowledge and skill they could gain the confidence of government actors. Communications skills that were learned in basic skills classes or in psychiatric nursing classes are critical in listening to the discussion of larger health issues and in being able to present nursing's agenda. Personal stories gained from professional nurses' experience anchor altruistic conversations with legislators and their staffs in an important emotional link toward policy design. Nurses' vast network of clinical experts produces nurses in direct care who provide persuasive, articulate arguments with people "on the Hill" during appropriations committee hearings and informal meetings.

Nurses began to participate in formal, short-term internship programs with elected officials and in bureaucratic agencies. Most of the programs were created by nurses' organizations that were convinced of the importance of political involvement. The interns and fellows learned how to handle constituent concerns, how to write legislation, how to argue with opponents and remain colleagues, and how to maneuver through the bureaucracy. They carried the message of the necessity of the political process to the larger profession, although the rank and file still were not active in this role.

As nurses moved into advanced practice and advanced practice demanded master's degree preparation, the role of the nurse in the policy process became clearer. Through the influence of nurses with their legislators, clinical nurse specialists, certified nurse midwives, certified registered nurse anesthetists, and nurse practitioners were named in several pieces of federal legislation as duly authorized providers of health care. The process was slow; however, the deliberate way of including more nurse groups over time demonstrated that to "get a foot in the door" is an effective method of allowing change within the seemingly slow processes of government. Some groups of nurses did not understand the political implications of incrementalism (the process of making changes gradually) and wanted all nurse groups named as providers at one time. They did not understand that most legislators do not have any idea what registered nurses do. Those nurse lobbyists who worked directly with legislators and their staff bore the brunt of discontent within the profession and worked diligently and purposefully to provide a unified front on the Hill and to expand the definition of *provider* at every opportunity. The designation of advanced practice nurses as providers was an entree to federal reimbursement for some nursing services, a major move toward improved client and family access and health care. Advanced practice nurses (APNs) became acutely aware of the critical importance of the role of political activist. Not only did APNs need the basic knowledge, they understood the necessity of practicing the role, developing contacts, working with professional organizations, writing fact sheets, testifying at hearings, and maintaining the momentum to move an idea forward.

However, most nurses still focus their political efforts and skills on the legislative process. They do not have an understanding of the comprehensiveness of the policy process, the much broader process that precedes and follows legislation. For APNs to integrate the policy role into the character of expert nurse, they must recognize the many opportunities for action. APNs cannot afford to "do their own thing," that is, just provide direct patient care. They cannot ignore the political aspects of any issue. Nurses who have fought the battles for recognition as professionals, for acknowledgment of autonomy, and for formal acceptance of clinical expertise worthy of payment for services have enabled APNs today to provide reimbursable, quality services to this nation's residents. The American Association of Colleges of Nursing (*Essentials,* 1996 and 1998) underscored the importance of understanding and becoming involved in policy formation, and the organization and financing of health care for the APN with its document on essential components of baccalaureate and master's education in nursing.

Finding a Foundation in Theory and Research

As nurses in the middle of the 20th century sought more education in institutions of higher learning, they found few nursing programs at the master's and doctoral levels. However, potential nurse scholars were exposed to an array of disciplines from which they could study. Many of those disciplines enjoyed an academic history and were respected for having a body of knowledge. Education, psychology, anthropology, and sociology were the most common academic fields entered by early nurse scholars, and the nurses soon adapted concepts, models, and theories to nursing practice. The process of teaching and learning, principles of adult education, and styles of leadership were drawn from the field of education. Psychology and sociology lent nursing a rational approach to studying behavior, helped nurses ascribe determinants of social and asocial conduct, and provided nursing with a theoretical foundation in interpersonal therapeutic communications. Through the study of anthropology, nurses learned about the customs and values of people different from themselves, the commonalities of human behavior, and the rigors of conducting field research. Aspects of these disciplines became integrated into nursing education, research, and practice.

Nurses became interested in the idea and applicability of theory and within a generation had begun considering the philosophical foundations and theories of nursing. Early nurse theorists, such as Peplau (1952), Orem (1971), and Henderson (1966), concentrated on organizing clinical practice as a deliberate, reasoned response by the nurse to sick people. This move toward intentional activity based on astute observations and thoughtful connections served nursing well. Nursing became "as much an intellectual activity as a physical endeavor" (Halloran, 1983, p. 17). Nursing theories were extrapolated from systems theory as Rogers (1970) and King (1971) developed and refined their thinking about the discipline. Watson (1979) and Benner (1984), building on humanistic concepts and examining the essence of the profession, furthered the theoretical foundation of nursing as they challenged others to conceptualize and redefine commonly held assumptions and relationships. Leininger (1978) confronted nursing's ethnocentricity and provided theoretical groundwork for cultural care from a global perspective. Nurse scholars in other countries, such as Grijpdonk in Belgium and Van de Brink Tjebbes in The Netherlands, developed theories that are being tested for applicability in their own and other cultures (R. Martijn, personal communication, November 12, 1997). These early nurse theorists, among others, changed the direction of nurses from dependent workers to autonomous thinkers.

The link between nursing research and advanced nursing practice became evident as nurses moved into graduate programs. Master's and doctoral education required research courses, practica, theses, and dissertations. The knowledge and skills that nurses developed served as a foundation for study in a wide array of disciplines and in as many areas of nursing as are available. Although much research was completed, not all of it added to the body of knowledge of clinical nursing. Early studies focused on attitudes and behaviors of nurses and nursing students. Inquiry into theories and models of education, instructional methods, and curriculum development and evaluation contributed to improved presentation of nursing in the academic setting and to the teaching/learning processes practiced by nurses in clinical settings.

Clinical nursing research became a focus area in the 1990s when outcome data were needed to defend nurse decisions. Clinical research cited in nursing journals moved from a few published studies to a wave of clinical trials in a variety of patient care areas. Brooten and Naylor (1995) referred to "nurse dose" (the amount and type of nursing needed to produce an effect of nursing care) as critical in determining outcomes. Blank (1997) named nursing case management as the vehicle through which health care will be restructured as the quality of nursing care is measured through clinical outcomes. Clinical pathways were espoused as a successful way to demonstrate the importance of outcomes to health care providers and payers (Porter-O'Grady, 1996; Zander, 1990). Hegyvary (1992) expanded the concept and proposed that patient outcomes reflect the economic, organizational, political, and social context within which they are studied. Far beyond local impact, the influence of nurse experts can never be overestimated for their work with the federal Agency for Health Care Policy and Research (AHCPR) in the development of clinical practice guidelines. As AHCPR evolved into the Agency for Healthcare Research and Quality (AHRQ), health services research took on an important role in further defining what nursing is and the value of nurses.

The initial link between nursing and policy can be viewed as beginning in the 1960s when nurses sought federal funding for research. The explosion of social programs and the raising of social consciousness that occurred in the 1960s and 1970s in the United States alerted nurses to the value of political activity. The professional association provided a structure for the voice of nursing and developed a cadre of nurses who contributed to policy formation and were committed to political activism.

Today's nurses have a much clearer understanding of what constitutes nursing and how nurses must integrate political processes into their practices to further the decisions made by policy makers. Nurses continue to focus on the individual, family, community, and special populations in the provision of care to the sick and infirm and on the activities that surround health promotion and the prevention of disease and disability. Advanced practice nurses have a foundation in expert clinical practice and can translate that knowledge into understandable language for elected and appointed officials as the officials respond to problems that are beyond the scale or impact of individual health care providers. As nurses continue to refine the art and science of nursing, forces external to the profession compel the nursing community to consider another aspect—the business of nursing—that is paradoxical to the long history of altruism.

A New Organizational Paradigm

The whole economic basis of capitalism, i.e., the manufacturing system, had become rapidly outdated by the beginning of the new millennium. Traditional organizational structures that were invented in the late 19th century to accommodate the move from a farm-and-feudal system to an urban-industrial system no longer fit a new age. Hierarchical, bureaucratic institutions had been the norm and centralized, top-down administration had been the method of control. Information was the new commodity, and communications systems were needed to create and disseminate the plethora of new material. The computer chip had replaced the printing press and forced a move to a new organizational model (Porter-O'Grady and Wilson, 1995). Efficiency and cost containment led to downsizing and rightsizing, which often were euphemisms for "smallsizing" that translated into firings and layoffs. Machine workers had been replaced by technologists, who were being replaced by "knowledge workers" (Drucker, 1959, p. 40). Knowledge workers required new structures and processes for doing their work.

The new paradigm for organizations in the 21st century begins with changes within one's head; that is, a move to a perspective that is outside the usual way of thinking. What work is done, where it is done, and how it is done are mundane questions that demand creative answers. Large manufacturing plants no longer are needed if merchandise can be made elsewhere and retailers can rely on just-in-time inventories. The very question of what product should be produced requires evaluation. The "where" of work has changed. Offices do not have to exist in a skyscraper, because a computer can be located at the beach, in a mountain retreat, or in a kitchen. However, the new worker cannot afford the isolation and detachment noted in the title character of Bartleby, the scrivener (Melville, 1853), who simply "preferred not to" be a part of the group. Drucker (1995) insisted that knowledge workers have two new requirements: (1) they work in teams and (2) if they are not employees, they must be affiliated with an organization. He emphasized that organizations are important because they provide a continuity that enables the worker to convert specialized knowledge into performance. Drucker (1999) also noted that productivity is an organization's greatest challenge. This is especially true in a company in which thinking and making decisions are the major processes. Systems thinking, a metaparadigmatic approach, is crucial to the effectiveness of an organization in the 21st millennium (Flood and Senge, 1999).

An organization must have a mission that is publicized and in which all workers (both traditional employees and managers) can invest their energies. Structures and processes should be constructed to facilitate the work of the institution (Wheatley, 1992). Part of the new paradigm is based on the assumption that prior worker-and-manager practices that evolved from the old bureaucratic model are outdated and must be replaced with collaborative communications that can mobilize and empower all people in the organization (Champy, 1995). People do not expect establishments to remain static or stable; organizations learn new lessons continuously or they fail (Senge, 1990). Peters (1988) addressed the chaotic nature of new companies as being patterned and dynamic, two characteristics of organizations in the new paradigm that provide direction for all levels of workers. Peters (1997) also noted that innovative organizations are inhabited by innovative people who seek affiliation with others in new, productive coalitions.

Partnerships are valued over competition, and the old rules of business that rewarded power and ownership have given way to accountability and shared risk. Reengineering the old systems to the new systems does not mean merely automating processes or restructuring the organizational chart. Reengineering involves a radical, cross-functional, futuristic change in the way people think (Porter-O'Grady and Malloch, 2002), a reframing or "discontinuous thinking" (Blancett and Flarey, 1995, p. 16). Long-term planning is replaced by strategic planning, and vertical work relationships are replaced with networks and webs of people and knowledge. All workers at all levels share a commitment to the organization and an accountability to define and produce quality work (Covey, 1991). All workers share responsibility for self-governance, from which both the organization and the worker benefit (Porter-O'Grady et al., 1997). Control is replaced by leadership. The new leader does not use policing techniques of supervision but enables and empowers colleagues through vision, trust, and respect (Bennis and Nanus, 1985; Kouzes and Posner, 1987; Porter-O'Grady and Wilson, 1999). Encouragement, appreciation, and personal recognition are celebrated together in an effective organization (Kouzes and Posner, 1999). Exhibit 1–1 presents a framework for organizations in this millennium.

| EXHIBIT 1-1 | **Framework for Effective Organizations in the 21st Century** |

- Mission: vision, product/outcome
- Structure: network, linkages, distribution of power, risk management
- Processes: production, challenge, correction
- Culture: communication, technology, access, recognition

Kennedy and Charles (1997) assert that, rather than the "authority" or blind obedience of the industrial establishment, the new leader must return to the origin of the word *author* and serve as coach and mentor by helping others learn. Much as Siddhartha learned that knowledge can be transmitted to others but wisdom must be experienced (Hesse, 1951), the worker of the 21st century needs the knowledge that is passed on from those who have learned over time in order to experience the wisdom necessary to be competent and fulfilled in the new organization.

The Changing Paradigm in Health Care

The impact of the enormous changes occurring in business and industry in the late 20th century was reflected in the health care delivery system. Hospitals faced a dinosaurlike future due to several changes. The traditional medical model of a complex hospital system of sick care, a profusion of technology, and ethical questions that could not have been anticipated at the beginning of the century were pointing to a serious need for reform in the health care system. The United States was spending 13 percent of its gross national product on health care, a figure that caused great concern to government officials and economists.

Cost containment began with congressional demand for prospective payment for Medicare recipients through diagnosis-related groups (DRGs). Government-funded Medicare, the largest payer of health care services to the elderly in the country, replaced the retrospective method of payment for primarily hospital services (i.e., nursing services) with a system that linked medical diagnoses to length of stay (Fuchs, 1993). Private insurance companies followed the government's lead and reinvented their methods of payment, changing to a prospective system.

Hospital administrators, faced with decreasing income, were forced to contain costs. Nursing care long had been considered by financial personnel as an expenditure, and nurses were not usually thought of as income generators. The actual cost of nursing care was unknown, and few nurses knew how to calculate it or even what factors to consider. Financial analysts and business executives who did not understand the value of quality care became focused on costs and profit. Nursing, a profession that had matured over a few short decades into a confident discipline, found itself confronted with assaults from business decisions that affected the type, setting, scope, and quality of nursing care. How nursing services are produced and calculated, how much nursing care is required for each recipient, and how to decide what mix of service providers is needed became very important questions.

A pecking order, which was especially noticeable in hospitals, had been established in which nurses were subservient to physicians. Rules were valued, and compliance with rules was the measure of success. "Doctors orders" were considered inviolate commands, and nurses' clinical knowledge and judgment were discounted. This arrangement generated physician-nurse games in which communication from nurses was couched in passive, circuitous language. Separation of disciplines occurred as health workers focused on distinct parts of the person's illness or problems. Compartmentalization served a pyramidal system but did not contribute to a holistic approach to providing comprehensive health care.

Nurses were confronted with a system that was changing around them and that sometimes produced subtle changes whose impact was not recognized immediately. Nurse managers found themselves dealing with budgets, variances, and other business-related activities for which they had not been educated. Nurses without appropriate education in management and community health were forced to seek referrals for patients who were being discharged after brief hospitalization and to ensure continuity of care in homes and other health care agencies.

Corporate mergers and acquisitions and other organizational arrangements resulted in a tumultuous hospital-cum-health care system in which layoffs, staff reductions, and elimination of positions and departments affected nurses in many ways. Nurse administrators encountered executive decisions to downsize when new systems and processes were not yet in place. For example, the position of nurse manager was eliminated in many hospitals in the 1990s with the expectation that staff nurses would assume responsibility and accountability for managerial activities, but the requisite education and training were not provided. Licensed nurses were replaced in many institutions with unlicensed assistive personnel who were given inadequate training in a short time and expected to provide comprehensive care with little supervision to ill patients with complex conditions. Staff nurses worried that patient and nurse safety was jeopardized.

The Pew Health Professions Commission (1995) studied the training and practice of health care professionals and recommended revolutionary changes in how the professions are regulated and educated. From interdisciplinary and multidisciplinary courses and programs to single professional licensure, the recommendations focused on preparing nurses, physicians, dentists, pharmacists, and other health care professionals for practice within the new health care paradigm. The Pew Commission encouraged cross training for multi-skilled allied health workers. Nurses understood early that the new definition of interdisciplinary means nursing, allied health, medicine, and other health professions. On the other hand, many physicians think "interdisciplinary" means specialists in orthopedics, cardiology, radiology, and pulmonology who work together, and allied health professionals believe the term means collaboration among occupational therapists, physical therapists, and physicians' assistants. There still is work to be done to convince all health care providers of the value of an interdisciplinary team for the patient and the provider.

Nurses who weathered drastic organizational changes were seldom acknowledged as having to face problems. Noer (1993) was one of the few authors who wrote about the guilt and depression felt by those who did not lose their jobs but were expected to carry on in sometimes deprived circumstances. Nurses took the lead in efforts to redesign nursing systems by proposing systems that replaced the industrial-age concept of responsibility that bred paternalism with accountability, in which empowerment, partnerships, and leadership are fostered (Porter-O'Grady and Wilson, 1995). Reengineering the workplace for nurses demanded a transformation to professional practice (Blancett and Flarey, 1995). Some health care systems did not integrate information technology into the new order, resulting in restructured old systems rather than new paradigms of health care, according to nursing informatics expert Roy Simpson (personal communication, June 6, 1998).

Health care in the 20th century was delivered most often through hospitals, although there was a major move to the community in the last decades (Aiken, 1990). In the 1990s, new systems of nurse empowerment were created by visionary nurse leaders such as Blancett and Flarey (1995), Porter-O'Grady and Wilson (1995), and Wolf and colleagues (1994a, b). Nursing responses to external forces of managed care centered on a system of case management in which the nurse, preferably an advanced practice nurse, brokered and coordinated care for clients before, during, and after hospitalization (Ethridge and Lamb, 1989; Genna, 1987; Maurin, 1990; Mundinger, 1984; and Zander et al., 1987). Models of case management were created for many organizational structures, acute care facilities, hospices, and community health enterprises (Bower, 1992). As case managers, APNs took the lead in including members of other disciplines in decisions about the health care of clients, families, and communities.

Early in the 21st century, hospitals were investing in corporate partnerships with other health care and business organizations. Many mergers and acquisitions resulted in staff cuts, and nurses and other health care professionals (e.g., pharmacists, physicians, physical therapists) were forced to rethink the way in which care was provided. Collaboration became a necessity, and whole departments have begun to build coalitions with each other to reduce complexity and improve communication. Health care report cards provided mixed response as to their utility in making informed choices about hospitals and physicians (Dranove et al., 2003). After the 1999 Institute of Medicine report (Koln et al.) noted the large number of medical errors in hospitals, over 90 major industries formed the Leapfrog Group (Milstead, 2003) that recommended urban hospitals adopt computerized physician order entry, evidence-based hospital referrals, and the use of intensivists. Evidence-based nursing practice developed at the same time and provided credibility for nursing interventions.

Venegoni (1996) identified five significant factors that influenced the changes in health care systems for the 21st century: (1) place (site of delivery); (2) people (who receives care); (3) preventive model (reward for health, not sickness); (4) paradigm (quality improvement and customer satisfaction); and (5) process (modern technology). The comparison of the old hospital paradigm and the emerging model, Exhibit 1–2, illustrates a practical expression of Venegoni's factors.

Nurses were taking on new positions in all types of health care systems and had become sophisticated providers of care. Beyond that, nurses were beginning

---

EXHIBIT 1–2   **Comparison of Old Health Care Paradigm with New Paradigm**

Old Paradigm	New Health Care Paradigm
Hospital based, acute care	Short-term hospital: same-day surgery, 23-hour stays; prehospital testing and precertification; telehealth/telemedicine; home health; mobile vans; school and mall clinics
Specialty units	Cross-training (multiskilled workers): LDRP, OR/PACU, CCU/telemetry
Hierarchical management	Decentralization (unit budget, scheduling, variance); shared governance; strategic plan
Physician as captain of ship; others are followers	Inter/multidisciplinary team, collaboration; case management (registered nurse/broker)
Nurse as employee; job focused, "refrigerator nurse"	Nurse as professional: career-focused clinical ladder; continuing credentials; tuition reimbursement, paid certification exam
Medical condition; focus on segment	Holistic person in family/community; pastoral care, parish nurse
"Sick" care; focus on cure	Health care, health promotion, prevention programs; focus on cure, care, and continuity of care; complementary health alternatives
Cost containment; focus on billing	Focus on patient and accountability of caregivers/ agency; electronic patient record, patient/continuous quality improvement, care maps
Written medical record	Integrated electronic records: smart card, bedside computers
Fee for service	Managed competition (HMO, PPO, IPA)
Physician as employer	Physician as employee; capitation system
One insurance plan	Variety of insurance options ("covered lives"): basic plan, dental, eye, long-term care, cancer, disability
80 to 100 percent	Greater deductible, lower percentage coverage, or copayment insurance

to integrate the roles of educator, researcher, administrator, and political activist. As client advocates, nurses speak out on issues of prevention of illness and disability, safety and environmental hazards, and informed consent. Nurses have come to realize the critical nature of involvement with legislators who make policies such as laws, regulations, and programs that affect nurses, patients, and the health care system. A more comprehensive understanding of the societal mandate for nursing services requires that nurses assume an active part of a complex system of sociocultural, economic, and political forces. Nurses, especially those in advanced practice, are expanding the scope of nursing in direct care by addressing health care issues that are a matter of public interest. Decisions that affect the public interest are made over time in the policy arena.

What Is Public Policy?

In this chapter, *policy* is an overarching term used to define both an entity and a process. Although there has not been a clear definition of policy in the nursing literature (Rodgers, 1989), scholars in political science have developed definitions and models from which nursing can benefit. The purpose of public policy is to direct problems to government and secure government's response (Jones, 1984). Although there has been much discussion about the boundaries and domain of government and the extent of difference between the public and private sectors, that debate is beyond the scope of this chapter.

The definition of *public policy* is important because it clarifies common misconceptions about what constitutes policy. In this book, the terms *public policy* and *policy* are interchangeable. The process of creating policy can be focused in many arenas and most of these are interwoven. For example, environmental policy deals with health issues such as hazardous material, particulate matter in the air or water, and safety standards in the workplace. Education policy, more than tangentially, is related to health—just ask school nurses. Regulations define who can administer medication to students; state laws dictate what type of sex education can be taught. Defense policy definitely is related to health policy when developing, investigating, or testing biological and chemical warfare. Health policy directly addresses health problems and is the specific focus of this book.

Policy as an Entity

As an entity, policy is seen in many forms as the "standing decisions" of an organization (Eulau and Prewitt, 1973). As formal documented directives of an organization, official government policies reflect the beliefs of the administration in power and provide direction for the philosophy and mission of government organizations. Specific policies usually serve as the "shoulds" and "thou shalts" of agencies. Some policies, known as *position statements*, report the opinions of organizations about issues that members believe are important. For example, state boards of nursing (government agencies created by legislatures to protect the public through the regulation of nursing practice) publish advisory opinions on what constitutes competent and safe nursing practice.

The term *policy* is used often to refer to goals, programs, and proposals. Although such substitution may be confusing in conceptualizing policy, the term may be seen as a type of verbal shorthand for colleagues who are discussing a specific program or program goal. For example, nurses who talk about the gag-rule policy of the Reagan administration understand that they are discussing programs, such as Title X of the Medicare program related to family planning that forbade health professionals from discussing abortion as an option to clients in agencies that received federal funding. A similar gag rule occurred in the 1990s when many health maintenance organizations forbade physicians to discuss treatment options with patients.

Agency policies can be broad and general, such as those that describe the relationship of an agency to other governmental groups. In the most narrow sense, policies can be specific announcements, such as operational procedures. Procedure manuals in government hospitals that detail steps in performing certain nursing tasks are examples of specific policy activities. Both general and specific policies serve as guidelines for employee behavior within an institution. Although policies and procedures often are used interchangeably, policies usually are considered more broad.

Laws are types of policy entities. As legal directives for public and private behavior, laws serve to define action that reflects the will of society—or at least a segment of society. Laws are made at the international, federal, state, and local levels and have the impact of primary place in guiding conduct. Lawmaking usually is the purview of the legislative branch of government in the United States, although presidential vetoes, executive orders, and judicial interpretations of laws have the force of law.

Judicial interpretation is noted in three ways. First, courts may interpret the meaning of laws that are written broadly or with some vagueness. Laws often are written deliberately with language that addresses broad situations. Agencies that implement the laws then write regulations that are more specific and that guide the implementation. However, courts may be asked to determine questions in which the law is unclear or controversial (Williams and Torrens, 1988). For example, the 1973 Rehabilitation Act prohibited discrimination against the handicapped by any program that received federal assistance. Although this may have seemed fair and reasonable at the outset, courts were asked to adjudicate questions of how much accommodation is "fair" (Wilson, 1989). Second, courts can determine how some laws are applied. Courts are idealized as being above the political activity that surrounds the legislature. Courts also are considered beyond the influence of politically active interest groups. The court system, especially the federal court system, has been called upon to resolve conflicts between levels of government (state and federal) and between laws enacted by the legislature and interpretation by powerful interest groups. For example, courts may determine who is eligible or who is excluded from participation in a program. In this way, special interest groups that sue to be included in a program can receive "durable protection" from favorable court decisions (Feldstein, 1988, p. 32). Third, courts can declare the laws made by Congress or the states unconstitutional, thereby nullifying the statues entirely (Litman and Robins, 1991). Courts also interpret the Constitution, sometimes by restricting what the government (not private enterprise) may do (Wilson, 1989).

Regulations are another type of policy initiative. Although they often are included in discussions of laws, regulations are different. Once a law is enacted by the legislative branch, the executive branch of government is charged with administrative responsibility for implementing the law. The executive branch consists of the president and all of the bureaucratic agencies, commissions, and departments that carry out the work for the public benefit. Agencies within the government formulate regulations that achieve the intent of the statute. On the whole, laws are written in general terms, and regulations are written more specifically to guide the interpretation, administration, and enforcement of the law. The Administrative Procedures Act (APA) was created to provide opportunity for citizen review and input throughout the process of developing regulations. The APA ensures a structure and process that is published and open, in the spirit of the founding fathers, so that the average constituent can participate in the process of public decision making.

All of these entities evolve over time and are accomplished through the efforts of a variety of actors or players. Although commonly used, the terms *position statement, resolution, goal, objective, program, procedure, law,* and *regulation* really are not interchangeable with the word *policy*. Rather, they are the formal expressions of policy decisions. For the purposes of understanding just what policy is, nurses must grasp policy as a process.

Policy as a Process

In viewing policy as a guide to government action, nurses can study the process of policy making over time. Milio (1989) presents four major stages in which decisions are made that translate to government policies: (1) agenda setting, (2) legislation and regulation, (3) implementation, and (4) evaluation. Agenda setting is concerned with identifying a societal problem and bringing it to the attention of government. Legislation and regulation are formal responses to a problem. Implementation is the execution of policies or programs toward the achievement of goals. Evaluation is the appraisal of policy performance or program outcomes.

Within each stage, formal and informal relationships are developed among actors both within and outside of government. Actors can be individuals, such as a legislator, a bureaucrat, or a citizen. Actors also can be institutions, such as the presidency, the courts, political parties, or special-interest groups. A series of activities occurs that brings a problem to government, which results in direct action by the government to address the problem. Governmental responses are political; that is, the decisions about who gets what, when, and how are made within a framework of power and influence, negotiation, and bargaining (Lasswell, 1958).

Even as this book explains each of the stages of the policy process and explores them for areas in which nurses can provide influence, one must recognize that the policy process is not necessarily sequential or logical. The definition of a problem, which usually occurs in the agenda-setting phase, may change during legislation. Program design may be altered significantly during implementation. Evaluation of a policy or program (often considered the last phase of the process) may propel onto the national agenda (often considered the first phase of the process) a problem that differs from the original. However, for the purpose of organizing one's thoughts and conceptualizing the policy process, the policy process is examined from the linear perspective of stages.

Even before the process itself can be studied, nurses must understand why it is so important to be knowledgeable about the components and the functions of the process and how this public arena has become an integral part of the practice of advanced nursing.

Why Nurses and Public Policy?

Registered professional nurses have studied the basics of how a bill becomes a law in their baccalaureate programs. An extension of the focus on legislation usually is provided in graduate schools. However, most nurses (and most nurse educators) do not have a clear understanding of the total policy process. To focus on legislation misses a whole range of governmental and political activities—activities in which professional nurses should have a central place. In the 1990s, the health care delivery system was the subject of a major thrust of reform. Reform is a political process in which priorities are determined and public policy decisions are made. Nurses, as the largest group of health care professionals in the country and as the providers of the most direct and continuous care to individuals and groups, were "at the table." That is, nursing was included in the short list of groups convened by a presidential mandate that were instrumental in assisting the government in the mid-1990s to make changes that would directly affect the health of citizens and the legal purview of the health care professions. The nursing presence was a direct result of the many years of leadership exerted by a few nurses (mostly through the professional association) who have understood the importance and have worked tirelessly to develop relationships, to suggest problems and alternative solutions, and to demonstrate willingness to compromise in the present to secure greater gain in the future. Although the federally directed process of reform did not result in substantial change, all of the issues that nursing brought to the discussion were still being addressed after legislation failed. These issues, such as universal access to health care, a basic services package, an emphasis on health promotion and disease prevention, catastrophic coverage for long-term care, and an initial emphasis on at-risk populations such as women and children (*Nursing's Agenda,* 1994), fell to the states for discussion.

Nurses and nursing are at the center of issues of tremendous and long-lasting impact, such as access to providers, quality of care, and reasonable cost. In addition, issues crucial to the profession are being decided, such as who is eligible for government reimbursement for services and what is the appropriate scope of practice of registered nurses in advanced practice. If nurses wait until legislation is being voted before they become involved, it will be too late to affect decisions. Nurses have learned the legislative process. Nurses have written letters and made visits to their legislators. Now nurses must move forward and apply the knowledge of the whole policy process by speaking out to a variety of appropriate governmental actors and institutions so that nursing can move issues onto the national agenda, lobby Congress with alternatives, and provide nursing expertise as policies and programs are being designed. In addition, nurses must be the watchdogs as programs are implemented so that target groups are served and services are appropriate. Nurses should be experts at program evaluation and continuing feedback to ensure that old problems are being addressed, new problems are being identified, and appropriate solutions are being considered. The opportunities for nursing input throughout the policy process are unlimited and certainly not confined narrowly to the legislative process. Nurses are articulate experts who can address both the rational shaping of policy and the emotional aspects of the process. Nurses cannot afford to limit their actions to monitoring bills; they must seize the initiative and use their considerable collective and individual influence to ensure the health, welfare, and protection of the public and health care professionals.

An Overview of the Policy Process

Most of the chapters in this book address specific components of the policy process in depth and from a theoretical perspective. However, at the outset, advanced practice nurses should have an overview of the total process so that they do not get stuck on legislation. Many useful articles and books have been written about policy in general and even about specific policies, but few have addressed the scope of the policy process or defined the components. The elements of agenda setting (including problem definition), government response (legislation, regulation, or programs), and policy and program implementation and evaluation are distinct entities but are connected as parts of a whole tapestry in the process of public decision making.

Agenda Setting

Getting a health care problem to the attention of government can be a tremendous first step in getting relief. The actual mechanism of defining a health care problem is a major political issue in which APNs can participate, especially in a collective manner as an interest group. Problem definition often is influenced by special-interest groups. When acquired immune deficiency syndrome (AIDS) was first diagnosed in the 1980s, the disease was perceived as a problem of homosexuals and intravenous drug users. Within this definition, assumptions were made by government officials that the disease might be confined to a small population. Federal health agencies were not likely to obtain a large budget for a disease that affected small groups, especially those considered outside the mainstream of American values. Gay rights activist organizations such as the Gay Men's Health Crisis (GMHC) and AIDS Coalition to Unleash Power (ACTUP) were special-interest groups that were instrumental in persuading the government to alter the definition of the AIDS problem by broadening it to include persons other than homosexuals. As AIDS became known in hemophiliacs, infants, and heterosexual men, the problem became redefined as a community health problem. From this perspective, AIDS was perceived as having an impact on a larger segment of the population, including mainstream Americans. Government officials in the administrative and legislative branches were pressured to assume responsibility for addressing an epidemic. Officials were able to identify a variety of departments and agencies beyond the traditional health and human services, such as the Department of Defense and the Bureau of Indian Affairs, that could seek funding for programs of research and treatment. Defining the problem differently increased access to the national agenda.

APNs must come to understand the concepts of windows of opportunity, policy entrepreneurs, and political elites. "Sound bites" and "word bites" are tools that were introduced by people who were invested in getting the AIDS crisis onto the national agenda (Milstead, 1993). Gay rights groups used radical political action tactics borrowed from the civil rights movement of the 1960s and 1970s to get their message heard by those in Washington, DC. Activists conducted sit-ins and marches, testified at hearings, ridiculed weak efforts to provide research and treatment, and held press conferences. During the press conferences, self-taught activists learned that although a person may be recorded by microphone or video camera during a speech, only a few seconds would be broadcast on the news. Activists prepared written scripts of selected material from their interviews in advance of the interviews and presented the scripts to the media people. This allowed the speakers to talk at length about their issues and yet focus the media replay to ensure that a specific message was promoted.

Government Response

The government response to public problems often emanates from the legislative branch and comes in three forms: (1) laws, (2) rules and regulations, and (3) programs. Because only senators and representatives can introduce legislation (not even the president can bring a bill to the floor of either house), these elected officials command respect and attention. The work of legislation is not clear cut or linear. Informal communication and influence are the coin of the realm when trying to construct a program or law from the often vague wishes of disparate groups. The committee structure of both houses is a powerful method of accomplishing the work of government. Conference committees are known as the "Third House of Congress" (How our laws, 1990) because of their power to force compromise and bring about new legislation. APNs must appreciate the difference between the authorization and appropriations processes and seek influence in both arenas. Becoming involved directly with legislators and their staffs has been a training ground for many APNs. Supporting or opposing passage of a bill often has served as the first contact with the political process for many nurses. However, this place often has been the stopping point for many nurses because they were unaware of other avenues of involvement, such as the follow-up process of regulations and rulemaking.

Lowi (1969) noted that administrative rulemaking often takes place as an effort to bring about order within environments that are unstable and full of conflict. Some regulations codify precedent; others break new ground and address issues not previously explicated. An example of the latter is the Federal Trade Commission's (FTC) Trade Regulation Rules. In 1964, the FTC, whose mission is to protect the consumer and enforce antitrust, wrote regulations requiring health warnings on cigarette packages. The tobacco industry reacted so fiercely that Congress quickly passed a law that nullified the regulations and replaced them with less stringent ones (West, 1982). Other ways to sanction agencies whose rules are viewed as too restrictive are to reduce budget allocations and increase the number of adjudications or trial-like reviews. Advanced practice nurses must become knowledgeable about the regulatory process so that they can spot opportunities to contribute or intervene prior to final rule making (The regulatory process, 1992).

Programs are concrete manifestations of solutions to problems. Program design often is a joint effort of legislative intent, budgetary expediency, and political feasibility (the latter meaning "an interest group arrangement hammered out in Congress" [Skocpol, 1995, p. 283]). There are many opportunities for nurses in advanced practice to become involved in the design phase of a program. Selecting an agency to administer the program, choosing the goals, and selecting the tools that will ensure eligibility and participation are all decisions in which the APN should collaborate.

Policy and Program Implementation

It is important that APNs keep reminding their colleagues that the phases of the policy process are not linear and that policy activities are fluid and move within and among the phases in dynamic processes. The implementation phase includes those activities in which legislative mandates are carried out, most often through programmatic means. The implementation stage also includes a planning ingredient. Problems occur in program planning if technological expertise is not available. This is particularly important to nurses, who are experts in the delivery of health care in the broadest sense.

If government officials do not know qualified, appropriate experts, then decisions about program planning and design often are determined by legislators, bureaucrats, or staff who know little or nothing about the problem or the solutions. As excellent problem solvers, APNs have many opportunities to offer ideas and solutions. One strategy is to employ second-order change to reframe situations and recommend pragmatic alternatives to implementors (de Chesnay, 1983; Watzlawick et al., 1974). Bowen (1982) used probability theory to demonstrate how program success could be improved. She suggested putting several clearance points (instances where major decisions are made) together so that they could be negotiated as a package deal. She also advocated beginning the bargaining process with alternatives that have the greatest chance for success and using that success as a foundation for building more successes, a strategy she referred to as a "bandwagon approach" (p. 10). In the past, nurses have done the opposite: focused on failure and perceived lack of nursing power. APNs have begun to note successes in the political arena and are building a new level of success and esteem. The nurse in advanced practice today uses the strategies of packaging, success begets success, and persistence in a deliberate way so that nurses can increase their effective impact in the implementation of social programs. Although nurses most often work toward positive impact, they have found that opposition to an unsound program can have a paradoxical positive effect. Although not in the public arena, an example of phenomenal success in the judicious use of opposition occurred when the professional body of nursing rose up as one against the American Medical Association's 1986 proposal to create a new type of low-level health care worker called a registered care technician. The power emerged as over 40 nursing organizations stood together in opposition to an ill-conceived proposal that would have placed patients in jeopardy and created dead-end jobs.

Policy and Program Evaluation

For nurses who have worked within the nursing process of clinical reasoning (Pesut and Herman, 1999), the process of evaluation seems to be a logical component of the policy process. Evaluation is the systematic application of methods of social research to public policies and programs. Evaluation is conducted "to benefit the human condition to improve profit, to amass influence and power, or to achieve other goals" (Rossi and Freeman, 1995, p. 6). Evaluation research is a powerful tool for defending viable programs, for altering structures and processes in order to strengthen programs, and for providing rationale for program failure. Goggin and colleagues (1990) proposed that researchers investigate program implementation within an analytical framework rather than a descriptive one. They argued that a "third generation" of research established within a sound theory would strengthen the body of knowledge of the policy process. APNs can contribute to both the theory and the method of evaluation.

Evaluation must be started early and continued throughout a program. An unconscionable example of a program that should have been stopped even before it was begun is the Tuskegee "experiment." From 1932 to 1972, a group of African-Americans was used as a control group and denied antibiotic treatment for syphilis even after treatment was known to be successful (Thomas and Quinn, 1991). Beyond evaluation research, this study clearly points out the moral and ethical concerns that are mandated when researchers work with human beings. Should a study or program be started at all? At what point should it be stopped? What is involved in "informed consent"? If a program involves experimental therapy, what are the methods for presenting subjects with relevant data so that participation preferences are clear (Bell et al., 1988)? These kinds of questions should be considered automatically by today's researchers, but it is the responsibility of APNs as consumer agents to ask the questions if they have not been asked or if there is any doubt about the answers.

A Bright Future

The multiple roles of the APN—provider of direct care, researcher, consultant, educator, administrator, consumer advocate, and political activist—reflect the changing and expanding character of the professional nurse. Today is the future; nursing action today sets the direction for what health care becomes for projected generations. As true professionals with a societal mandate and a comprehensive body of knowledge, nurses function as visionaries who are grounded in education, research, and experience. APNs serve as the link between human responses to actual and potential health problems and the solutions that may be addressed in the government arena. Full integration of the policy process becomes evident when professional nurses discern early the social implications of health problems, seize the opportunity to inform public officials with whom the nurses have credible relationships, provide objective data and subjective personal stories that help translate big problems down to a level of understanding, propose alternative solutions that acknowledge reality, and participate in the evaluation process to determine the effectiveness and efficiency of the outcomes.

Educating Our Political Selves

Nurses in advanced practice should be expert in the knowledge and skills of political activity. Basic content in undergraduate nursing programs must be reexamined in light of the needs of the profession. Educators must do more than plant the seeds of interest and excitement in baccalaureate students. Educators must model activism by talking about the bills they are supporting or opposing, by organizing students to assist in election campaigns, and by demanding not only that students write letters to officials but that they mail them and provide follow-up. Educators can develop games in which students maneuver through a virtual bureaucracy to move a health problem onto the agenda. Brainstorming techniques can lead students to discover innovative alternative solutions. Baccalaureate students can analyze policy tools to discover how and when to use them. Teachers of research methods and processes can use political scenarios to point out how to phrase clinical questions so that legislators will pay attention. Program effectiveness can be studied in research and clinical courses. The theoretical components taught in class and followed by practical application through participation in political and legislative committees in professional organizations must serve as "basic training" for the registered nurse.

Graduate education must demand demonstrated knowledge and application of more extensive and sophisticated political processes. Nursing must increase the total of those with master's degrees and doctoral degrees beyond 9.6 percent and 0.6 percent, respectively, of nearly 2.7 million registered nurses (Spratley et al., 2000). All graduate program faculty should serve as models for political activism. The atmosphere in master's and doctoral programs should heighten the awareness of students who are potential leaders. Faculty will motivate students by displaying posters that announce political events and by including students in discussions of nursing issues framed in a policy context. Students who spot educators at rallies and other political and policy occasions are learning by example. Faculty should advertise their experiences as delegates to political and professional conventions. A few faculty will serve as mentors for students who need to move from informal to sustained, formal contact with policy makers and who have a policy track in their career trajectories. Both faculty and students should consider actual experience in government offices as a means of learning the nitty-gritty of how government functions and of demonstrating their own leadership capabilities. *The Nurses' Directory of Capitol Connections* (Bull et al., 2000) is an excellent resource for identifying a wide range of opportunities for participation of nurses who work in the policy arena.

If students hesitate and seem passive about involvement, educators must help these nurses determine where their passions are. This may help students focus on where they might start. Often the novice can be enticed by centering on a clinical problem.

Identifying Problems

Advanced practice nurses, by definition, are "professional nurses who have successfully completed a graduate program in nursing or a related area that provides specialized knowledge and skills that form the foundation for expanded roles in health care" (ANA House of Delegates, 1993, p. 5). According to this denotation, APNs function in the provision of direct clinical care; as educators, administrators, and researchers; in consultative and counseling roles; and with a variety of titles. Within this broad interpretation, APNs have the capacity and opportunity to identify and frame problems from multiple sources.

Clinical Problems   The choice of a clinical problem on which to focus one's energy is a major decision. A nurse may be working in a specialized area and may see a need for more research or alternatives to treatment. For example, those who work with patients and families with breast cancer already may have a passion for issues critical to this area. Other current topics receiving attention include diabetes, obesity, AIDS, early detection and treatment of prostate cancer, child and parent abuse, cardiac problems in women, and empowering caregivers (Hash and Cramer, 2003; Pierce and Steiner, 2003). Professional problems that are especially critical to nurses in advanced practice include reducing barriers that prevent practice autonomy and reimbursement for nursing services. Workplace issues include advocacy for workplace safety and management strategies for training and redeploying nurses as work sites change. Related social problems that affect nurses include the increase of street violence and bioterrorism. There is a plethora of problems and "irritations" that can arouse the passion of a nurse in advanced practice.

Funding for Education   Preparing nurses at the graduate level, either with master's or doctoral degrees, has been a problem on several levels. The first concern was with a cyclical shortage of nurses, especially during war time when nurses left hospital employment and entered the armed forces. The Social Security Act of 1935 and, a decade later, the National Mental Health Act of 1946 provided some federal funding for graduate education and research (Lash, 1986). By the 1950s, nurses were seeking graduate degrees, but there were not enough programs in nursing. Part of the problem was that not enough nurses held doctoral degrees and could teach in graduate programs (Aiken, 1986). Organized nursing knew that federal legislators had initiated a GI bill that provided money to attend college for those who served in World War II. Nursing advocates convinced legislators that nurses were a scarce national resource, and funds were appropriated for nursing education through the Nurse Training Acts (NTAs) that began in 1943. Funding encouraged the initiation of new graduate nursing education programs, such as nurse-practitioner programs. By 1966, an amendment created grants for students, and the 1972 bill awarded capitation grants to nursing education programs to expand enrollment and increase graduations. With the infusion of federal dollars, the quantity and quality of educators and education improved (Kelly and Joel, 1995).

Nursing education as a functional area lost ground with the expansion of technology, the explosion of knowledge, and the increase in clinical master's degrees that began in the 1990s. Nursing's heritage of experienced teachers (education majors were acceptable routes for women/nurses who pursued higher education in the first half of the 20th century) was supplanted with clinically competent APNs who often were not schooled in principles of teaching and learning. Funding for nurses who sought baccalaureate and master's degrees focused on clinical nursing. Although this was appropriate in order to accommodate new knowledge about genetics, immunology, pharmacology, ethics, and other important content, teaching was slowly squeezed out. In the first decade of the 21st century, academic institutions face not only a shortage of faculty, but a shortage of faculty who have backgrounds in the principles of education. A few colleges and universities have begun doctoral programs with a focus on teaching, and many master's programs offer an education track. Funding for scholarships and loans in the early 2000s reflects a beginning recognition of the need for adequately prepared nurse-teachers.

Support for Nursing Administration   The only area in which federal funding was not provided directly was in nursing administration. Even though NTA criteria for student qualifications clearly eliminated those studying nursing administration by denying their eligibility, potential leaders in that specialty became very important as managed care schemes replaced traditional fee-for-service arrangements. Nurses' need for knowledge about budgets, organizations, change theory, human resource strategies, and other formerly tangential material became critical in the 1990s. Federal money for education in that area had not been a priority, and nurse administrators have had to shoulder the burden of their education alone with the hope of executive and entrepreneurial opportunities through which they could recoup some of their financial investment. Federal nurse traineeships did change the eligibility in the late 1990s to include nurses with administration majors, but the funding competed with that for clinical scholarships.

Investment in Nursing Research   From early nurse scientist programs that encouraged research training in physical and behavioral science programs to later grants that allowed nursing education programs to develop researchers in nursing, federal funds have provided the impetus for scientific inquiry into nursing concerns. Pre- and postdoctoral fellowships for nurse scientists and new investigator awards fostered research activity and the education of future researchers. Faculty development grants and research conferences made it possible to study and disseminate findings. The creation of the National Center for Nursing Research and its later elevation to the National Institute of Nursing Research (NINR) were outgrowths of struggles within the profession and between nursing and federal officials in efforts to secure funding for nursing research, especially clinical research (Brown, 1986). Although funding increased slowly over the years, NINR remains the lowest-funded institute of National Institutes of Health (NIH).

Government responds to social problems that either are too big for the private sector or are particular to the mission of government. The leadership role of government has been pictured by Osborne (1992) as "steering" rather than "rowing" in the 1800s with the provision of land grants for colleges and in the 1990s with funding for advanced practice nurses. Nurses must steer the course as health care experts by staying involved in the political process and influencing health policy. All registered nurses, especially those in advanced practice, have an extraordinary investment in the new structures and processes that will continue to be negotiated to provide health care to the citizens and residents of the United States.

Expanding the Framework

Nurses were central players in early discussions of a new health care delivery system (Backer et al., 1993). The 1990s nursing agenda for health care reform was a timely and fresh approach that rejected the traditional medical model and instead focused on the consumer as well as the provider. Nurse practitioners, clinical nurse specialists, and those in the new paradigm of the blended role in advanced practice spoke out as agents of patients and families to ensure that critical elements that affect health care cost, quality, and access are incorporated into current and future organizational arrangements for the delivery of care. Nurses and nursing were a strong political force in discussions of what health care delivery should be.

Practice the Rules of Debate   Nurses absolutely must "get their act together" and work toward a unified voice on issues that affect the public health and the nursing profession. Whatever their differences in the past—anger from entry-into-practice arguments that have dragged on for over half a century; disparagement and animosity among those with varied levels of education; cerebral and pragmatic concerns about gaps between education and practice, practice and administration, or administration and education—nurses must put these kinds of divisive, emotional issues behind them if they expect to be taken seriously as professionals by elected and appointed public officials and policy makers. Nurses cannot afford to stop arguing critical issues internally, but they must learn how to argue heatedly among themselves—and then go to lunch together. Nurses can learn lessons from television shows such as *Crossfire, The McLaughlin Group,* and *The Capital Gang* about how to challenge, contest, dispute, contend, and debate issues passionately and then shake hands and respect the opponent's position. Passionate issues must not polarize the profession any longer and, more important, must not stand in the way of a unified voice to the public.

Strengthen Organized Nursing   The most productive and efficient way to act together is through a strong professional organization. As organizations in general have restructured and reengineered for more efficient operation, so will the professional associations. APNs have a knowledge base that includes an understanding of how organizations develop and change. This theoretical knowledge must serve as a foundation for leadership in directing new organizational structures that are responsive to members and other important bodies. National leaders must talk with state and local leaders as new configurations are conceived. States must confer among themselves to share innovations and knowledge about what works and what does not.

The Nursing Organizations Alliance (Saver, 2003), composed of the presidents and executive directors of over 50 major nursing organizations, held an inaugural meeting in 2003. The alliance is a loose collection of groups that provides a forum to discuss and debate issues important to a wide range of perspectives. Time will tell how effective this organization will be in serving as an internal medium for airing differences and coming to consensus.

Issues such as the role of collective bargaining units within the total organizational structure, the position of individual membership vis-à-vis state membership, the political role of a specialized interest group (nurses) in creating public policy, and the issue of international influence in nursing and health care require wisdom and leadership that APNs must exert as the American

Nurses Association addresses its place as a major voice of this country's nurses. One united voice is necessary to carry nursing's messages to the public. For example, the Tri-Council of Nursing (ANA, American Association of Colleges of Nursing, American Organization of Nurse Executives, and the National League for Nursing) took a single message to Congress to increase funding for NINR and to authorize and appropriate funding for the Nurse Reinvestment Act (to create scholarships for students and faculty).

Issues inherent in multistate licensure are being debated today, and the outcome will reflect the extent to which nurses will use concepts of telehealth in their practices. Because APNs already are eligible for Medicare reimbursement for telehealth services that are provided in specified rural areas (Burtt, 1997), these nurses are rich resources and must be included in reasoned discussions on this issue. State boards of nursing in every state and jurisdiction face issues of appropriate methods of recognizing advanced nursing practice, the role of the government agency in regulating nursing and other professions, and the analysis of educationally sound and legally defensible examinations for candidates.

Nurses who have been reluctant to become "political" cannot afford to ignore their obligations any longer. Each nurse counts, and, collectively, nursing is a major actor in the effort to ensure the country's healthy future. Nurses have expanded their conception of what nursing is and how it is practiced to include active political participation. A nurse must choose the governmental level on which to focus: federal, regional, state, or local. The process is similar at each level: Identify the problem and become part of the solution.

Advanced practice nurses understand the scope of service delivery, continuity of care, appropriate mix of caregivers, and the expertise that can be provided by multidisciplinary teams. By being at the forefront of understanding, nurses have a moral and ethical mandate to participate in the public-policy process. Dynamic political action is as much a part of the advanced practice of nursing as is expert direct care.

Work with the Political System   By now, many APNs have developed contacts with legislators, and have appointed officials and their staffs. A new group that holds great potential for nurse interaction is the Congressional Nursing Caucus in the U.S. House of Representatives, begun in 2003 by Representatives Lois Capps (D-CA) and Ed Whitfield (R-KY). This bipartisan group assembles to educate Congress on all aspects of nursing—education, practice, research, leadership. Members will hold briefings on the nurse shortage, patient and nurse safety issues, preparedness for bioterrorism, and other relevant and pertinent issues and concerns. The caucus will serve as a "clearinghouse for information and a sounding board for ideas brought forth by the nursing community" (American Nurses Association Commends, 2003, p. 1). APNs must stay alert to issues and be assertive in bringing problems to the attention of policy makers. It is important to bring success stories to legislators and officials—they need to hear what good nurses do and how well they practice. Sharing positive information will keep the image of nurses in an affirmative and constructive picture. Legislators must run for office (and U.S. Representatives do this every 2 years), so media coverage with an APN who is pursuing noteworthy accomplishments is usually welcomed eagerly.

Conclusion

Nurses in advanced practice must have expert knowledge and skill in change, conflict resolution, assertiveness, communication, negotiation, and group process to function appropriately in the policy arena. Professional autonomy and collaborative interdependence are possible within a political system in which consumers can choose access to quality health care that is provided by competent practitioners at a reasonable cost. Nurses in advanced practice have a strong, persistent voice in designing such a health care system for today and for the future.

The policy process is much broader and more comprehensive than the legislative process. Although individual components can be identified for analytical study, the policy process is fluid, nonlinear, and dynamic. There are many opportunities for nurses in advanced practice to participate throughout the policy process. The question is not whether nurses should become involved in the political system, but to what extent. In the whole policy arena, nurses must be involved with every aspect. Knowing all of the components and issues that must be addressed within each phase, the nurse in advanced practice finds many opportunities for providing expert advice. APNs can use the policy process, individual components, and models as a framework to analyze issues and participate in alternative solutions.

Nursing has a rich history. The professional nurse's values of altruism, respect, integrity, and accountability to consumers remain strong. In some ways, the evolution of nursing roles has come full circle, from the political influence recognized and exercised by Nightingale to the influence of current nurse leaders with elected and appointed public officials. The APN of the 21st century practices with a solid political heritage and a mandate for consistent and powerful involvement in the entire policy process.

Discussion Points

1. Read Nightingale's *Notes on Nursing* and other historical sources of the mid-1800s and discuss how Nightingale used personal and family influence to move her agenda for the Crimea and for nursing education.
2. Read articles about Mildred Montag's proposal for associate degree nursing education and discuss the implications of moving nursing out of hospitals and into institutions of higher learning.
3. Read the 1965 ANA *Position Paper on Educational Preparation for Professional Nursing* and articles in response to the position paper before discussing the impact among nurse educators and among types of nursing programs.
4. Compare the definition of nursing according to Nightingale, Henderson, the ANA, and your own state nurse practice act. What is the difference in a legal definition

and a professional definition? What are the similarities? What did definitions include or not include that reflected the state of nursing at the time? Construct a definition of nursing for today and 10 years from now.

5. Discuss the role of research in nursing. What has been the focus over the past century? What is the pattern of nursing research vis-à-vis topic, methodology, relevance? To what extent do you think nursing research has had an impact on nursing care? Cite examples.

6. Trace the amount of federal funding for nursing research. Do not limit your search to federal health-related agencies; that is, investigate departments (commerce, environment, transportation, etc.), military services, and the Veterans Administration. What opportunities does this present for nurse scientists?

7. Read books (e.g., Blancett and Flarey, Covey, Noer, Porter-O'Grady and Wilson) and articles (e.g., Curtin, Milstead, O'Malley, Wolf) about the changing paradigm in health care delivery systems. Discuss the change in nursing as an occupation and nursing as a profession. What does this mean in today's transformational paradigm?

8. Consider a thesis, graduate project, or dissertation on a specific topic (e.g., clinical problems, health care issues) using the policy process as a framework.

9. Identify policies within public agencies and discuss how they were developed. Interview members of an agency policy committee to discover how policies are changed.

10. Have faculty and students bring to class official governmental policies. What governmental agency is responsible for developing the policy? For enforcing the policy? How has the policy changed over time? What are the consequences of not complying with the policy?

11. Identify nurses who are elected officials at the local, state, or national level. Interview these officials to determine how the nurses were elected, what their objectives are, and to what extent they use their nursing knowledge in their official capacities. Ask the officials if they tapped into nursing groups during their campaigns. If so, what did the nurses contribute? If not, why not?

12. Discuss the major components of the policy process and discuss the fluidity of the process. Point out how players move among the components in a nonlinear way.

13. Using Exhibit 1–1 as a framework, construct a health care organization in which access is provided and quality care is assured.

14. Develop an assessment tool by which students can determine their own level of knowledge and involvement in the policy process. Reminder: Stretch your thinking beyond legislative activity.

15. Watch *Crossfire, The McLaughlin Group, The Capital Gang,* or a similar television program and analyze the verbal and nonverbal communication patterns, pro-and-con arguments, and other methods of discussion. Discuss your analysis within the framework of gender differences in communication and utility in the political arena.

16. Construct a list of ways in which nurses can become more knowledgeable about the policy process. Choose at least three activities in which you will participate. Develop a tool for evaluating the activity and your knowledge and involvement.

17. Select at least one problem or irritation in a clinical area and brainstorm with other APNs or graduate students on how to approach a solution. Discuss funding sources; be creative.

18. Attend a meeting of the state board of nursing, the district or state nurses association, or a professional convention. Identify issues discussed, resources used,

EXHIBIT 1-3	**Requirements for the New Paradigm of Health Care Delivery for the 21st Century**	
Skill	*Teaching Technique*	*Evaluation Measure*

communication techniques, and rules observed. Evaluate the usefulness of the session to your practice.

19. Using Exhibit 1–2 as a guide, write in activities and practices that you see or are involved within the new paradigm.

20. Discuss what skills (task, interpersonal, etc.) and attitudes are required for the nurse in the new paradigm. Who is best prepared to teach these skills, and what teaching techniques should be used? How will they be evaluated? Develop a worksheet (see Exhibit 1–3) to facilitate planning.

21. Discuss at least five strategies for helping nurses integrate these skills into their practices.

References

Aiken, L. H. (1990). Charting the future of hospital nursing. *Image: Journal of Nursing Scholarship* 22(2), 72–78.

Aiken, L. H. (1986). Nursing education: The public policy debate. In J. C. McCloskey and H. K. Grace (Eds.), *Current Issues in Nursing* (2nd ed., pp. 680–696). Boston: Blackwell Scientific Publications.

American Nurses Association commends Reps. Capps, Whitfield for forming congressional nursing caucus (2003). Retrieved from http://www.nursingworld.org. G:releases03\caucus_rel_319.wpd.

ANA House of Delegates. (1993). *Regulation of advanced nursing practice* (action report). Washington, DC: American Nurses Publishing Co.

Argyris, C. (1962). *Interpersonal Competence and Organizational Effectiveness.* Homewood, IL: Dorsey Press.

Backer, B. A., Costello-Nikitas, D., and Mason, D. J. (1993). Power at the policy table—when women and nurses are involved. *Revolution* 3(2), 68–71, 74–76.

Bell, D. E., Raiffa, H., and Tversky, A. (1988). *Decision Making.* Cambridge, MA: Cambridge University Press.

Benner, P. G. (1984). *From Novice to Expert: Excellence and Power in Clinical Nursing Practice.* Menlo Park, CA: Addison-Wesley.

Bennis, W. and Nanus, B. (1985). *Leaders.* New York: Harper and Row.

Blancett, S. S. and Flarey, D. L. (1995). *Reengineering Nursing and Health Care: The Handbook for Organizational Transformation.* Gaithersburg, MD: Aspen Publishers, Inc.

Blank, A. E. (1997). Linking the restructuring of nursing care with outcomes. In E. L. Cohen and T. G. Cesta (Eds.), *Nursing Case Management* (2nd ed., pp. 261–273). St, Louis, MO: Mosby.

Bowen, E. (1982). The Pressman-Wildavsky paradox: Four addenda on why models based on probability theory can predict implementation success and suggest useful tactical advice for implementers. *Journal of Public Policy 2*(1), 1–22.

Bower, K. A. (1992). *Case Management by Nurses.* Washington, DC: American Nurses Publishing.

Brooten, D. and Naylor, M. D. (1995) Nurses' effect on changing patient outcomes. *Image: Journal of Nursing Scholarship 27*(2), 95–99.

Brown, B. J. (1986). Past and current status of nursing's role in influencing governmental policy for research and training in nursing. In J. C. McCloskey and H. K. Grace (Eds.), *Current Issues in Nursing* (2nd ed., pp. 697–712). Boston: Blackwell Scientific Publications.

Bull, J., Sharp, N., and Wakefield, M. (2000). *Nurses' Directory of Capitol Connections* (5th ed.) Fairfax, VA: George Mason University Center for Health Policy, Research and Ethics.

Burtt, K. (1997, Nov./Dec.). Nurses use telehealth to address rural health care needs, prevent hospitalizations. *The American Nurse 29*(6), 21.

Champy, J. (1995). *Reengineering Management.* New York: Harper Business.

Covey, S. R. (1991). *Principle-Centered Leadership.* New York: Summit Books.

de Chesnay, M. (1983). The creation and dissolution of paradoxes in nursing practice. *Topics in Clinical Nursing 5*(3), 71–80.

Dranove, D., Kessler, D., McClellan, M., and Satterthwaite, M. (2003). Is more information better? The effects of "report cards" on health care providers. *Journal of Political Economy 3*(11), 555–585.

Drucker, P. F. (1999). Knowledge worker productivity: The biggest challenge. *California Management Review 4*(21), 79–94.

Drucker, P. F. (1995, Feb.). The age of social transformation. *Quality Digest,* pp. 36–39.

Drucker, P. F. (1959). *Landmarks of Tomorrow.* New York: Harper.

Erickson, J. R. and Sheehy, C. (1998). Clinical research in the advanced practice role. In C. M. Sheehy and M. McCarthy (Eds.), *Advanced Practice Nursing: Emphasizing Common Roles* (pp. 242–263). Philadelphia: F.A. Davis Company.

Essentials of Baccalaureate Education for Professional Nursing Practice (The). (1998). New York: American Association of Colleges of Nursing.

Essentials of Master's Education for Advanced Practice Nursing (The). (1996). New York: American Association of Colleges of Nursing.

Ethridge, P. and Lamb, G. (1989). Professional nursing case management improves quality, access, and cost. *Nursing Management 20*(3), 30–35.

Eulau, H. and Prewitt, K. (1973). *Labyrinths of Democracy.* Indianapolis, IN: Bobbs-Merrill, p. 465.

Feldstein, P.J. (1988). *The Politics of Health Legislation.* Ann Arbor, MI: Health Administration Press.

Flood, R.L. and Senge, P.M. (1999). *Rethinking the Fifth Discipline: Learning Within the Unknowable.* London: Routledge.

Fuchs, V.R. (1993). *The Future of Health Policy.* Cambridge, MA: Harvard University Press.

Genna, J. (1987, Nov./Dec.). AIDS management. *Healthcare Forum Journal,* pp. 18–48.

Goggin, M.L., Bowman, A. O'M., Lester, J.P., and O'Toole, L.J., Jr. (1990). *Implementation Theory and Practice: Toward A Third Generation.* New York: HarperCollins Publishers.

Haas, J.E. (1964). *Role Conception and Group Consensus.* (Research monograph No. 17); Columbus, OH: The Ohio State University, Bureau of Business Research.

Halloran, E.J. (1983). Staffing assignment: By task or by patient. *Nursing Management* *14*(8), 17.

Hash, K.M. and Cramer, E.P. (2003). Empowering gay and lesbian caregivers and uncovering their unique experiences through the use of qualitative methods. *Journal of Gay and Lesbian Social Services. Issues in Practice, Policy and Research 15*(1/2), 47–64.

Hawkins, J. and Thibodeau, J. The role of research in advanced practice. In J. Hawkins and J. Thibodeau (Eds.), *The Advanced Practitioner: Current Practice Issues.* New York: Tiresias Press.

Hegyvary, S. (1992). Outcomes research: Integrating nursing practice into the world view: National Institutes of Health, *Patient Outcomes Research: Examining the Effectiveness of Nursing Practice* (17–24). (DHHS publication No. 93-3411).

Henderson, V. (1966). *The Nature of Nursing: A Definition and its Implications for Practice, Research, and Education.* New York: Macmillan.

Hesse, H. (1951). *Siddhartha.* New York: Bantam Books.

How our laws are made. (1990). United States Government Printing Office, House Document 101–139, 4.

Jones, C.O. (1984). *An Introduction to the Study of Public Policy* (2nd ed.). Monterey, CA: Brooks/Cole.

Kelly, L.Y. and Joel, L.A. (1995). *Dimensions of Professional Nursing* (7th ed.). New York: McGraw-Hill, Inc., p. 399.

Kennedy, E. and Charles, S.C. (1997). *Authority.* New York: Simon & Schuster.

King, I.M. (1971). *Toward a Theory for Nursing.* New York: John Wiley and Sons, Inc.

Koln, L.T., Corrigan, J.M., and Donaldon, M.S. (Eds.) (1999). To err is human: Building a safer health system. A report from the Committee on Quality of Healthcare in America, Institute of Medicine, National Academy of Sciences. Washington, DC: National Academy Press.

Kouzes, J. and Posner, B. (1999). *Encouraging the Heart: A Leader's Guide to Rewarding and Recognizing Others.* San Francisco: Jossey-Bass.

Kouzes, J. and Posner, B. (1987). *The Leadership Challenge.* San Francisco: Jossey-Bass.

Lash, A.A. (1986). Federal financing and its effect on higher nursing education. In J.C. McCloskey and H.K. Grace (Eds.), *Current Issues in Nursing* (2nd ed., pp. 663–679). Boston: Blackwell Scientific Publications.

Lasswell, H.D. (1958). *Politics: Who Gets What, When, How.* New York: Meridian Books.

Laws governing nursing in South Carolina. (1994). Columbia, SC: South Carolina Department of Labor, Licensing, and Regulation.

Leininger, M. (Ed.) (1978). *Transcultural Nursing: Concepts, Theories and Practices.* New York: John Wiley & Sons.

Litman, T. J. and Robins, L. S. (1991). *Health Politics and Policy* (2nd ed.). Albany, NY: Delmar Publishers, Inc.

Lowi, T. (1969). *The End of Liberalism.* New York: Norton.

Making sense of the new reimbursement laws. (1997). Washington, DC: American Nurses Association.

Manier, J. (July 7, 2002). U.S. quietly OKs fetal stem cell work. *Chicago Tribune.* Retrieved from http://www.chicagotribune.com/technology/local/chi-0207070379jul07. 0.18011553.story.

Maurin, J. (1990). Case management: Caring for psychiatric clients. *Journal of Psychosocial Nursing 28*(7), 8–12.

Melville, H. (1853). Bartleby, the scrivener: A story of wall street. *Putnam's Monthly Magazine 2*(911), 546–577.

Milio, N. (1989). Developing nursing leadership in health policy. *Journal of Professional Nursing 5*(6), 315.

Milstead, J. A. (2003). Leapfrog group: A prince in disguise or just another frog? *Nursing Administration Quarterly 26*(4), 16–25.

Milstead, J. A. (1993). The advancement of policy implementation theory: An analysis of three needle exchange programs. (doctoral dissertation). University of Georgia.

Mundinger, M. (1984). Community-based care: Who will be the case managers? *Nursing Outlook 32*(6), 294–295.

National Institutes of Health. (1996). *Capitol Update 11*(24), 6.

Noer, D. M. (1993). *Healing the Wounds.* San Francisco: Jossey-Bass.

Nursing Facts. (1994). Washington, DC: American Nurses Association.

Nursing's Agenda for Health Care Reform. (1994). Washington, DC: American Nurses Publishing, Inc.

Orem, D. E. (1971). *Nursing: Concepts of Practice.* Scarborough, Ontario: McGraw-Hill.

Osborne, D. E. (Ed.) (1992). *Reinventing Government: How the Entrepreneurial Spirit Is Transforming the Public Sector.* Reading, MA: Addison-Wesley.

Peplau, H. (1952). *Interpersonal Relations in Nursing.* New York: Springer.

Pesut, D. and Herman, J. (1999). *Clinical Reasoning: The Art and Science of Critical and Creative Thinking* (2nd ed.). Albany, NY: Delmar Learning.

Peters, T. J. (1997). *The Circle of Innovation: You Can't Shrink Your Way to Greatness.* New York: Knopf.

Peters, T. J. (1988). *Thriving on Chaos.* New York: Knopf.

Pew Health Professions Commission. (1995, Nov.). *Critical Challenges: Revitalizing the Health Professions for the Twenty-First Century* (3rd report.). San Francisco, CA: UCSF Center for the Health Professions.

Pierce, L. and Steiner, V. (2003). The male caregiving experience: Three case studies. *Stroke* 34(1), 315.

Pierce, L., Steiner, V., and Govoni, A. (2002). In-home, on-line support for caregivers of persons with stroke: A feasibility study. *CIN: Computers, Informatics, Nursing* 20(4), 157–164.

Porter-O'Grady, T. (1996). Accountability and the role of advanced practice. In C. E. Loveridge and S. H. Cummings (Eds.), *Case Management in the New Paradigm* (pp. 477–480). Gaithersburg, MD: Aspen Publishers, Inc.

Porter-O'Grady, T., Hawkins, M. A., and Parker, M. L. (1997). *Whole-Systems Shared Governance: Architecture for Integration.* Gaithersburg, MD: Aspen Publishers, Inc.

Porter-O'Grady, T. and Malloch, K. (2002). *Quantum Leadership: A Textbook of New Leadership.* Gaithersburg, MD: Aspen Publishers, Inc.

Porter-O'Grady, T. and Wilson, C. K. (1999). *Leading the Revolution in Health Care: Advancing Systems, Igniting Performance,* 2nd edition. Gaithersburg, MD: Aspen Publishers, Inc.

Porter-O'Grady, T. and Wilson, C. K. (1995). *The Leadership Revolution in Health Care: Altering Systems, Changing Behaviors.* Gaithersburg, MD: Aspen Publishers, Inc.

Rodgers, B. L. (1989). Exploring health policy as a concept. *Western Journal of Nursing Research* 11(6), 694–702.

Rogers, M. E. (1970). *An Introduction to the Theoretical Basis for Nursing.* Philadelphia: F. A. Davis Company.

Rossi, P. H. and Freeman, H. E. (1995). *Evaluation a Systematic Approach* (5th ed.). Beverly Hills, CA: Sage Publications.

Saver, C. (2003). Alliance takes another step. *Nursing Spectrum Midwestern Edition* 4(1), 12.

Senge, P. (1990). *The Fifth Discipline: The Art and Practice of the Learning Organization.* New York: Doubleday.

Skocpol, T. (1995). *Social Policy in the United States.* Princeton, NJ: Princeton University Press.

Spratley, E., Johnson, A., Sochalski, J., Fritz, M., and Spencer, W. (2000). The registered nurse population, March 2000. U.S. Department of Health and Human Services, Health Resources and Service Administration, Bureau of Health Professions, Division of Nursing. Retrieved at http://bhpr.hrsa.gov/healthworkforce.

The regulatory process. (1992, Dec. 4). *Capitol Update* 10(23), 1.

Thomas, S. B. and Quinn, S. C. (1991). The Tuskegee syphilis study, 1932 to 1972: Implications for HIV education and AIDS risk reduction education programs in the black community. *American Journal of Public Health* 8(11), 1498–1505.

Venegoni, S. L. (1996). Changing environment of healthcare. In J. V. Hickey, R. M. Ouimette, and S. L. Venegoni (Eds.), *Advanced Practice Nursing: Changing Roles and Clinical Applications* (pp. 77–90). Philadelphia: Lippincott.

Watson, J. (1979). *Nursing: The Philosophy and Science of Caring.* Boston: Little, Brown.

Watzlawick, R., Weakland, C. E., and Fisch, R. (1974). *Change.* New York: WW Norton & Co.

West, W. F. (1982, Sep./Oct.). The politics of administrative rulemaking. *Public Administration Review,* pp. 420–426.

Wheatley, M. (1992). *Leadership and the New Science.* San Francisco: Berrett-Koehler.

Williams, S.J. and Torrens, P.R. (Eds.) (1988). *Introduction to Health Services* (3rd ed.). Albany, NY: Delmar Publisher, Inc.

Wilson, J.Q. (1989). *American Government Institutions and Policies* (4th ed.). Lexington, MA: D.C. Heath and Co.

Wolf, G., Boland, S., and Aukerman, M. (1994a). A transformational model for the practice of professional nursing—Part I: The model. *Journal of Nursing Administration 24*(4), 51–57.

Wolf, G., Boland, S., and Aukerman, M. (1994b). A transformational model for the practice of professional nursing—Part II: Implementation of the model. *Journal of Nursing Administration 24*(5), 38–46.

Zander, K., Etheredge, M., and Bower, K. (Eds.) (1987). *Nursing Case Management: Blueprints for Transformation.* Boston: New England Medical Center.

Zander, K. (1990). The 1990s: Core values, core change. *Frontiers in Health Service Management 2*(1), 39–43.

Agenda Setting

Elizabeth Ann Furlong, JD, PhD, RN

2

Key Terms

Contextual dimensions   Studying issues in the real world, in the circumstances or settings of what is happening at the time.

Iron triangle   Legislators or their committees, interest groups, and administrative agencies that work together on a policy issue that will benefit all parties.

Stakeholders   Policy actors, policy communities, and policy networks; people and groups that have a say in what goes on.

Streams   Kingdon's concept of the interaction of public problems, policies, and politics that couple and uncouple throughout the process of agenda setting.

Window of opportunity   Limited time frame for action.

Introduction

"And, we must persist to eliminate the words *collaboration* and *supervision* from every statute and regulation in the country. Though frustrating and time-consuming, each time legislators open the Nurse Practice Act for revision, they become better informed of our issues" (Pearson, 2003a, p. 8). This advanced nurse practice concern is one of many political and legislative concerns faced by nurse practitioners in 2003. This chapter will emphasize the agenda-setting aspect of policy by using an exemplar case study of how the National Institute of Nursing Research moved onto the political agenda. Agenda setting is the process of moving a problem to the attention of government so that solutions can be considered. APNs can apply the knowledge from this case study to the many current concerns they face such as the just-listed scope of practice issues.

"At the end of my pilgrimage, I have come to the conclusion that among the sins of modern political science, the greatest of all has been the omission of passion" (Lowi, 1992, p. 6). This criticism does not apply to public policy researchers' current scholarly interest in agenda setting, policy design, and alternative formulation, nor does it apply to certain policy communities who push for selected public policies. The passion of the former group, the researchers, is seen in their search and inquiry for a better understanding of public policy. The passion of the latter, policy communities, is reflected in their tenacity on policy design, in pushing to make sure that a policy is put into practice as was intended.

Advanced practice nurses, as well as policymakers and citizens, are interested in the best public policy to address society's concerns. In the past, political science researchers have mostly studied the latter steps of policymaking—implementation and evaluation—to gain an understanding of public policy and a knowledge that could be used by policymakers to create better public policy. Although all stages of the policy process have been studied, the need for more research on the earlier parts of policymaking—agenda setting, policy formulation, and policy design—has drawn more discussion in recent years (Bosso, 1992; Ingraham, 1987; May, 1991). Thus, research interest in these latter areas grew during the 1980s and 1990s and it continues into the 21st century.

The National Center for Nursing Research Amendment

Victor Hugo wrote "Greater that the tread of mighty armies is an idea whose time has come" (Kingdon, 1995, p. 1). For nurses, one example of this was the initiation of legislation in 1983 that has increased the funding base for nursing research. An amendment to the 1985 Health Research Extension Act, which created the National Center for Nursing Research (NCNR) on the campus of the National Institutes of Health, is the focus of this chapter's research information.

Creation of the NCNR came about because of a goal of a group of nurse leaders during 1983 and 1984 to create a national institute of nursing. In order to pass the legislation in 1985, a political compromise was made with legislators to create a center instead of an institute. However, in 1993, the NCNR was changed to an institute. Today the agency continues as the National Institute of Nursing Research (NINR).

Discussion in this chapter of the NCNR amendment focuses on agenda setting and policy formulation that occurred from 1983 to 1985. This chapter also discusses the policy design that led to the policy change in 1993 when the center became an institute. And, finally, this chapter will include updates of what this legislation has meant for the nursing profession and for patient care.

The Influence of National Nursing Groups

The creation of the National Center for Nursing Research (NCNR) on the campus of the National Institutes of Health (NIH) was a policy victory for national nursing organizations. Despite the victory, those nursing organizations still need a better understanding of agenda setting, policy formulation, and policy design as they work for other policy changes in the future. Although nurses' groups traditionally have not been considered strong political actors, these groups recognize the importance of political activity to bring about public policies that enhance patient care (Warner, 2003). However, in the last decade of the 20th century, nurses' groups were just emerging as actors in policy networks. "Yet a full cadre of nurse leaders who are knowledgeable and experienced in the public arena, who fully understand the design of public policy, and who are conversant with consumer, business and provider groups does not yet exist" (DeBack, 1990, p. 69).

In a study of significant national health organizations that play a key role in the health policy-making area (Laumann et al., 1991), no nursing organizations were cited. The scope and nature of nursing care and certain restrictions to providing that care are closely related to public policy. APNs are well aware of this as state legislative activity daily affects their professional practice. Raudonis and Griffith (1991) and Warner (2003) are three of many nurse leaders who challenged nurses to be more knowledgeable about health policy. These leaders also urged nurses to become more empowered on health policy issues. If that were to happen, public policy could better reflect the contributions of nursing to patient care, to the health of citizens, and to cost-effective quality solutions for the financial crisis of the health care system. Nagelkerk and Henry echoed this concern: "To date, few studies in nursing can be classified as policy research. Leaders in our field, therefore, have identified this type of undertaking as a priority" (1991, p. 20).

Research on the NCNR amendment is important because it studies political actors who are not generally studied, i.e., nurses' interest groups. This research contributes to public policy scholars' knowledge of all actors in policy networks. Laumann et al. acknowledged that "we may even run a risk of misrepresenting the sorts of actors who come to be influential in policy deliberation" (1991, p. 67). The significance of this research becomes obvious when the Schneider and Ingram model of "social construction of target populations" in policy design is applied to the nurse interest groups (1993a). For example, how nurses were viewed by policymakers—the social construction of nurses as a target population—influenced not only the policy that nurses were interested in, but also passage of the total NIH reauthorization bill.

Dohler (1991) compared health policy actors in the United States, Great Britain, and Germany and found that it is much easier to have new political actors in the United States because there are multiple ways to become involved. He has written of the great increase in new actors since 1970. Baumgartner and Jones (1993) also described multiple paths of access to becoming involved.

Gender Bias Issue

Because 97 percent of nurses are women, the NCNR example is relevant to concerns about the gender issue in nursing and political science research.

"Even short of arguing that political science concepts and theories have been developed from a male-only perspective, it is all too easy to point to examples of gender bias in political science research, such as failure to focus on policy issues of importance to women, assuming that findings apply to everyone when the population studied was predominantly male . . ." (Johnson and Joslyn, 1991, p. 29).

The policy involved in the NCNR example was important to the predominantly female nursing interest groups. The policy also was important for other women. The amendment to create the NCNR was part of a larger women's issue within the political context that had significant bearing on why this issue was put on the agenda. Another indicator of the concern with gender bias is the research conducted by Kelly and Fisher. "The [American Political Science Review] *APSR* . . . published a mere 24 articles related to women from 1906 through . . . 1991" (1993, p. 544). Further, the bill discussed in the NCNR case was politically significant in that it was one of only six vetoes in which Congress overrode President Reagan during his two terms.

Overview of Models

Several researchers have developed models of agenda setting and policy formulation (Baumgartner and Jones, 1993; Cobb and Elder, 1983; Kingdon, 1995). Several political scientists are developing theoretical modeling of policy design (Hedge and Mok, 1987). Ingraham is one of several authors who have noted the lack of one design, one theory, or one model in policy design (1987). Meanwhile, public policy scholars are pushing for more empirical study of agenda setting, alternative formulation, and policy design (Schneider and Ingram, 1993a).

Data analysis reveals the importance of the Schneider and Ingram model (1993a) of the social construction of target populations and of the Kingdon model (1995) for an understanding of the agenda-setting process of this amendment to the NIH reauthorizing legislative bill. Analysis of this legislation over a period of a decade also underscores the importance of the Dryzek (1983) definition of policy design. An analysis of the legislation supported the importance of studying the contextual dimension that has been advocated by Bobrow and Dryzek (1987), Bosso (1992), deLeon (1988–1989), Ingraham and White (1988–1989), May (1991), and Schneider and Ingram (1993b). The value of other models—institutional, representational communities and institutional approach, and the congressional motivational model—is addressed as these models contribute to an understanding of this example. Finally, during the study of interest groups opposed to this legislation, the researcher noted two occurrences of iron triangles in the early 1980s. These findings will be discussed in more detail.

Some models of agenda setting and policy design did not help to explain this example, such as May's model of policies without publics, Cobb and Elder's model of agenda setting, policy design models that emphasize the study of policy instruments and tools, and Baumgartner's model.

Kingdon Model

Kingdon (1995) tries to answer two public policy questions: How do issues get on the political agenda? And once the issues are there, how are alternative solutions devised? In describing his model, Kingdon identifies both participants and processes that explain the emergence of the agenda and the alternatives. The participants can be actors inside or outside of government. The processes are conceived as three streams that he labels policy streams, problem streams, and political streams. Finally, these processes are affected by a window of opportunity that allows for the merger of these streams and the setting of an agenda. He distinguishes between items on the nongovernmental-systemic agenda and the governmental-formal agenda. The formal agenda consists of those issues that governmental officials are actively discussing and trying to resolve. Kingdon's research shows that the two types of agendas are affected differently by the three streams.

Of the actors in the federal government who are participants, the ones most influential in agenda setting are the administration (the president and his or her advisors), members of Congress, and, to a lesser extent, congressional staff. In the overall ranking, members of Congress ranked second to the administration in importance in agenda setting. This was true despite all the barriers that Congress members face. The ability of a member of Congress to set agendas is furthered if he or she is a committee chairperson, a ranking minority member on a committee, or viewed as a powerful representative.

Kingdon notes that members of Congress become involved in agenda setting to initiate policy to meet constituent needs, to enhance members' reputation in Washington regarding their ability and power, and to put sound public policy into effect. Although congressional staff members are not viewed as having as important a role as the administration and Congress members, the interdependence of the staff and the member is noted. Staff frequently are conduits of ideas and issues to the representative or senator. Staff are in a position, by virtue of their ready access to important members of Congress, their ability to concentrate all their energies on given subjects, and their straddling of political and technical worlds, to have considerable impact on the alternatives considered by important people and even on the agendas of those people. It is important to remember, however, that staffers do all of these things within the limits that are set by the senators and representatives who hire and can fire them (Kingdon, 1995).

Kingdon suggests that elected officials are more important to agenda setting while staffers are more important to alternative formulation. In comparing governmental versus nongovernmental actors, he finds that the former are more instrumental in agenda setting. He finds that the latter (especially interest groups) sometimes play more of a key role in blocking agendas than in promoting agendas. Further, nongovernmental actors are more important in formulating alternative solutions to problems than in agenda setting.

An interest group is most influential if it can "convince governmental officials that it speaks with one voice and truly represents the preferences of its members. If the group is plagued by internal dissension, its effectiveness is seriously impaired . . ." (Kingdon, 1995, p. 55). In discussing this idea, Kingdon alludes to different groups being treated differently by elected officials depending on the group's organizational unity, income, and education. Although the language is different, this is similar to what Schneider and Ingram (1991) investigate in more detail with their model of the social construction of target populations—and the importance of such when analyzing policy. APNs will be more effective when they are united and speak with one voice. A current example is how all four groups of APNs in Nebraska are organizing in a unified manner to change state legislation in 2004 relative to scope of practice.

Although Kingdon studied the various participants who are responsible for agenda setting, he also emphasized that an idea can come from anywhere and that in some ways its source of origin does not matter. He emphasized that it is essential for an idea to land on fertile soil and be nurtured. "Thus the key to understanding policy change is not where the idea came from but what made it take hold and grow" (Kingdon, 1995, p. 76). His research focuses on an idea that suddenly takes off, "an idea whose time has come" (p. 1). His model is adapted from the Cohen-March-Olsen model of organizational decisions. Both models see decision making as a dynamic, fluid process rather than a linear, sequential process. "A problem is recognized, a solution is available, the political climate makes the time right for change, and the constraints do not prohibit action" (Kingdon, 1995, p. 93).

A problem stream can be marked by systematic indicators of a problem, by a sudden crisis, or by feedback that a program is not working as intended. In Kingdon's research, 50 percent of the interviewees reported on the importance of systematic indicators (such as studies and reports) in getting an issue on the agenda. He differentiates between a condition and a problem: conditions become problems when people believe that something ought to be done about them. Thus, APNs can convert conditions of concern into problems.

The second stream, policy, is characterized by the policy community, the presence of ideas, the "softening-up" phase, criteria for the survival of ideas, and the presence of available alternatives. Policy communities are those groups of specialists who have a concern and expertise in certain areas, such as health. This fluid group of both governmental and nongovernmental actors is known to each other by their writings, their professional organizations, and their networking.

In some policy areas, there are specific policy entrepreneurs who are willing to invest "their resources—time, energy, reputation, and sometimes money—in the hope of a future return" (Kingdon, 1995, p. 129). John Wennberg is evaluated by Gray (1992) as an entrepreneur in the setting of a health services research agenda. Although such entrepreneurs sometimes solve problems, Kingdon suggests that many times such individuals are looking for problems to which they can attach their pet solution. APN policy entrepreneurs can identify problems to which they can apply their health policy solutions.

To be placed on an agenda, an idea must have been "softened up." The principle here is that people have to get used to new ideas, and then someone must build support and acceptance for new proposals. This can be done by policy entrepreneurs, policy communities, or agenda-setting participants through education or by freeing "trial balloons" and making speeches. This phase is known as "getting your ducks in a row," "greasing the skids," and "get people to talking" (Kingdon, 1995, p. 135–136).

The third stream of Kingdon's model is the political stream, which consists of the public mood, pressure group campaigns, election results, partisan or ideological distributions in Congress, and changes of administration. Factors that can be influential in this stream include committee jurisdictional boundaries and turf concerns among agencies and government branches. APNs must understand that in the political stream, it is necessary to study coalition building by government officials. Negotiation and persuasion are effective techniques. In wanting a winning coalition, elected officials may more likely say, "You give me my provision, and I'll give you yours" rather than, "Let me convince you of the virtue of my provision" (Kingdon, 1995, p. 167).

Finally, agenda setting occurs as a coupling of streams during a critical time when a window of opportunity appears. "Policy windows open infrequently, and do not stay open long" (Kingdon, 1995, p. 166). Thus it is important for policy entrepreneurs or policy communities to be alert to opportunities. Agendas are affected more by the problem and political streams, whereas alternatives are affected more by the policy stream. Windows of opportunity open because of changes in the political stream or because new problems capture officials' attention.

Examples of changes in the political stream include a new administration or a shift in the partisan or ideological distribution of seats in Congress. Bosso (1992) has included election years as potential windows of opportunity. Hall (1987) writes about the importance of the status of certain congressional members, such as the ranking minority member. In alternative formulation, the policy stream and the policy community are very important.

Data show that the policy option of a national center for nursing research came from the political stream. The amendment arrived on the agenda both as part of substitute NIH legislation to Rep. Waxman's (D-CA) bill and as good public policy for a target population that would be helpful to Rep. Madigan's (R-IL) reelection chances. Data indicated that this policy option surfaced very quickly and then was pursued on the formal agenda as the only policy option. Thus, Kingdon's model about policy alternatives does not apply here.

Although other policy alternatives were discussed at different times, the first policy option, the National Institute of Nursing (NIN) amendment, was the only one pursued on the formal agenda until fall 1985, when a compromise was reached. In this research, the political stream became the important stream. The initial discussion by congressional staffers that led to the acceptance of this issue and its placement on the formal agenda by Rep. Madigan with the support of nursing's Tri-Council (the American Nurses Association [ANA], the American Association of Colleges of Nursing [AACN], the National League for Nursing [NLN], and the American Organization of Nurse Executives [AONE]) prevented the serious consideration of other policy alternatives.

Kingdon wrote "Many times, proposals and ideas float around . . . for some time, without being taken very seriously" (1995, p. 31). Although the idea for the NIN arrived on the formal agenda in 1983 because of Rep. Madigan, the data indicated a 5-year history of the idea.

One of Kingdon's congressional staff interviewees said this about information and communication patterns on the Hill: "It's interesting, dealing with the Hill. It's very informal. Most of it is oral, most of it among friends. . . . On the Hill, there are no channels. It's who knows whom, which friends you develop" (1995, p. 41). This fluidity of interpersonal interchange was mentioned by one of the interviewees for this study in her analysis of how the idea of a national institute emerged on the agenda. This was evident in the data about the initial agenda-setting process for this research—congressional staffers had knowledge about a recent Institute of Medicine (IOM) report that indicated a funding problem for nurse researchers. The staffers and the congressman combined this knowledge with their analysis of how politically feasible such a policy would be. They did this among themselves and also by contacting their Senate counterpart staff member, Dr. Sundwall. This is an example of how the policy community works.

This issue's placement on the formal agenda by a congressman fits with Kingdon's model of the importance of such actors in agenda setting. His research found that members of Congress were the significant actors in agenda setting 91 percent of the time. Kingdon further stated: "But members of Congress, in contrast to most other actors, have the unusual ability to combine some impact on the agenda with some control over the alternatives" (1995, p. 38). The importance of this ability was seen in this example. The initial policy option, once decided by Rep. Madigan, the nursing interest group and later through Rep. Madigan's negotiations with Rep. Waxman and his staff, was faithfully pursued during the legislative process. Once Rep. Madigan and Rep. Waxman completed their negotiations with each other, Rep. Madigan kept control of the policy alternative (the original NIN amendment) that he wanted.

Kingdon discussed three incentives for senators and representatives to set agendas with policies—the same reasons that Fenno (1986) and Hall (1987) have identified. The interview data showed that Rep. Madigan's agenda-setting NIN policy met all three of these incentives. The first incentive of meeting present and future constituent needs was a major reason not only for Rep. Madigan, but also for his calculation of winning the support of other congressional members. This was the importance of the Schneider and Ingram model of the perceptions of the social construction of target populations; there were nurses in Rep. Madigan's district and in every district in the country. Congressional staff interview data reflected that Madigan pursued this policy because it also met the two other incentives: It was sound policy, and it enhanced his congressional reputation.

Kingdon's research found that congressional staff members were important 41 percent of the time in getting issues on the agenda. Although congressional staff gave the credit to Rep. Madigan for setting the agenda, the data indicate the importance of the staff in initiating this policy option. Kingdon noted that staff can have "a considerable impact on the alternatives considered" (1995, p. 44). This was evident from the interview data; the staff had brainstormed several alternatives and decided on one, the NIN policy, then pursued that with Rep. Madigan. However, it was acknowledged by staffers that there were many issues that Rep. Madigan could have put on the agenda and, once on the agenda, that he had the choice to support or not support. The fact that he initiated this agenda item and then tenaciously supported it demonstrated his commitment to the issue. A congressional staffer gave examples of issues after 1986 that were important to nurses but which Rep. Madigan chose not to support. Kingdon's research points up the interdependence between the congressional staffers and the member (1995). To succeed with public policy, APNs must know elected officials *and* their staff (Warner, 2003).

Whether discussing the executive or legislative branch of government as agenda setters, Kingdon distinguishes between the visible and the invisible participants. He notes that the "generation of alternatives occurs more in the hidden cluster . . . and that the process of generating alternatives is less visible than the agenda-setting process" (1995, p. 73). Although two articles identified Dr. Heller, a congressional staffer and an IOM Robert Wood Johnson Health Policy Fellow, as the initiator of the idea, the interview data revealed the invisible participants who played a part in the generation of ideas and policy alternative discussion. Research by DeGregorio and Snider (1993) also attest to staff influence. "In closing, these findings corroborate something staff alumni have been reporting for years through numerous, published legislative case histories. Some staffers play important leadership roles in the formulation of consequential, national policy . . ." (1993, p. 25). Mueller also noted the importance of congressional staff to all aspects of policy development (1988).

In the Kingdon model, interest group influence on agenda setting has been described more as blocking than promoting agendas. Data from this research found the NIH and the American Association of Medical Colleges (AAMC) as interest groups that tried to block the formation of an NIN. On the other hand, the nurse interest group actively promoted the policy. Kingdon wrote of interest group resources that have a bearing on agenda setting, alternative formulation, and the legislative process. The importance of these resources was evident in this research data. The geographical distribution of nurses in all congressional districts was an electoral advantage to Rep. Madigan and to all congresspeople whose support he wanted for this NIN legislation.

A second factor is the degree of unity that an interest group displays to congressional members. "Part of a group's stock in trade in affecting all phases of policy making—agendas, decisions, implementation—is its ability to convince governmental officials that it speaks with one voice and truly represents the preferences of its members" (1995, p. 55). Although nurse leaders were very concerned about showing unity because of initial decision making that caught the nursing community off guard, the evidence demonstrated that the nursing interest group consistently displayed such unity with Rep. Madigan. (Nursing journals in 1983 reflected some difference of opinion about the feasibility of initiation of the NIN.) Nurses demonstrated unswerving follow-through with the direction set by Rep. Madigan. Congressional staffers frequently cited this factor as one of the reasons the bill was successful.

Another dimension that Kingdon found that affected agenda setting was elections, cited as only moderately important to setting the agenda in 30 percent of the interviews. As just discussed, Rep. Madigan's reelection concerns influenced his introduction of this amendment. In applying the social construction of target population model to this legislative example, one can evaluate the importance of this population (nurses in every district) to both his and other congressional members' reelections. Further, most nurses were female, and promoting a policy for women addressed the gender gap, a perceived disparity in the attention given to women by politicians.

In his model of agenda setting, Kingdon discusses the problem of infinite regress—the difficulty of determining the origin of an idea. Part of this is because of the fluidity of ideas and of communication that occurs among all political actors—the administration, individuals on Capitol Hill, interest groups, and the news media. What is important is that an agenda idea lands on fertile soil. Kingdon wrote that it was futile to specify the exact origin of an idea. Interview data indicated that the proposal had been an idea from Sen. Kennedy (D-MA) and Rep. Pursell (R-MI) but was never pursued. Further, when the idea was initiated by Rep. Madigan and quickly accepted by the ANA, it caught the nursing interest group by surprise. Indicators that this idea did not land on totally fertile soil included data about the policy alternatives discussed by nurses and the concern voiced about keeping nurses united in focusing on the NIN option and not switching to another policy alternative. This agenda idea did not go through the "softening-up" period of which Kingdon writes. This lack of "softening up" is what made the nursing interest group so concerned about not losing unity within the nursing community.

Coupling of the three streams occurred because of the timing of the reauthorization of the NIH bill. All nurses did not recognize this as a window of opportunity. For an idea to get on the agenda, the three streams are coupled at a certain time. Different factors influence each of the three streams and, in turn, each stream affects agendas and alternatives differently. Beginning with the problem stream, ideas can get on the agenda if there are indicators of a problem or if there is inequity in distribution of resources among groups. For this example, the importance of the 1983 IOM report was consistently cited as such an indicator. This study, released by the IOM in January 1983, alerted Dr. Heller to the problem of a lack of funding for nursing research. The importance of the IOM report as an indicator of a problem also relates to research by Feldman, Putnam, and Gerteis (1992). They had researched the positive effect that foundation-funded commissions' studies have had on health policy in this country. The IOM was such a funded report. The NIN policy as an agenda idea was enhanced because of the great inequity in how health research money was spent: $5 million for nursing research compared to several billion for NIH. Kingdon wrote: "It takes time, effort, and mobilization of many actors, and the expenditure of political resources to keep an item prominent on the agenda" (1995, p. 109). Many interviewees spoke of the commitment that Rep. Madigan made to this policy. At any time, he could have given it up.

In the second policy stream, Kingdon noted that officials pursue initiatives because of electoral reasons. However, he also wrote that officials pursue policy because of its sound substantive content. Interview data revealed both of these reasons for Rep. Madigan's initiating the idea. Within the policy stream, five criteria must be met for a proposal to survive:

1. technical feasibility
2. value acceptability within the policy community
3. tolerable cost
4. anticipated public agreement
5. a reasonable chance for elected decision makers to be receptive to it

Although the NIN option met the latter three criteria, the first two factors played a role when policy alternatives were considered. For example, the concern of those nurses who questioned having this proposal at this time related to two factors: Was nursing ready from a scientific, intellectual perspective to move to the prestigious NIH campus? And was a critical mass of nurse researchers available? In addition to the question of feasibility, there was a question of values: Would nursing education suffer financially because its federal location was being separated from nursing research? Did nurses value nursing research to the possible harm of nursing education? Nursing research might be at NIH, while nursing education programs would remain at the Department of Health and Human Services. Some leaders thought that would diminish the power of nursing.

The third stream, the political stream, consists of factors such as electoral periods, partisan distribution, and ideological concerns in Congress and national moods. All of these factors influenced the setting of this agenda. The national mood of concern about gender had a bearing on the target population of nurses being selected. This was important for Republicans because they were not garnering as many women's votes as were Democrats. By advocating for a policy that affected a profession that was predominantly female, Republicans hoped to attract more women voters. Because there were nurses in every congressional district in the country, this sound public policy also had very positive political implications for all Republicans.

Kingdon speaks specifically to jurisdictional questions and territorial turf battles. The importance of these issues was seen in this example. Rep. Waxman was pursuing policy because he wanted more power for his subcommittee. Rep. Madigan pursued policy because of his concern about who controlled NIH turf—NIH officials or Congress. Consensus building is important in the political stream. "Here, coalitions are being built through the granting of concessions in return for support of the coalition . . ." (Kingdon, 1995, p. 167). Data described the coalition building between Rep. Waxman and Rep. Madigan. Rep. Waxman accepted Rep. Madigan's NIN policy option, and then Madigan worked with Waxman in promoting the total NIH bill.

In summarizing these findings in relation to the Kingdon model, this example validated the importance of the political and problem streams. However, the NCNR amendment was passed without meeting the policy stream processes described by Kingdon.

Advanced practice nurses may be able to apply the Kingdon model to ongoing priority practice issues with which they are concerned. For example, they can be attentive to the three streams (policy, problem, and political) and a window of opportunity in which to move their agenda. Every year a legislative update is printed in *The Nurse Practitioner*. This is one way to recognize the advances made in state policies in the areas of scope of practice, prescriptive authority, reimbursement practices, title protection, and emerging issues (Pearson, 2003b).

Although the exemplar case study used in this chapter is that of the National Institute of Nursing Research getting on the political agenda and passing as national legislation, APNs also need to be aware of taking political activity in regulatory agencies when that is the best way to problem solve. Nurse practitioners are finding increased difficulty in having mail-order pharmacies recognize and fill their prescriptions (Edmunds, 2003). Two nurse practitioners from New York and South Carolina addressed this problem stream by working with the Food and Drug Administration and the Federal Trade Commission because they recognize the venue of working through regulatory agencies is the best initial solution for this problem (Edmunds, 2003).

Another successful legislative victory for nurses has been the creation of the Vietnam Women's Memorial that was dedicated in 1993. In applying Kingdon's model to this situation, the problem stream was the most important. This monument, which recognizes the contributions of nurses in the Vietnam War, moved onto the agenda and was tenaciously pursued at the legislative and regulatory processes for 10 years by Diane Carlson Evans, RN, Army nurse (Carlson Evans, 2002). She attended the 1982 dedication of the Vietnam Veterans Memorial "and it did not feel right; it did not resonate the total truth" (personal communication, April 2003). That reaction was the problem stream, i.e., the 1982 Vietnam

Veterans Memorial did not genuinely constitute or reflect the total truth of what a Vietnam memorial should convey. It did not express any of the contributions or suffering of women and nurses who also had a part. This legislative and regulatory victory was initiated by an interest group first by Ms. Carlson Evans and later by the many coalitions she engaged to assist her in this endeavor. This example shares the trait of tenacity with the NINR example; in both cases, nurses were tenacious about accomplishing their goals.

Importance of Contextual Dimensions

Some authors, notably Bobrow and Dryzek (1987), Bosso (1992), deLeon (1988–1989), Ingraham and White (1988–1989), May (1991), and Schneider and Ingram (1993b), have emphasized the need to analyze the political context in which policies get on the agenda, alternatives are formulated, and policies are put into effect. Although neither a definitive nor an exhaustive list, five contextual dimensions are suggested by Bobrow and Dryzek (1987) for studying the success or failure of any designed policy: (1) complexity and uncertainty of the decision-system environment; (2) feedback potential; (3) control of design by an actor or group of actors; (4) stability of policy actors over time; and (5) the audience must be stirred into action. DeLeon says that sometimes researchers, because of their unstructured environment, have chosen to study approaches and methodologies that may meet scientific rigor better, but in doing so come "dangerously close to rendering the policy sciences all-but-useless in the real-life political arenas" (1988–1989, p. 300).

DeLeon notes that it is difficult to impossible for researchers to "structure analytically the contextual environment in which their recommended analyses must operate" (1988–1989, p. 300). Researchers have to work in a world with great social complexity, extreme political competition, and limited resources. Of these writers, Bosso and May are especially strong in their advocacy of this contextual approach to the study of public policy. Bosso (1992) echoes deLeon's concern:

> In many ways, the healthiest trend is the admission, albeit a grudging one for many, that policymaking is not engineering and the study of policy formation cannot be a laboratory science. In policy making contexts do matter, people don't always act according to narrow self-interest, and decisions are made on the basis of incomplete or biased information. (1992, p. 23)

Data from congressional documents, archival sources, and personal and telephone interviews show the importance of the political context to all aspects of policy design—how the policy arrived on the agenda, how policy alternatives were formulated, the legislative process, implementation, and redesign of the legislation 8 years later resulting in new legislation within 2 years to accomplish the original goal (Bobrow and Dryzek, 1987; Bosso, 1992; deLeon, 1988–1989; Ingraham and White, 1988–1989; May, 1991; Schneider and Ingram, 1993b).

Examples of Political Contextual Influence

First, partisan political party conflict within Congress influenced the initial agenda setting of the amendment and the legislative process throughout the 2 years. Opposition to Rep. Waxman's NIH bill in the spring and summer of 1983 resulted in Rep. Madigan's initiating a substitute policy. As noted by two congressional staffers, this was an example of partisan conflict. Another example of partisanship, noted by an interviewee, was that the appointment of Dr. Ada Sue Hinshaw as the first director of the NCNR was made easier because she was Republican. (The administration at the time was Republican.)

Second, a U.S. Representative's concern with his reelection chances influenced the initial agenda setting because of the congressional perception that nurses were a "target population" that could help his reelection chances. Several respondents noted that this was an important factor in the initial decision for this type of public policy.

A third contextual dimension was the bipartisan negotiation to enact policy. Such negotiations by Rep. Waxman and Rep. Madigan in early fall 1983 resulted in a firm resolve during the 97th and 98th Congresses to stay with the proposed NIN policy and during the 99th Congress to accept a compromise of an NCNR. Another example of bipartisan negotiation was the early committee work by Rep. Madigan, Rep. Broyhill (R-NC), and Rep. Shelby (D-AL) to forge a simple bipartisan amendment that was four lines long. The bipartisan effort of these three representatives smoothed the way for passage of this amendment by the subcommittee.

Fourth, interest group unity on a policy was a factor. Such unity by nurse groups was considered by many interviewees to be an important factor in the bill's passage. This factor also was important in explaining why no other policy alternatives were pursued. Because the decision to support Rep. Madigan was officially made by the Tri-Council in the summer of 1983, and although other policy alternatives were considered after that, the priority of presenting unity with Rep. Madigan was maintained.

Dohler's research (1991) reported on the importance of the unity of policy communities. He concluded that the deregulation of two organizations, the Professional Standards Review Organization and the Health Systems Agencies, occurred because of the "weakened stability of the network segment" (1991, p. 267). He determined that if there is not a stable united policy community, programs falter. If there is such stability (as with the nursing community in this research), there is an increased chance of success.

Fifth, lack of interest group unity with a congressperson was seen as a negative factor. Such behavior by the AAMC had disillusioned Rep. Madigan and increased his interest in initiating the NIN policy.

Sixth, partisan conflict between the White House and an interest group (nursing) that supported Democratic presidential and vice presidential candidates had an influence on this legislation's history. This campaign support by the ANA for the Democratic candidates was evaluated as the reason for the

1984 Republican presidential veto of the NIN amendment and the NIH bill that had passed Congress. Interviewee data showed one congressperson's concern with how the ANA Political Action Committee (PAC) distributed its money—mainly to Democratic candidates. Research by Makinson (1992) a decade later on the 1990 election reflected that the ANA PAC gave 85 percent of its money to Democratic candidates (1992). Similar trend lines are true in 2003.

Seventh, ideological and partisan conflicts over other issues within the larger NIH bill affected the bill's legislative history. Concerns about fetal tissue research and animal rights research caused much difficulty in the early 1980s. Concerns about immigration laws and HIV-infected immigrants raised concerns in the 1990s and affected compromises and passage of the bills. Such other issues, although not about the NIN amendment, had a major effect on the bill's legislative history. APNs need to understand bills in their holistic content and the many pressures on a particular bill.

Eighth, concerns with the federal deficit influenced discussion of the bill and decision making. The creation of new federal entities was opposed because of the deficit concern. President Reagan consistently used this argument as a reason not to create an NIN.

Ninth, legislation passed during a "lame-duck" presidential term was a factor. The NIH bill with the NCNR amendment was passed in 1985 when President Reagan was beginning his second term. Republican congresspeople did not feel as constrained to vote along party lines, and that was reflected in the 1985 legislative vote and the override vote. Thus, the timing of this vote in President Reagan's lame-duck term helped the bill's passage.

Tenth, the history of Congress with selected administrative agencies influenced the political context. Rep. Waxman's attempted control of NIH was a factor in Rep. Madigan's initiation of NIH legislation during the summer of 1983. Data support the analysis that of all administrative agencies, the NIH consistently was regarded positively by Congress members. This was reflected in ample funding levels on a consistent basis.

Contrary to this usual positive regard was the negative situation between Rep. Dingell (D-MI) and the NIH. He had "captured" letters sent by NIH officials to research scientists asking them to lobby their Congress members for increased funding. Rep. Dingell reminded NIH officials that this activity violated law. Further, this situation led Rep. Dingell and other Congresspeople to ask: Who was and who should be in charge of the NIH?

Eleventh, the interaction of Congress, administrative agencies, and the Office of Management and Budget (OMB) also influenced the political context. The congressional funding pattern identified in the 10th factor changed somewhat in the early 1980s. NIH officials became anxious when OMB dictated that NIH make a last-minute revised budget to honor a 1980 promise to fund 5,000 new grants yearly. This mandated division of NIH's economic pie contributed to NIH officials' not wanting new research entities on their campus that would further erode current programs and projects. A second similar budgetary crisis occurred at NIH in spring 1985 that again caused much consternation for NIH officials and research scientists.

Twelfth, the internal political dynamics of Congress also influenced this legislation. Rep. Waxman was a member of the congressional class of 1974, when the dynamic in Congress was a decentralization of power and increased congressional staff. The data revealed that Rep. Waxman was interested in gaining more power and control over NIH. Although his committee had authorizing power over NIH, it did not have the greater power of the appropriations committee that was responsible for funding. However, with his ability to authorize legislation, Rep. Waxman had leverage to gain more power. His attempt to micromanage NIH resulted in Rep. Madigan's initiating substitute policy.

Thirteenth, interaction between the White House and Congress affected the legislation. For example, President Reagan publicly vetoed the legislation in 1984, although he could have done it quietly by not signing the bill. This was done to alert the Congress to expected conflict the following year if the bill's provisions were kept the same.

An example of the negative relationship between the White House and Congress related to the override vote in 1985. Data showed that members of Congress (and many of the president's party) felt betrayed over their work on this legislation and over what they thought their communication had been with the president about passing this policy and putting it into effect. This sense of betrayal spurred their work in securing the veto override vote. Another example of the relationship between the White House and Congress was the number of presidential vetoes by President Reagan of congressional legislation and the few veto-override votes. Since his inauguration, President Reagan had vetoed 41 legislative bills; this override of the NIH bill veto was the fifth successful override vote since 1981 (*Congressional Quarterly*, 1985).

Fourteenth, even international political relations were a consideration. During fall 1985, the Senate waited until the Geneva Summit was finished before beginning the veto-override vote. This was done to keep President Reagan from losing any credibility during the summit meeting because the Soviet leader would be aware of the veto-override vote.

Fifteenth, the skills and abilities of an interest group in furthering its intended policy had an influence on the context of legislation. Data revealed that in the early 1980s many factors influenced the ability of the nursing interest group to promote this policy once it was on the agenda. These influences were: (1) the formation of the Tri-Council; (2) a special interest in public policy of the executive director of the NLN; (3) the coming need to reauthorize the Nurse Education Act; (4) many deans of nursing education programs who were policy oriented; (5) a combination of people who saw the need; (6) much networking by nurses; (7) the presence of highly motivated people who were interested in furthering the nursing profession; (8) nurses appointed to positions within the White House; (9) more nurses working on the Hill; and (10) the study conducted by Dr. Joanne Stevenson (personal communication, 1990) on nurse researchers' inability to obtain NIH grants. These factors were obtained from interview data.

Sixteenth, the adage that "all politics is personal" influenced the legislation at various points. Data revealed the importance of personal relationships in getting the idea on the agenda, in gaining strategic information, in sharing needed information, and in asking for requests. For example, strategic networking at certain cocktail parties helped, as did carpooling with selected political actors.

Finally, the importance of congressional staffers to the initiation and passage of legislation must be noted. Several interviewees spoke of the importance of certain staffers in their tenacity to ensure that the NCNR amendment was passed. Other staffers noted the importance of the professional education background and socialization of staffers in influencing the types of policy options that are initiated and worked on with vigor. Interview data attested to the tenacity of one Capitol Hill staffer during the conference committee.

Two of Bobrow and Dryzek's (1987) five contextual dimensions were in evidence and contributed to the success of this policy, both because the NCNR was passed as legislation in 1985 and because the NCNR became a national institute of nursing research in 1993. The two criteria are related in this instance: the control of design by an actor or group of actors and the stability of policy actors over time. Once this policy was on the agenda and once nurses were united, the nursing interest group was committed to it: "control of design by an actor." The nursing interest group showed unity in working with Rep. Madigan and staying the course. Thus, although there were other policy alternatives discussed, they were never vigorously pursued by the nurse interest group. Once the compromise for NCNR was made in 1985, the nurse interest group found that acceptable because they knew they had a "foot in the door" and because they planned to accomplish their original design (a NINR) at a later date.

The second dimension, stability of policy actors, also relates to the nurse interest group. This group of nurse leaders was stable over a decade and kept tenaciously to its goal. Although the policy arrived on the formal agenda because of Rep. Madigan, once the policy was there, a very stable group of nurse actors worked over a decade to see that the original policy design eventually was enacted (change from a NCNR to a NINR).

May (1991) writes that regardless of how one defines policy design there is the "emphasis on matching content of a given policy to the political context in which the policy is formulated and implemented" (p. 188). This statement describes the contextual dimension of how this public policy arrived on the formal agenda. Rep. Madigan was going to introduce substitute legislation for Rep. Waxman's NIH bill. Rep. Madigan's NIN amendment was based on an appraisal of what policy content would best work in that political context.

Ingraham and White wrote: "Politics can influence both design process and design outcome in a number of ways. It can constrain problem definition and the range of alternative solutions available for consideration. . . . It can, in fact, eliminate the process of design altogether" (1988–1989, p. 316). Data indicate that this happened. Partisan politics and reelection politics influenced the design process—the policy option that was chosen (the NIN proposal). That policy option moved quickly to the formal agenda, where it then moved forward in the legislative process. The politics of that option kept other alternative solutions from being seriously considered. Although the data (archival and interview) reveal that other policy alternatives were discussed, they were never pursued. Thus, the politics of this situation influenced the design process and the selection of the policy option and constrained the availability of other policy alternatives.

Schneider and Ingram Model

In addition to the political context emphasis, Schneider and Ingram (1991, 1993a, 1993b) specifically push for empirical research that studies the social construction of target populations (those groups affected by the policy). They propose that one can best understand agenda setting, alternative formulation, and implementation by knowing how elected officials perceive different target populations; in other words, by knowing the "social construction"—images, symbols, and traits of such populations.

In their beginning work in this area, Schneider and Ingram model a theory in which there is a continuum of target populations categorized as the advantaged, contenders, dependents, and deviants. Their model suggests that there are pressures to initiate beneficial policy that help those groups that are seen positively, while groups that are seen negatively will receive punitive policy. They argue that groups that are viewed positively are the "advantaged" and the "dependents" while the negatively perceived groups are the "contenders" and the "deviants." This is a beginning categorization, and they call for empirical research in this area. They admit that their theory needs three items:

1. a definition of target populations and of social constructions
2. an explanation of how social constructions influence public officials in choosing agendas and designs of policy
3. an explanation of how policy agendas and designs influence the political orientations and participation patterns of target populations

The idea of target population is taken from the policy design literature and refers to policy that is goal oriented, purposeful, and aimed at change in people's behavior. The social construction of target populations includes two factors: (1) an awareness of the shared traits that make a particular group socially meaningful and (2) specific values, symbols, and images that one associates with that target population. In discussing the second point, the researchers describe a link between the social construction of target populations and the behavior of elected officials in their agenda-setting behaviors.

To better understand the idea of social construction of target populations, examples are given from the model proposed by Schneider and Ingram.

Positively viewed target populations (the advantaged and the dependents) could be on a continuum of being viewed with and without power. For example, the elderly, business people, military veterans, and scientists (the advantaged) would be examples of target populations who are viewed positively and with power. Target populations who are considered more dependent, such as children, mothers, and the disabled (the dependent), are viewed positively but with less power.

Likewise, there is category of negatively viewed target populations (the contenders and the deviants). Again, these groups can be viewed with and without power. Examples that Schneider and Ingram (1991) provide of negatively perceived target populations include the rich, big unions, minorities, cultural elites, and the moral majority (the contenders). Target populations viewed negatively and without political power include criminals, drug addicts, communists, flag burners, and gangs (the deviants). The authors describe how this model could be applied to understand agenda setting. Social constructions of target populations help provide better answers to Lasswell's (1936) enduring question: Who gets what, when, and how? Conventional political science hypotheses about the characteristics that determine groups' influence in setting policy agendas and influencing policy content become significantly more robust when augmented by assessments of social constructions. Further, understanding social construction of target populations helps to explain how elected officials behave, and why—in some circumstances—officials will support policy provisions that distribute benefits at odds with their apparent self-interest, as determined by their assessment of interest group and constituency opinion (Schneider and Ingram, 1993b).

Because research (Hall, 1987; Kaji, 1993) shows that important motivations for congressional members are their interests in winning reelection and in initiating sound policy that addresses social problems, Schneider and Ingram's model of congressional members' perception of groups is relevant to the agenda setting, alternative formulation, and legislative action in which they participate. This model predicts that certain types of policy tools will be used more frequently with certain types of target populations. The need for empirical research in this approach to public policy study provides a ripe area for APNs. For example, a 1997 study by Declercq and Simmes examined how "drive-through deliveries" got on the state legislative agendas and were passed as legislation by several states quite quickly. This clinical issue has implications especially for nurse practitioners and nurse midwives. Some of the findings correlate with similar findings in this NINR case study examination—use of Kingdon's model, importance of contextual dimensions, and importance of symbols.

The Schneider and Ingram theory, together with Kingdon's research, provides the best explanation for understanding the process of the NCNR legislation. Schneider and Ingram (1991, 1993a, 1993b) say that one can best understand agenda setting, alternative formulation, and implementation by knowing how elected officials see different target populations; and by knowing the social construction, or images, symbols, and traits of such populations. The data consistently revealed that this NCNR policy was initiated by Rep. Madigan because of the social construction of this target population of nurses. Proposing public policy for this target population would help him pass his substitute NIH legislation. In the model developed by Schneider and Ingram (1991), nurses, as a target population, would be on the continuum of positively viewed groups. Although Schneider and Ingram acknowledge that theirs is an emerging model that needs empirical testing to refine and define several of its phenomena, this author found it to be of explanatory value and extreme importance.

Mueller (1988) wrote: "Politicians must be convinced that they will gain from new policies—either through political success or through program effectiveness" (p. 443). The selection of nurses as a target population when Congress members, especially Republicans, needed the female vote contributed to a convincing argument for potential political success for them.

Other Models and Theories

Cobb and Elder Model   The concepts of the Cobb and Elder model (1983) include a distinction between the systemic and the formal or institutional agenda. The systemic agenda includes those concerns that are "more abstract, general and broader in scope and domain" (p. 14). On the other hand, formal or institutional agenda items are those that are "explicitly up for the active and serious consideration of authoritative decision makers" (p. 86). This means items that are specific and concrete and that are proposals before any governmental body for action. These theorists identify six traits that help explain why an issue expands, gains public attention, and moves from the systemic agenda to the formal agenda:

1. the concreteness or specificity of the issue
2. the social significance or breadth of the effect on society
3. the temporal relevance or the long-term implications of the issue
4. the complexity or the technical intricacy of the issue
5. the categorical precedence or how similar issues were previously resolved
6. the interval of time or how rapidly an issue develops public attention

Steckenrider (1991) is one of many researchers who has used the Cobb and Elder model to better understand a policy. Steckenrider's research found that the issue of Alzheimer's disease met the six characteristics that Cobb and Elder had identified that move an item from the systemic to the formal agenda. Sharp's study of policy making concerning illicit drugs (1992) has extended an earlier model of agenda setting to a new network type of agenda setting. A network model of agenda setting presumes that an issue does not arise from one single easily identifiable source. Rather, the concern springs from the interactions among actors from many locations. In her case study research, Sharp concluded that this occurred either because actors in different settings were responding to the same dramatic events or because they independently recognized political opportunities. Thus, APNs need to be alert to the application of such a network model of agenda setting.

Policies With and Without Publics Model   Besides his concern with contextual factors, May's research (1991) in policy design is focused on the difference between "policies with publics" and "policies without publics." He asserts that there are different design and implementation challenges depending on whether or not the policy is characterized as having few or many interest groups favoring or challenging the policy. DeLeon (1988–1989) had stated that a concrete definition of context and its effect upon policy would ease the design, selection, implementation, and evaluation of policies. May's work is a beginning step in this direction.

Institutional Model   Yet another dimension to the study of policy design is that advocated by Krane (1993). Although he is proposing that more attention be paid to federalism and intergovernmental relations in understanding public policy, he also supports more emphasis being given to the effects of institutions on policy. "The 'new institutionalism' and the nascent theory of policy design share a theoretical concern with understanding the effects of different institutional structures on the behavior of individuals" (p. 189).

Bosso (1992) and Brandl (1988) are other writers who argue for more research on how institutions shape and influence policy. For example, Bosso notes the institutional structure of Congress with the expected rhythm of reelection periods. He applies Kingdon's theory of agenda setting and observes that reelection periods can bring windows of opportunity. Another example of the effects of institutions on agenda setting is the division of authority between national and subnational jurisdictions. Problems at the subnational level may or may not make it on a national agenda.

As stated in an earlier section of this chapter on contextual influences, institutional structures affected Rep. Waxman. He was influenced by being in the congressional class of 1974 and was influenced by how power was distributed in committees. Many new congresspersons were elected over incumbents in 1974 because of cynicism following the Watergate scandal. Americans wanted a "change of face." This also was the time of decentralization of power within Congress, i.e., more power was given to committees and subcommittees versus a few individuals. Rep. Waxman had a reputation for enhancing his power with these changes. These institutional characteristics influenced Waxman's behavior in trying to gain more control over NIH. Kaji (1993) said that the Committee on Energy and Commerce was "affectionately known on the Hill as 'Energy and Conquest' for the strong personalities and battles which are common there" (p. 4). Bosso (1992) wrote of the institutional structure of Congress with its expected rhythm of reelection periods and how that rhythm influences windows of opportunity for agenda setting. The data reflected this institutional characteristic. Rep. Madigan was concerned about his reelection and this affected the policy option he chose to introduce: the NIN amendment.

Representational Communities and Institutional Approach   The most recent work by Peterson (1993) studies policy from two important dimensions: (1) the representational community of organized interests and (2) the structural context of institutions. In his study of health policy, he says that representational communities have changed from iron triangles to policy networks. Iron triangles are beneficial relationships among individuals in an interest group, members of Congress, and governmental employees in a bureaucratic agency. They work together for a certain policy that benefits all of them. Policy networks, more fluid communities of policy experts in a specific area, have come to replace iron triangles.

Peterson further notes that in the past 20 years the types of interest groups in this representational community or policy network have changed. He uses the language of stakeholder and stake-challenger to describe those interest groups that benefit from status quo policy and those interest groups that do not benefit from such policy or are harmed by it—or both. APNs are stake-challengers in this changing health care system.

Changes also have occurred in government structures. Congressional changes starting in 1971 have contributed to this changed policy environment. These changes include: (1) decreased power and autonomy of committee chairs, (2) increased power to subcommittees, (3) expanded professional staff resources on Capitol Hill, (4) more open meetings because of sunshine laws, and (5) decentralization of Congress and an entrepreneurial spirit (Peterson, 1993; Woods, 1993).

Congressional Motivation Model   Other aspects of the literature that have an effect on agenda setting include the work by Fenno (1973, 1978, 1986), Hall (1987), and Kaji (1993) on the motivations of congressional members regarding their initiation and pursuit of selected policies. Fenno (1973) found that these members were motivated by the goals of reelection, influence within Congress, and enacting good public policy as they advanced certain ideas. Fenno's model (1973) applied to this example. Data from several interviewees showed these motivational reasons to explain why Rep. Madigan initiated the NIN policy and why he tenaciously pursued it.

Hall studied decision making in the House Education and Labor Committee during the 97th Congress (1987). He found that members of Congress were actors advancing their political goals. Four goals influenced their behavior on that committee:

1. serving their district's interests
2. making good policy
3. making a political mark
4. promoting the president's agenda

Understanding an official's behavior can be challenging and is underscored by the following:

> Not only are congressmen not, in Mayhew's phrase (1974), "single-minded seekers of reelection," to characterize them as single-minded seekers of any goal does considerable injustice to the complex set of motives that shape their behavior, even on a single committee and a small sample of bills. (Hall, 1987, p. 121)

Hall further discusses the barriers and constraints that members have depending on their freshman or senior status and their position as a committee chairperson. Hall's research offers important implications because committee and subcommittee representation is not reflective of the larger body; rather, it is biased and dependent on members' interests in policies. He writes: "The range of interests, values and geographic constituencies thus expressed on any given issue is likely to be even more narrow, the bias of interests represented more severe, than the study of committee assignments can reveal" (Hall, 1987, p. 122).

Hall (1987) found that effective action in subcommittees was linked to the ranking minority member. Data from the NIN example revealed the same pattern: Rep. Madigan, as ranking minority member on the committee, was effective in pursuing substitute legislation. Hall also said that the 97th Congress, for the first time in three decades, was characterized by Republican control of the Senate and the White House. This had positive consequences for House Republicans. As a minority House staffer said, "Because we have the Senate, the committee majority [of the House] has come to recognize the value of getting the minority on board" (Hall, 1987, p. 120). The House Democratic majority knew they needed the Senate to pass legislation. In the NIN case, these bipartisan dynamics and recognition were evident in the summer and fall of 1983, when Rep. Madigan and Rep. Waxman completed their negotiations.

Mouw and Macken (1992) describe the 1980s as a period of divided government with a conservative president and "an organized and savvy Democratic House leadership" (p. 88). They also noted the shift in House membership in 1982 because of the recession, which resulted in liberal Democrats replacing conservative Republicans. The center of the political landscape had moved to the left.

Kaji studied the Clean Air Act of 1990 and developed a game theory view of advocacy in which congressional efforts to advance an issue is related to the utility of the issue, the utility of other objectives, the behavior of other relevant actors, available resources, and the opportunity for compromise. The results of his research were that Congress members pushed certain issues when acceptable compromises were unavailable and when advocacy of those issues was an efficient use of their resources. In their respective states and in national concerns, APNs must study issues to best apply this efficient use of their congressional resources.

Punctuated Equilibrium Model   Baumgartner and Jones (1993) have studied several policies (nuclear power, child abuse, smoking, pesticides) over time and have created what they call the *punctuated equilibrium model*. This is a model in which issues emerge and then cause changes in institutions. Such institutional changes may remain for decades, only to be replaced by changes as other issues arise on the agenda. There are long periods of relative stability, equilibrium, or incrementalism punctuated by short dramatic changes. However, these bursts of change affect future institutional policymaking. This agenda-setting research is unique in that it combines a cross-sectional and longitudinal design.

Bosso (1992) acknowledged that there was "no single model, no grand theory of policy design," (p. 21) and he argued for "more case studies upon which good mid-level theories can be built" (p. 21). He further called for longitudinal case studies that would give insight on how problems, policies, and policy communities evolve. Sabatier (1988) also advised studies that span a decade so one can better understand policy subsystems and policy change.

The Influence of Policy Design   The policy-design model that best contributes to an understanding of this legislative amendment is the middle-ground definition of policy design by Dryzek: "the process of inventing, developing and fine-tuning a course of action with the amelioration of some problem" (1983, p. 346). The data that support this analysis are the interview data that describe how the policy got on the formal agenda: Rep. Madigan introduced a policy to solve the problem of limited research money for nursing. This policy-design model also is especially evident in the tenacity of the nursing interest group. It persevered over a decade and "fine-tuned a course of action" so that the group's goal of an institute finally was fulfilled in 1993. The nursing interest group's dedication to its goal was seen in its lobbying over the 2-year period in the early 1980s and then again in the early 1990s.

Heitshusen (1993) has written of the importance of the lobby effort at all stages of legislation. The nursing lobby's effectiveness was described by a congressional staffer who said this about the ANA members: "They did things right . . . they were united. . . ." Although such nursing unity was not unprecedented, it was noteworthy. Nursing has not always been unified on issues, and this has been harmful to the profession. However, in this instance it was a major variable that led to the success of this policy. This "fine-tuning of a course of action" also is reflected in the other outcomes noted during the decade. Once the NCNR was established in 1986, positive changes occurred from then until 1993 as measured by increased research funding, increased grants, and increased research training positions.

Berman's work on the politics of federal technology policy in the 1980s shows the importance of key interest group constituencies and supportive bureaucracies to such policy development and implementation (1991). Data revealed that the lobbying effort by the nurse interest group from 1983 to 1985 and 1991 to 1993 and the commitment of nurse researcher employees in the newly established NCNR in 1986 had such an effect on policy development and implementation.

Iron Triangles   Public policy researchers have written of the change over time from the existence of iron triangles to the more fluid policy networks and policy communities (Heclo, 1978). Kingdon (1995) wrote of iron triangles and gave an example from his research of such an iron triangle with NIH. In this NINR example, data were found in the scientific media, as well as from a congressional staffer who demonstrated that in 1982 and 1983 the concept of the iron triangle was reported in NIH-related policy. The first example was with the revised 1983 NIH budget that Dr. Wyngaarden (director, NIH), had to develop quickly. The second example, as told by an interviewee, also was concerned with budgetary concerns. In both examples, lobbying was done through the close collaboration of the three corners of an iron triangle: (1) the interest group of research scientists, (2) the governmental agency of NIH, and (3) the congressional subcommittee responsible for the agency's funding. The importance of this finding is for APN researchers to be alert to the possibility that iron triangles may not have been totally replaced by policy networks and policy communities.

NINR: 20 Years after Agenda Setting

Agenda setting of the NINR has resulted in positive outcomes for the profession of nursing. In 2001 the NINR celebrated a fiscal milestone when their budget exceeded the $100 million mark (Grady, 2001b). This contrasts with $16 million which is how much the National Center for Nursing Research had in its budget in 1986 after the NCNR was first established (Grady, 2001b). The $100 million budget is also noteworthy given the $5 million dollars that nurses were receiving in research in 1983 prior to this agenda-setting legislation. In conjunction with national goals of decreasing health disparities, the NINR has specific research goals and strategies in this area; i.e., to fund those research projects that address those goals (Phillips and Grady, 2002). In addition, in 2001 the NINR along with the National Center on Minority Health and Health Disparities began a pilot project that enhanced partnerships between minority-serving nursing schools and more research-intensive university nursing research programs (Grady, 2001a). Other research goals include research in the areas of management of chronic pain, cachexia, and informal caregiving in noninstitutional settings (Grady, 2002b). Another indicator of success has been the increase in percentage of research grants getting funded. The NINR success rate jumped from 14 percent to 31 percent; the average success rate for other NIH grants is 31 percent. The increase in the number of research grants received at NINR is a healthy indicator, not only of the success rate but also of the increased research practices of nurses and their submission of grants for funding. At NIH, NINR has become the lead institution for end-of-life issues and is recognized in research in chronic illness, caregiver research, genetics, and telehealth (Grady, 2002a). Other indicators include a change from funded, small pilot studies to full-scale clinical intervention studies, doctoral graduates conducting postdoctoral fellowships, competition for continuations of grants, increased publications because of funded research, and the dissemination of knowledge into clinical practice and application by staff nurses (Grady, 2001b).

The importance of agenda setting of the NINR to the growth of nursing research in the 1980s and since then is best summed up by Stolley, Buckwalter, and Garand: "Perhaps the most important factor was the creation in 1986 of the National Center for Nursing Research" (2000, p. 13).

Conclusion

"No data are ever in themselves decisive. Factors beyond only the data help decide which policy is formulated or adopted by the people empowered to make the decision to form policy" (James, 1991, p. 14). James (1991) is referring to data in a problem stream as described by Kingdon. The accuracy of this quote was seen in this research because the Schneider and Ingram theory of the "social construction of target populations," together with the Kingdon model and the contextual dimension, explained the policy process.

The contextual dimension influenced all aspects of the policy, from agenda setting in 1983 through policy redesign in 1991 with passage of the amended legislation in 1993 that accomplished the original 1983 goal. The importance of studying the political context was demonstrated by the 17 contextual dimensions that influenced this legislative policy process.

Of particular explanatory value in the early agenda-setting and policy-alternative formulation of this legislation were the Schneider and Ingram model and the Kingdon model. The particular amendment was pursued because of application of the "social construction of target populations." That is, the target population of nurses was chosen because they would help Rep. Madigan's and other Congress members' chances for reelection. With this model, the Kingdon theory adds to the further understanding of this legislation. Within Kingdon's model, neither the problem stream nor the policy stream was decisive for the process of this legislation; rather, it was the political stream. The factors of the political stream (reelection chances for Rep. Madigan and other congresspeople, partisan ideology in Congress, the public mood about gender issues, and turf concerns between government agencies) all strongly influenced the setting of this issue on the agenda. The following hypotheses supported by this empirical research include policy is more likely to be initiated for those target populations who are positively viewed by Congressmen; issues are more likely to reach the formal agenda when the political stream factors are related to positively viewed target populations; and policy process is best understood in a contextual perspective.

In summary, for APN scholars this research contributes to an understanding of agenda setting and policy design by having evaluated the importance of the Schneider and Ingram model, the Kingdon model, policy design, and the contextual dimension to policy initiation, development, implementation, and policy redesign in the creation of the National Institute for Nursing Research.

Discussion Points

1. How did the Kingdon model explain the NCNR getting on the political agenda?
2. How can APNs become aware of factors in the problem stream to which Kingdon alluded?
3. What are examples of policy streams that APNs could be advancing relative to their practice?
4. How can APNs be involved in the political stream?
5. How can APNs anticipate windows of opportunity?
6. According to Schneider and Ingram, to which of the four target populations do nurses belong? Discuss the relevance to agenda setting.
7. What are ways that APNs can network with congressional members and their staffers?
8. How can APNs promote unity among themselves and with other nurses?
9. What current contextual dimensions can promote APN practice?
10. How can APNs use the Kingdon model and the Schneider and Ingram model?

References

Baumgartner, F. R. and Jones, B. D. (1993). *Agendas and Instability in American Politics.* Chicago: University of Chicago Press.

Berman, E. M. (1991). The politics of federal technology policy: 1980–1988. *Policy Studies Review 10*(4), 28–41.

Bobrow, D. B. and Dryzek, J. S. (1987). *Policy Analysis by Design.* Pittsburgh, PA: University of Pittsburgh Press.

Bosso, C. J. (1992). Designing environmental policy. *Policy Currents 2*(4), 1, 4–6.

Brandl, J. (1988). On politics and policy analysis as the design and assessment of institutions. *Journal of Policy Analysis and Management 7*(3), 419–424.

Carlson Evans, D. (2002). Transforming vision into reality: The Vietnam women's memorial. In D. J. Mason, J. K. Leavitt, and M. W. Chafee (Eds.), *Policy and Politics in Nursing and Health Care* (4th ed.) pp. 185–200. St. Louis, MO: Saunders.

Cobb, R. W. and Elder, C. D. (1983). *Participation in America: The Dynamics of Agenda-Building* (2nd ed.). Baltimore: Johns Hopkins University Press.

Congressional Quarterly (1985, July 27), p. 1493. Washington, DC: U.S. Printing Office.

DeBack, V. (1990). Public policy—nursing needs health policy leaders. *Journal of Professional Nursing 6*(2), 69.

Declercq, E. and Simmes, D. (1997). The politics of "drive-through deliveries": Putting early postpartum discharge on the legislative agenda. *The Milbank Quarterly 75*(2), 175–202.

DeGregorio, C. and Snider, K. (1993, April). *Proximity and Power: Staff Elite in the U.S. House of Representatives.* Paper presented at the Midwest Political Science Association, Chicago, IL.

deLeon, P. (1988–1989). The contextual burdens of policy design. *Policy Studies Journal 17*(2), 297–309.

Dohler, M. (1991). Policy networks, opportunity structures, and neo-conservative reform strategies in health policy. In B. Main and R. Mayntz (Eds.), *Policy Networks:*

Empirical Evidence and Theoretical Considerations (pp. 235–296). Frankfurt am Main: Campus Verlag.

Dryzek, J. S. (1983). Don't toss coins in garbage cans: A prologue to policy design. *Journal of Public Policy 3*(4), 345–368.

Edmunds, M. (2003). Advocating for NPs B go and do likewise. *The Nurse Practitioner 28*(2), 56.

Feldman, P. H., Putnam, S., and Gerteis, M. (1992). The impact of foundation-funded commissions on health policy. *Health Affairs 11*(4), 208–225.

Fenno, R. F. (1986). Observation, context, and sequence in the study of politics. *APSR 80*(1), 3–15.

Fenno, R. F. (1978). *Home Style: House Members in Their Districts.* Boston: Little, Brown & Co.

Fenno, R. F. (1973). *Congressmen in Committees.* Boston: Little, Brown & Co.

Grady, P. A. (2001a). News from NINR: Research partnership program to address health disparities. *Nursing Outlook,* p. 237.

Grady, P. A. (2001b). News from NINR: Happy birthday, NINR. *Nursing Outlook 49*(2), 66.

Grady, P. A. (2002a). News from NINR: NINR's fifteenth anniversary symposium. *Nursing Outlook 50*(1), 1.

Grady, P. A. (2002b). News from NINR: FY 2002 budget increase for NINR. *Nursing Outlook 50*(2), 56.

Gray, B. H. (1992). The legislative battle over health services research. *Health Affairs 11*(4), 38–66.

Hall, R. L. (1987). Participation and purpose in committee decision making. *American Political Science Review 81*(1), 105–127.

Heclo, H. (1978). Issue networks and the executive establishment. In A. King (Ed.), *The New American Political System.* Washington, DC: American Enterprise.

Hedge, D. M. and Mok, J. W. (1987). The nature of policy studies: A content analysis of policy journal articles. *Policy Studies Journal 16*(1), 49–62.

Heitshusen, V. (1993, April). Strategic Lobbying by Interest Groups: The Role of Information and Institutional Change. Paper presented at the annual meeting of the Midwest Political Science Association meeting, Chicago, IL.

Ingraham, P. W. (1987). Toward more systematic consideration of policy design. *Policy Studies Journal 15*(4), 611–628.

Ingraham, P. W. and White, J. (1988–1989). The design of civil service reform: Lessons in politics and rationality. *Policy Studies Journal 17*(2), 315–330.

James, P. (1991). Bravo to the nursing emphasis on policy research. *Reflections 17*(1), 14–15.

Johnson, J. B. and Joslyn, R. A. (1991). *Political Science Research Methods.* Washington, DC: CQ Press.

Kaji, J. T. (1993). A Simple Theory of Legislative Advocacy. Paper presented at the annual meeting of the Midwest Political Science Association, Chicago, IL.

Kelly, R. M. and Fisher, K. (1993). An assessment of articles about women in the "top 15" political science journals. *PS: Political Science & Politics 26*(3), 544–558.

Kingdon, J. W. (1995). *Agendas, Alternatives, and Public Policies*. New York: Harper Collins College Publishers.

Krane, D. (1993). American federalism, state governments, and public policy: Weaving together loose theoretical threads. *PS: Political Science and Politics 26*(2), 186–190.

Lasswell, H. (1936). *Who gets what, when and how?* New York: McGraw-Hill.

Laumann, E. O., Heinz, J. P., Nelson, R., and Salisbury, R. (1991). Organizations in political action: Representing interests in national policy making. In B. Marin and R. Mayntz (Eds.), *Policy Networks: Empirical Evidence and Theoretical Considerations* (pp. 63–96). Frankfurt am Main: Campus Verlag.

Lowi, T. J. (1992). The state in political science: How we become what we study. *American Political Science Review 86*(1), 1.

Makinson, L. (1992). Political contributions from the health and insurance industries. *Health Affairs 11*(4), 120–134.

May, P. J. (1991). Reconsidering policy design: Policies and publics. *Journal of Public Policy 11*(2), 187–206.

Mouw, C. J. and Macken, M. B. (1992). The strategic agenda in legislative politics. *American Political Science Review 86*(1), 87–105.

Mueller, K. J. (1988). Federal programs to expire: The case of health planning. *Public Administration Review 48*(3), 719–725.

Nagelkerk, J. M. and Henry, B. (1991). Leadership through policy research. *Journal of Nursing Administration 21*(5), 20–24.

Pearson, L. (2003a). NPs stand ready for 2003. *The Nurse Practitioner 28*(1), 8.

Pearson, L. (2003b). Fifteenth annual legislative update. *The Nurse Practitioner 28*(1), 26–58.

Peterson, M. (1993). Political influence in the 1990s: From iron triangles to policy networks. *Journal of Health, Politics, Policy, and Law 18*(2), 395–438.

Phillips, J. and Grady, P. A. (2002). Reducing health disparities in the twenty-first century: Opportunities for nursing research. *Nursing Outlook 50*(3), 117–120.

Raudonis, B. M. and Griffith, H. (1991). A model for integrating health services, research, and health care policy formation. *Nursing & Health Care 12*(1), 32–36.

Sabatier, P. A. (1988). An advocacy coalition framework of policy change and the role of policy-oriented learning therein. *Policy Sciences 21*(2), 129–168.

Schneider, A. L. and Ingram, H. (1993a). How the social construction of target populations contributes to problems in policy design. *Policy Currents 3*(1), 1–4.

Schneider, A. and Ingram, H. (1993b). Social construction of target populations: Implications for politics and policy. *American Political Science Review 87*(2), 334–347.

Schneider, A. and Ingram, H. (1991). The Social Construction of Target Populations: Implications for Citizenship and Democracy. Paper presented at the annual meeting of the American Political Science Association in Washington, DC.

Schneider, A. and Ingram, H. (1990). Behavioral assumptions of policy tools. *Journal of Politics 52*(2), 510–529.

Sharp, E. B. (1992). Agenda setting and policy results: Lessons from three drug policy episodes. *Policy Studies Journal 20*(4), 538–551.

Steckenrider, J. S. (1991). *Agenda Building on Health Issues: A Focus on Alzheimer's Disease.* Paper presented at the annual meeting of the American Political Science Association in Washington, DC.

Stolley, J. M., Buckwalter, K. C., and Garand, L. (2000). The evolution of nursing research. *Journal of the Neuromusculoskeletal System 8*(1), 10–15.

Warner, J. R. (2003). A phenomenological approach to political competence: Stories of nurse activists. *Policy Politics, and Nursing Practice 4*(2), 135–143.

Woods, P. D. (1993). *The Dynamics of Congress.* Washington, DC: The Woods Institute.

Government Response: Legislation

Mary Wakefield, PhD, RN, FAAN

3

Key Terms

Caucus An association of members of Congress, a political party, or other group created to advocate a political ideology or a regional or economic interest.

Constituents Residents of a geographic area who can vote for a candidate and whom a member of Congress represents.

Interest group An organized group with a common cause who work to influence the outcome of laws, regulations, or programs.

Issue specialists A loose network of researchers, academics, and government staff who are knowledgeable about a particular topic and who often discuss ideas and critique or suggest policy solutions.

Legislative assistant (LA) An employee of a senator or representative who is responsible for keeping the member apprised of legislative proposals, negotiations, and hearings. LAs often draft reports and serve as liaisons among elected and appointed officials. LAs may be politically neutral or partisan advocates of an issue.

Member An elected participant of a lawmaking body.

Staff Personnel hired to work in an agency, committee, or other organization. These employees carry out the day-to-day business of the office.

Introduction

The purpose of this chapter is to provide advanced practice nurses (APNs) and others with an understanding of the multiple factors that influence the development of public policy through the legislative branch of government. Many of the factors considered in this chapter are operationalized in both state and federal legislative arenas. Consequently, this discussion is relevant to nurses interested in affecting policy in state capitols or the nation's capitol.

In today's environment, an understanding and ability to influence policy development is critically important. The health policy work undertaken in the legislative arena directly or indirectly impacts virtually every facet of the APN's work—whether it is the medication one prescribes, the license one holds, the telehealth technology used to access a specialist, or the level of reimbursement received for providing care. Given the pervasive effect of policy on nursing practice, it is imperative that those in advanced practice know how to influence the policy that ultimately affects their practice and their patients. The policy-making process, in general, and the development of legislation, specifically, can be likened to a murky river that runs its course through many twists and turns. On the surface, the river may appear almost placid, inviting, hardly moving. However, beneath the surface, subtle, then strong currents push and pull, doing much of the work of moving the water and sweeping whatever is within it downstream. This chapter explores some of the currents that are often unseen, yet pivotal, in moving policy initiatives through the legislative process.

The Players

Six general categories of players exert notable influence in the legislative process. Although other categories can be named, individuals in the categories discussed here commonly engage in public health policy development and exert considerable influence throughout the process. The six categories include:

1. member of Congress
2. congressional staff
3. special interest groups and their lobbyists
4. the executive branch
5. constituents
6. the media

These categories are not listed in order of importance or ability to influence legislation. For example, a powerful lobbyist can often exert far more influence than a freshman member of the House of Representatives, especially if the latter is a member of the minority party. Rather, the influence of individuals from each of these categories ebbs and flows, varying with the policy issue at hand.

Members of Congress

Currently, there are 535 members of Congress: 100 senators and 435 representatives. The political party with control of the majority of seats wields considerable influence in significant ways, ranging from setting the legislative agenda to chairing all congressional committees. The identification of problems and possible solutions largely emanate from the political ideology of the party in control. Because of this, statements of belief and priorities expressed by the majority party serve as an important framework for subsequent legislation.

With few exceptions, tradition dictates that members of Congress with the greatest seniority move into positions of influence and are more likely than their junior counterparts to be given the committee assignments they desire. For example, a senior senator from an agricultural state who wishes to obtain a committee assignment on the Agricultural Appropriations Subcommittee is more likely to be given that assignment than a newly elected senator interested in the same position. Seniority is an important factor in determining who is at the table when key decisions are made by legislative bodies. It comes as no surprise, then, that discussion of the power incumbents wield by virtue of seniority or a committee assignment important to constituents back home frequently constitutes a major theme in incumbents' political advertising and campaigning during reelection time.

Though there is often a direct relationship between seniority and ability to wield power, personal characteristics tend to influence the degree of attention that members choose to give legislative issues. Some of these personal characteristics include the member's occupation prior to election, the home state or district the member represents, personal experience with the health care system, and even the gender and ethnic background of the legislator. Personal factors are important enough that effective lobbyists, such as APNs interested in obtaining the support of a legislator, will have reviewed the legislator's biography before the first meeting occurs. The significance of these characteristics is readily exemplified. For example, two senators with backgrounds in health care, one a social worker and the other a cardiac surgeon, are extremely active in a range of health policy initiatives. They frequently draw on their personal experiences in the health care field when, in committee meetings or on the floor of the Senate, members make a case for the importance of proposed legislation. Clearly, health legislation is not the sole prerogative of legislators who are former health care professionals. However, drawing on personal experience, their explanations speak volumes to their less knowledgeable colleagues when critical decisions about complex health legislation are being made. In cases where members have specific health care backgrounds, lobbyists will often seek out the guidance or assistance of members whose professional backgrounds are similar to the organizations they represent. Beyond the professional background of the member, it is not uncommon for lobbyists to know of any ties to health care that the legislator's family may have. For example, knowing that the spouse of a member is a nurse is often useful information to nurse lobbyists, while knowing that an influential senator has a son-in-law who is a chiropractor may be useful information to chiropractic lobbyists. One can assume that, at the very least, such members would be more knowledgeable about these health care providers than many of their congressional counterparts. In the best of all worlds, members with family who have ties to the health care field may be favorably predisposed toward policy supportive of similar provider groups.

It is also generally the case that members of Congress reflect the interests of their home district or state. For example, a senator from a tobacco-producing state is much more likely to oppose strict regulation of the tobacco industry than is a senator from a non-tobacco-producing state. However, personal phone calls from a senate colleague or a promise to provide support for an initiative important to the non-tobacco-state senator at some future date can often result in support from members who, on the surface, might appear to have no particular interest or stake in tobacco legislation. Because passage of legislation requires a majority vote, it is quite common for members to "buttonhole" their colleagues on the floor of the Senate, at a reception, or by phone at home in the evenings in order to enlist support or opposition. Likewise, it is not uncommon for members working with lobbyists to target uncommitted members, bringing pressure to bear on them from both inside and outside Congress. Working in tandem with congressional offices, nursing organizations frequently use grassroots efforts, meetings, and other strategies to sway uncommitted policy makers in order to obtain sufficient support or opposition for proposed legislation.

Even personal experience with the health care system can affect a member's views. For example, both Senator Inouye (D-HI) and former Senator Dole (R-KS) underwent lengthy rehabilitation following life-threatening wounds received in battle while serving in the military. Both men often publicly credited the nurses who cared for them with being instrumental in their successful recoveries. Senators with immediate family members with mental illnesses have been staunch advocates of parity in health insurance coverage for this category of illness.

Finally, although the vast majority of members of Congress are white males, there is an increase in ethnically diverse and female legislators elected to office. While members of Congress are sent to Washington, DC, to represent all of their constituents as well as the interests of the country at large, race and gender are factors that can unify members around policy activities. For example, the Congressional Black Caucus is an informal group of black members of the House of Representatives who meet to discuss shared interests. Likewise, female members of Congress have banded together to push for increased federal funding for breast cancer, and male members of Congress have cosigned and circulated letters urging support for prostate cancer research. Knowledge of these fundamental characteristics and how they may be brought to bear on legislation helps to guide nurse lobbyists who solicit support for policy positions. Although it is important to be familiar with the positions policy makers take on various issues, it is equally important to look for cues as to why they have taken or whether they are likely to take certain positions. Identifying these personal characteristics that extend beyond political party affiliation will help APNs determine how malleable an individual's position may be in the future.

Congressional Staff

Personal Office Staff Members of Congress employ a number of professional staff in their Washington, DC offices. Over the past 30 years, Congress has greatly expanded the number of staff in response to increasing workloads brought about by the complexity and breadth of policy issues about which members are expected to be knowledgeable. In congressional offices, there is usually a chief of staff or administrative assistant responsible for overseeing the press, political and public relations activity; directing office and personnel management; and maintaining oversight of the legislative operations. It is not uncommon for this individual to have political ties to the member, perhaps even having served as the campaign manager for the member's election to office. Congressional offices also have legislative directors who are responsible for day-to-day legislative activities. These individuals tend to have more policy expertise and less political involvement than the administrative assistant. Offices also have a press operation with at least one press secretary responsible for interacting with the media and disseminating information regarding the member's policy-related activities. The press secretary writes and distributes press releases about the member's work, organizes press conferences, and arranges interviews with media representatives. Specific legislative work is done by legislative assistants (LAs). Also worth noting is the fact that many offices welcome interns (often college students), fellows (often professionals with expertise in particular fields such as medicine or psychology) who may be participating in policy fellowship programs, or volunteers interested in learning about the legislative process or acquiring policy-related experience. The latter two categories may consist of university faculty, corporate executives, or any number of professionals, including advanced practice nurses.

On the staff of every member of Congress is an LA responsible for health policy. Legislative assistants generally assume responsibility for a number of issues. For example, in one congressional office, an LA may handle health, transportation, and banking while an LA in another congressional office may be responsible for health, welfare, education, and social security. Because of smaller office budgets, there tend to be fewer LAs in the offices of members of the House of Representatives than in the Senate offices. Also, Senate staff tend to receive higher salaries than their House counterparts. Senate positions are generally more sought after and filled with more experienced individuals. The average tenure for legislative assistants is 2 to 3 years after which many staff capitalize on their Hill experience by moving to higher paying lobbying positions for special interest groups. The majority of health LAs are in the mid to late 20s and, increasingly, are women. Even though legislative assistants are usually extremely influential in terms of crafting legislation, few have an educational background in health care. Nevertheless, because these positions are highly competitive, individuals who fill them are motivated, intelligent, and learn quickly. Given this description, clearly APNs, as their first task, must ascertain the knowledge level of the LA on policy issues of importance to the nursing community. Nurses in advanced practice cannot assume that legislative assistants have even a rudimentary knowledge of the education and practice of the APN. Quite unintentionally, LAs unfamiliar with the scope of practice of these nurses can exclude advanced practice nurses from health-policy initiatives.

As the key health advisor to members of Congress, these staff are influential in a number of ways. Health LAs are responsible for "staffing" members at committee hearings that focus on health policy, often writing the members' statements for them as well as crafting questions to ask witnesses who testify at hearings. Health LAs generally accompany members to meetings with lobbyists or constituents and are responsible for briefing the member prior to the meeting as well as completing any staff work necessary to implement decisions or commitments the member may make during the meeting. Health LAs may be responsible for writing speeches or drafting letters to the editor of a local newspaper to be submitted under the member's name. LAs (or their assistants, referred to as *legislative correspondents*) draft responses to constituent letters that will go out under the member's signature. Perhaps most importantly, the health legislative assistant advises the member on health-policy issues. These issues can range from a request for federal support for a health-related research project conducted at a clinic in the member's home state to a request for cosponsorship of a bill that would increase the utilization of telehealth technology. The LA's advice may be provided in a briefing memo or verbally to the member. In terms of legislation alone, hundreds of health-related bills are introduced in each session of Congress. It is the LA's responsibility to track those that might be of greatest interest to the member or viable during the session. Because of the tremendous demands on the member's schedule, it is not uncommon to see an LA providing "last-minute" information and advice while accompanying the member to the floor of the Senate for a vote on the health-related bill. It is the LA's responsibility to work with the office referred to as Legislative Council to draft bill language incorporating policy ideas that the member wishes to pursue.

Almost without exception, legislative assistants are pivotal to informing and influencing policy makers. An astute LA provides guidance based on knowledge of how a member's position will likely be greeted by constituents (e.g., nurses in the home state or district may oppose a particular stance while hospital administrators may support it and consumers may not have a strong opinion). This kind of legwork by the health LA is critically important in helping to keep the member informed of positions his or her constituents have and the related risks of antagonizing certain constituencies. Silence on an issue may be interpreted as indifference. Consequently, APNs must make their views known if they are to exert influence on policy initiatives under consideration. Legislative assistants generally craft initiatives or advise their members based on information the LAs receive, not on personal experience with health care. Consequently, LAs welcome information and recommendations from nurses who are constituents of the member for whom they work. Initiating and

maintaining communication with the health LAs of one's congressional delegation enhances the likelihood that an APN will be sought out for policy advice
on proposed legislation. The goal of individual APNs and their associations
should be to have the LA view them as a content expert and as an available
resource for a range of reasons, from eliciting ideas for legislation to critiquing
provisions of health-related bills.

While the health LA in Washington, DC, is a pivotal link, members maintain
offices in major cities in their districts or states that are staffed by assistants who
serve as conduits of information between the district or state office and the
Washington, DC office. Despite the fact that these offices are readily accessible,
they are often underutilized. The staff in local offices have a number of responsibilities, and nurses in advanced practice can access staff for a host of reasons.
Requests for a meeting with the member or health LA, information about bills,
the member's position on a specific piece of legislation, or an invitation to
address a nurses' conference can generally be routed through the local office.
Local staff are aware of the member's schedule when back in the district or state
and often accompany the member on tours, meetings, and other events. Consequently, staff in local offices can be an excellent resource, are accessible, and are
often less harried than their Washington, DC counterparts.

Committee Staff   In addition to personal staff, Congress employs hundreds of
experienced professional staff responsible for supporting the work of congressional committees. Committees generally have separate staff responsible to the
majority and the minority committee members, with a smaller number allocated to the minority. Although personal staff are responsible for a wide range
of issues (e.g., in addition to nonhealth legislative issues, even within the
health portfolio, personal staff may advise on Medicare, Medicaid, NIH appropriations, the Public Health Service, and numerous other federal health
programs), committee staff tend to have a narrow focus. For example, on the
Senate Finance Committee with jurisdiction over Medicare and Medicaid, one
staff member working for the chairperson and majority members may be
responsible only for Medicaid. Generally, committee staff are older than the
personal office staff and have significant expertise emanating from either
advanced educational degrees or professional experience in the content area
for which they are responsible. Previously, committee staff may have worked in
personal offices of members of Congress or as lobbyists. Committee staff may
also come from or move to federal agencies over which the committee has
responsibility. Committee staff who are seasoned in the work of the committee
become highly valuable to the committee chair and members, and often exert
influence directly related to their expertise. While members of Congress tend
to be generalists, responsible for an array of issues, committee staff function as
specialists. Because of the depth of knowledge in specific areas, committee
staff can usually command high salaries once they leave Capitol Hill.

Committee staff are usually responsible for planning the committee agendas, coordinating hearing schedules and witnesses, and preparing legislation

for committee and floor action. They gather and analyze information upon which policy is based and they draft committee reports. They staff the committee chair and ranking member in meetings and when the committee's legislation is considered in the full House or Senate chamber.

Personal office staff interact closely with committee staff, communicating their member's requests related to legislation before the committee. Committee staff tend to be most responsive to requests from their committee members. Consequently, lobbyists will always seek support for legislative provisions from committee members first and only if necessary will seek out the help of other members of Congress to intercede with the committee. To facilitate moving legislation, the committee staff in one chamber are in frequent contact with their counterparts in the other chamber, working out details and compromises. In fact, "Committee staff are expected to maintain continuous contact with their counterparts on other House and Senate committees, with executive agency officials responsible for programs, and with private sector organizations and groups and knowledgeable staff in the congressional support agencies" (Rundquist et al., 1992, p. 13). Because committees almost always serve as the gateway through which legislation must pass, committee staff are in pivotal positions to influence legislative products.

Special Interest Groups and Their Lobbyists

Interest groups are defined as "individuals who have organized themselves around some common interest and who seek to influence public policy. . . . They clarify and articulate citizens' preferences, warn policy makers of problems with their proposals, and suggest ways to make them more palatable . . ." (Weissert and Weissert, 1996, p. 102). Lobbyists represent interests ranging from academic institutions to the balloon industry to flight attendants. With approximately 20,000 lobbyists in Washington, DC (deVries and Vanderbilt, 1992), it is likely that an APN walking through the halls of a Senate or House office building is passing by individuals who are neither constituents nor members of Congress but, rather, are lobbyists. Furthermore, though congressional offices may be inundated with correspondence from constituents, much of the mail delivered to offices is produced by special-interest groups. The mail takes many forms, ranging from study-and-opinion poll results to analysis of a bill to magazines or videotapes presenting policy information. "Lobbying is the art of persuasion—attempting to convince a legislator, a government official, the head of an agency, or a state official to comply with a request . . ." (deVries and Vanderbilt, 1992, p. 1). In addition to sending unsolicited information, it is not uncommon for lobbyists to produce specific data at the request of a congressional office or even to write statements that can be incorporated into speeches given by the member.

In addition to meetings, mailings, conversations with LAs, and other strategies applied locally, lobbyists augment their efforts as necessary with grassroots campaigns; that is, to bring additional pressure to bear on a member, special interest groups often orchestrate phone and letter campaigns that involve voters from the member's home district or state. When statements, postcards, or telephone calls convey identical verbatim messages, it quickly becomes clear that the contacts are organized. However, volume often matters, regardless of whether the message appears organized or not. It is common for members to inquire about the number of letters and phone calls coming in that support or oppose a particular piece of legislation.

Directly related to congressional and presidential elections, it is important to note that many special-interest groups exert influence through political action committees (PACs). For example, in 1974 the American Nurses Association established a PAC "to support candidates who share ANA's views on health care quality and access issues and to advance nursing's political agenda." (What is ANA-PAC? p. 1). The ANA-PAC has been successful in amassing contributions from ANA members and converting them into financial support for political candidates.

Special-interest groups with shared views often combine resources through temporary coalitions to wield greater influence. For example, in 1997 over 10 nurse organizations worked together to track legislative proposals related to graduate medical education. Within the profession, the nursing community must speak with a unified voice. For policy makers to act, not only must the message be communicated, it must be consistent. Strategies employed by coalitions include meeting with members and/or LAs with a few representatives of the coalition and sending letters that are signed by multiple associations. These strategies convey broad support and not infrequently represent hundreds of thousands of members of associations.

It is not uncommon to find organizations coalescing around one policy issue and assuming opposing positions on another policy issue. It is vital that APNs learn to focus on issues and not take it personally if a person or group is supportive on one issue and not on another. The APN must recognize that an opponent in one circumstance may be an essential ally in another.

The Executive Branch

Even though regulatory agencies are dealt with elsewhere, it is important for APNs to note that considerable interaction occurs formally and informally between the legislative and executive branches of government and, consequently, the latter merits mention in the development of legislation. A few examples readily highlight this relationship. During the appropriations process, heads of federal agencies appear at appropriations committee and subcommittee hearings to present the administration's funding proposals for the coming fiscal year. For example, the head of the National Institute for Nursing Research appears before both the House and Senate Appropriations Subcommittees for Labor, Health and Human Services, and Education and related agencies. The testimony presented generally highlights major initiatives underway as well as activities that are being planned. Frequently, the agency head is knowledgeable of particular issues of concern to committee members, in particular the chairperson. For example, if the chair is known to have a special interest in mental health, references will be made to planning, implementation, evaluation, or research of any programs in that area. Although these hearings are often poorly attended by committee members, and the development of proposed funding levels may be well underway prior to the hearing, it is nevertheless an important opportunity for federal agency representatives to use this forum to bring their cases to both the Congress as well as the public, as the work of federal agencies is not automatically embraced (Gray et al., 2003).

Informally, there is significant contact between members, congressional staff, and agency officials. This contact is frequent in cases where the executive branch and members are of the same political party affiliation and between the executive branch and House and Senate leadership offices and chairs of congressional committees. Requests for information and negotiation on legislative proposals are common interactions. Likewise, although relatively few invitations can be filled, federal agency heads often will be invited by the member to the home state or district for tours, conferences, and other events. Appointed officials generally are accompanied by members of the congressional delegation, and their visits are often related to federal policy that has local implications. For example, in 2003 the head of the Centers for Medicare and Medicaid Services (CMS) attended public meetings in the home districts of the cochairs of the House Rural Healthcare Coalition to hear concerns about perceived Medicare payment inadequacy in those rural regions.

Constituents

Opinions may be held that Washington politicians are "bought and paid for" by special interests and, in truth, special interests can wield tremendous influence. However, ultimately voters send individuals to Washington, DC, and voters can replace them. Much of the legislation considered in the nation's capital is debated without stirring considerable interest by most constituents. However, in circumstances where it appears that a proposal may negatively affect constituents, informed consumers may be quick to respond. The 1994 debate over the Clinton Health Security Act, an effort to enact sweeping health care reform, is one illustration. Typically the purview of health care providers and other special-interest groups, this legislation prompted a widespread reaction. Bankers, restaurant owners, veterans, and farmers all had opinions about the proposal and freely expressed their views to elected representatives.

Most members of Congress go to great efforts to stay informed regarding the views of their constituents. Even members who represent states at great distances from Washington, DC, make frequent trips home to meet with individuals and participate in local activities. Likewise, major newspapers from the area a policy maker represents serve as an extremely important source of information about views back home. Even letters to the editor that reflect policy concerns are usually scanned by appropriate staff. Talk radio shows may be monitored on occasion by district or state staff to learn the views of individuals who call in as well as the program guests.

While the average voter's view is important, a professional with expertise and knowledge of a particular issue often brings added value to the message. Consequently, advanced practice nurses who serve as resources, highlight health problems affecting constituent groups, and propose policy solutions can be very effective with their own congressional delegation. In communicating with members or their staff, national data that describe the problem are helpful (e.g., projected shortages of registered nurses). However, members are most interested in descriptive information about the impact of a problem on the constituents they represent. Presented in conjunction with data, an anecdote about the effect of a particular problem helps to illustrate its significance.

Generally, there is no better source of information on health policy concerns than health care professionals who reside in a member's home district or state. Although health issues deliberated by Congress are national in scope, members of Congress place a high priority on protecting and promoting the health and welfare of their constituents. Consequently, an APN's opinions matter.

Nurses are most powerful when their elected representatives serve on committees with jurisdiction over health programs. That is, on any particular legislative proposal, nurses may be much more influential in one state than in another, depending on their representatives' committee assignments.

The Media

An APN may be surprised by the activity underway early in the morning in most congressional offices. Walking past staff desks, many individuals can be found taking a few moments to review copies of articles from morning newspapers published in the home state or district. Legislative assistants commonly review articles relevant to their issue portfolio at the same time that constituents are reading their local newspapers over breakfast. One of the first tasks of the day in the member's local office is to review and fax all newsworthy articles to the Washington, DC, office. These articles are then packaged by the press staff and distributed to legislative assistants. Likewise, the member is frequently provided with a packet of articles drawn from home state newspapers to review. It is not uncommon to find staff in local offices responsible for videotaping local evening news shows and reviewing them for information that may be useful to the congressional office. Using these mechanisms, staff stay well informed about which issues are highlighted in the press and how they are reported. The media, then, serve as an important conduit of information and opinion. Furthermore, news stories often serve as the catalyst for policy-related initiatives. Stories that focus on negative outcomes of medical errors have prompted significant legislation designed to address the identified problems. In addition to influencing policy, congressional members invest significant time in communicating directly or through their press secretaries with the media back home. Press releases are faxed to media outlets, and videotape of the member is fed back to television stations in the hope that a position taken or a vote cast will become a positive story on the local evening news or in the next morning paper. Therefore, the media can serve as both a catalyst for legislative initiatives and also as a method for communicating to constituents about legislative activity. The information presented by the press influences not just the public but policy makers and their staffs as well. This important function is one that can be capitalized on by knowledgeable nurses who use the media to express their views about particular health issues. It is important to note that when health-related stories run in the press and the stories do not reference nurses, the profession is invisible to both the public and policy makers. Often, views expressed by large numbers of individuals will have greater impact on policy makers than those that are expressed by a few. This simple principle underscores the importance of widespread engagement by nurses in advanced practice in the policy-development process. Although many voices, using various channels and strategies, are heard by policy makers and their staff, strength in communicating a message comes from a chorus of voices clearly articulating the problem and proposing policy solutions.

The Process

While expert nurses need to know who the major stakeholders are in policy development, they also must know how the policy-making process works and what strategies can be used to influence the product of this process. Just as health care providers have a common lexicon, individuals interested in public policy must understand terms and processes commonly used. Although entire textbooks are written describing in detail facets of the policy-making process, the purpose of this section is to facilitate an understanding of a few selected aspects of the policy-making process.

Legislation may be introduced at any time that the House or Senate is in session. Proposed legislation is termed a bill until it is passed in identical form by both the House and the Senate and is either signed by the president or becomes law without the president's signature. Hundreds of bills are often introduced in the first few days of a legislative session and may be offered through the final hours prior to adjournment, resulting in about 5,000 bills introduced annually (deVries and Vanderbilt, 1992). Bills are assigned numbers in the order in which they are introduced during the congressional session. Once introduced in the House or Senate chamber, the bill is then referred to the committee with jurisdiction over the substance of the bill.

Complicating consideration of a bill are referrals that are made to multiple committees. This occurs when different provisions of the bill are the purview of different committees. For example, a bill that includes public health service programs as well as malpractice provisions may be considered by both the Senate Judiciary Committee and the Committee on Health, Education, Labor, and Pensions. APNs must note that significant health policy is often developed in committees not thought of as having jurisdiction over health programs. For example, the Agriculture Appropriations Committee funds the Food and Drug Administration of the Department of Health and Human Services. Knowing the committee of jurisdiction is important in order to target members with the most influence over the bill.

There are three general types of committees in Congress: oversight, appropriations, and authorization committees. Each merits a brief description. Oversight committees do not act on legislation. Instead, they hold hearings to illuminate issues related to the committee focus. For example, the Senate Special Committee on Aging does not act on legislation related to the aged. However, it does play an active role in examining issues related to the elderly that can help inform members. For example, this committee may hold a hearing on the use of multiple prescription medications by nursing home residents or compromised quality in long-term care. Recommendations by individuals testifying before the committee could eventually be incorporated into bills considered by other health committees.

Authorizing committees are responsible for establishing or making changes in federal programs as well as setting a limit on the amount of federal funding that can be spent to implement the particular program. Most federal programs are evaluated by the committee of jurisdiction through a reauthorization process that usually occurs every 3 to 5 years. The time frame for evaluation is set in the authorizing legislation. Generally, bills authorizing the establishment or continuation of a federal program are enacted before money is appropriated to support the particular program. For example, the Nurse Education Act is authorizing legislation that established the Division of Nursing. At established time intervals, this law is reevaluated by the committees of jurisdiction. If agreement cannot be reached on provisions in reauthorizing legislation, a federal program such as the Division of Nursing, may be allowed to continue without the benefit of current authorization. When this situation occurs, it is often viewed as problematic. For example, an unauthorized program can be more susceptible to decreased funding or even elimination.

Appropriations committees are responsible for allocating federal funding on a fiscal year basis to support programs. Membership on these "purse-string" committees is often highly sought because the committee can serve as a conduit of funds to support programs important to constituents back home. For example, a legislator from a farm state will often seek membership on the Agriculture Appropriations Committee, an assignment of significant importance to constituents back home. Appropriations bills originate in the House, and funding levels may not exceed the ceilings established by the authorizing legislation. Likewise, the appropriations committee may choose to fund a particular program at a level significantly below that set by the authorizing committee. Although appropriations bills should only address funding levels, it is not uncommon for members of Congress to insert provisions that "authorize on an appropriations bill." This means that members may make significant programmatic changes by including related legislative language in appropriations bill that should be reserved for authorizing bills.

The appropriations process is an annual event, and fiscal year (FY) funding begins on October 1 and ends on September 30 of every year. A fiscal year is identified by the prefix "FY" followed by the last two digits of the ending year. For example, U.S. government FY04 means that the funding year began October 1, 2003, and ended September 30, 2004. Determining funding levels can be especially arduous when the executive branch and the legislative branch are controlled by members of different political parties with differing views about the importance of various programs, e.g., funding for defense versus funding for health care. As a result, it is not uncommon for Congress to fund federal programs after the start of the fiscal year through bills called "continuing resolutions" until such a time as the appropriations bills are finalized.

Of hundreds of bills that may be referred to an authorizing committee in any given legislative session, committee chairs determine which will be considered by the committee. For those bills that are considered, hearings usually are held to obtain information from individuals or organizations with interest in the legislation. This information is referred to as testimony and may be presented verbally during the hearing or in written form. Individuals wishing to comment on a particular bill may forward their views directly to the committee. However, communication can be most effective when a member of one's congressional delegation serves on the committee and constituents share their views with that elected representative. Following committee consideration, bills may be "reported out," which means sent to the floor of the Senate or House for a vote. Both chambers must act on proposed legislation in order for a bill ultimately to be enacted into law. After a vote by each chamber, successful bills are forwarded to a conference committee composed of members from both the Senate and the House. This committee is responsible for negotiating any differences in the bills as they were passed by the two chambers. Although the conference committee is not allowed to introduce new provisions for consideration at this point in the process, such action does occur on occasion. Finally, successful bills are reported out of the conference committee and final votes are cast by both the full Senate and the full House. With congressional work completed, the bill is forwarded to the president for signature and, thereby, is enacted into law. This brief description highlights some of the main events in the process of enacting legislation. Although there are nuances and considerable complexity not reflected in this description, understanding the basic processes is integral to nurses who wish to influence the policy-making process.

With the legislative process in mind, specific strategies that may be effective in influencing the process merit consideration. Nurse involvement in political and policy-making activity can consist of a range of activities along a continuum from paid membership in a nursing organization that has an active government-relations department to running for elective office. The question for APNs today is not whether to become involved in influencing policy, but, rather, the question is how and to what extent each nurse expert will operationalize his or her involvement. A menu of activities are described in the remainder of this chapter, most of which can be conducted without ever traveling to Washington, DC.

Practical Activities for APN Involvement

Research

Concrete efforts should be made by individual nurses and professional associations to link health policy with the activities in which nurses are involved. For example, the policy implications of nursing research should be delineated, whether the research is a master's thesis or a study conducted by a seasoned nurse researcher. Too frequently health policy is developed without the benefit of research-based knowledge. Nurses producing or even just reviewing research can help inform public health policy by linking findings to policy initiatives. Even though APNs find it important to share research findings with colleagues through professional journals, other equally important audiences for much of nursing research are consumers and policy makers. APNs may themselves be researchers, but equally important is the role of translating research findings to meaningfully inform public-health policy. For example, research findings described in a Centers for Disease Control and Prevention report may be useful to help illustrate a concern of a public-health nurse. Furthermore, citing such findings in correspondence to a policy maker and in a letter to the editor of a local newspaper are useful strategies for informing both the public and policy makers. As data accumulate, policy makers become increasingly aware of problems and their potential solutions, whether these data are numbers of uninsured or increasing costs associated with home health care. Based on data, policy may be revised to more effectively address particular problems. Using every available opportunity, advanced practice nurses need to conduct and present research so that it serves the public and influences the development of sound public policy. Beyond individual nurses, nurse organizations also give voice to the work of nurse researchers and disseminate relevant findings to policy makers.

Putting Issues in Context

Most health policy initiatives are designed to address a triad of concerns that includes cost, access, and quality. For example, concerns regarding increasing costs of prescription drugs and decreasing access to drug therapy for Medicare beneficiaries put this provision in the centerpiece of Medicare reform legislation introduced in 2003. APNs interested in getting an issue on the policy agenda need to consider and package their issue within the context of cost, access, and/or quality. Ideally, the proposed policy can be depicted as part of a solution to one or more of these major catalysts for health care policy. This is especially true when the policy sought appears to primarily benefit APNs. For example, the expansion of Medicare reimbursement for all nurse practitioners included in the Balanced Budget Act of 1997 lent itself to being described as a mechanism for increasing access of the elderly to health care providers in underserved urban, as well as rural, areas. Health legislative assistants considering legislative proposals almost always view requests in two ways.

First, what is the impact of the proposal on the interest group or individual requesting legislative change? Second, and more important, what is the impact of the proposal on the public's health? The policy recommendation may well meet the needs of both groups. For example, when flight attendants lobbied for a ban on smoking on all domestic flights, their actions were designed to benefit the members of their profession. However, the ban also limited exposure to smoke by nonsmoking passengers. When interacting with policy makers, the benefits that may be derived from a legislative proposal by constituents back home or the broader public need to be thoroughly described.

APNs can be most effective when they take positions on issues that are priority concerns for segments of the public. For example, if domestic violence and teenage smoking are community concerns, nurses should engage in discussing elements of the problem as well as proposing solutions. Being in touch with and responding to the health concerns of the community is no different from responding to the needs of a patient. Applying the APN's expertise to community concerns, whether the health concerns emanate from the local chapter of the AARP or the business community, results in two important benefits. Nurses' expertise contributes to the health of the community as well as to increasing the visibility of the profession.

Visibility

To increase the likelihood that policy makers will incorporate nurses' views into health policy initiatives, APNs need to ensure that their views are visible. For example, at health-related events where the media, policy makers, and the public meet, APNs also need to be represented. Nurses can bring informed opinions to most discussions regarding health care, whether the topic is health-professions workforce trends in a state or the health problems of school-age children. Using public forums, whether it is a city council meeting or a town meeting held by a member of one's congressional delegation, nurses in advanced practice should use these important opportunities to educate the public and policy makers about both the topic discussed as well as the role of the APN. Only by capitalizing on and creating new opportunities that enhance the visibility of the profession will nurses increasingly be viewed as content experts, better represented in news stories, and more readily incorporated into policy initiatives.

Effective Communication

To be effective in their work, nurses need to be adept at tailoring their communications in ways that will be readily understood. Nurses are very effective at conveying information, whether the audience is a fifteen-year-old or an eighty-five-year-old, a high school dropout or a nuclear physicist. Communication with policy makers, whether oral or written, also needs to be targeted and free of terminology unique to medicine and nursing. With multiple competing requests and demands, messages conveyed in the jargon of the discipline

frequently are lost on policy makers too busy to seek clarification or not sufficiently clear on the merits of the issue.

Because scores of problems are competing for the attention of members
and staff at any point in time, how nurses present an issue is critically important. Identifying one's expertise with the issue is the first place to start. In both
written and oral communications, nurse experts first need to briefly describe
their education and experience. This is an opportunity to educate the policy
maker about the work and expertise of APNs and also convey the fact that the
information being shared is grounded in professional experience. In addition,
the relevance of the issue to individuals beyond nursing should be identified.
Providing information regarding the impact of the issue on the member's constituents enhances the likelihood that the policy maker will act. All information that is presented must be accurate. Credibility and interest is quickly lost
when lobbyists or constituents oversell or inaccurately depict a particular problem. Advanced practice nurses need to convey information in an organized,
thorough, and concise form that reflects data when available and anecdotes
that clearly illustrate the concern.

Effective Communication

Written Communication   Individuals write to policy makers to express opinions,
acknowledge the member's work either positively or negatively, follow up on
meetings or phone calls, or share knowledge about a particular problem and
recommend policy solutions. A few rules should guide the development of written correspondence. The letter should be typed, no longer than two pages, and
focused on one or two issues at most. The purpose of the letter should be stated
at the beginning. Compelling rationale for the writer's concern or position on
an issue must be clearly presented. If the purpose of the letter is to express dis-
appointment regarding a stance on an issue or a vote that has been cast, the
letter should be as positive as possible. Conversely, writing letters thanking a
member for taking a particular position on an issue and public acknowledgment
of the policy maker's work is very important. A letter to the editor of the local
newspaper or a nursing newsletter lauding a member's position (with a copy forwarded to the member) is welcome publicity, especially during an election year.

Letters should always be sent following meetings or even conversations
that occurred in passing at large events. Correspondence should include a
reiteration of the major points covered in person as well as answers to questions that were raised during the course of the conversation. Business cards
should be included and the member and staff encouraged to contact the APN
or the professional association for further information.

Oral Communication   Regardless of whether a meeting is held in the member's
Washington, DC, office or at a health care facility, the first question to raise is
to determine the amount of time the staff or member is able to allocate. Too
frequently, constituents engage in small talk at the beginning of the conversation

only to find out that additional appointments have been added to the schedule or a vote on the floor is imminent. Also, the time available needs to be structured so that the issue can be succinctly presented followed by an opportunity for the staff or member to seek clarification or raise questions. The APN must not assume that the staff or member is as well informed on the issue as the nurse. Given the scores of policy concerns ranging from foreign affairs to transportation, members cannot keep abreast of every policy concern. If the meeting concludes and confusion exists regarding important aspects of the issue, the chance of a policy maker acting on the information is markedly diminished. To help ensure understanding, a one-page summary that underscores key points should be provided at the conclusion of every meeting. Finally, in letters and in meetings, numbers count. Noting that the views expressed are shared by a local nurse's organization, nurses employed at a health care facility, or even better, represent concerns of a coalition of groups, brings added clout to an issue.

Advanced practice nurses should not hesitate to invite members and their staff to conferences, meetings of nurses' organizations, or tours of nursing education or clinical facilities. The likelihood that the member will incorporate the request into a scheduled trip back home increases markedly when the policy makers are told that they will have the opportunity to meet with large numbers of nurses, patients, and/or other constituents. Also, if appropriate, invite the media and let the member know. If a member or his or her staff are unable to accept one invitation, do not hesitate to send future invitations. The likelihood of acceptance can increase with the size of the audience and proximity to an upcoming election.

Conclusion

Former Majority Leader Newt Gingrich (2003, p. 35) notes that "health and health care is the largest problem in American domestic policy today." With this level of attention, public policy in the health arena is an important vehicle for influencing professional nursing practice as well as the health of individuals, families, and communities. With an understanding of the players and factors that can influence the policy-making process, APNs can play a pivotal role in shaping the future of health care. At the start of the 21st century, competition for resources is serious and the need to find new solutions to complex problems is great. When policy makers acknowledge problems, potential solutions are identifiable, and when favorable political circumstances exist, a window of opportunity opens, although often only briefly (Longest, 1998). Recognizing this dynamic, when nurses in advanced practice communicate their contributions (i.e., solutions) to increased quality, enhanced access, and decreased cost of health services (i.e., problems), health policy makers should be responsive. Knowledge coupled with action can assure that responsiveness.

Eleven Lessons Learned from Nine Years on Capitol Hill

After serving as a legislative assistant to one U.S. Senator and as chief of staff to three Senators, the author left "The Hill" in 1996. Since then, she has served on multiple health committees that are advisory to either the U.S. Congress, executive branch agencies, or both. The following are prescriptions for other nurses in advanced practice who choose to engage actively in the exciting, rewarding, and frequently stressful world of public-health policy.

1. **You can gain a lot by giving a little.** Within a few years of graduating from my baccalaureate nursing program, I became very involved in my state nurses' association. The opportunities available through membership in a professional association allowed me to build communication and leadership skills, increase my knowledge about a range of professional issues, and expand and strengthen my professional network. Serving on committees and in elected positions provided an opportunity for real-world application for much of what I learned in my formal education.

2. **A lot of what you can accomplish does depend on who you know.** In my view, although financial support for campaigns in Washington, DC, does enhance access to policy makers, the real currency in the nation's capitol is relationships. Furthermore, nurses need to build relationships, not just within the profession, but also with representatives of public and private sector organizations with an interest in health care.

3. **Politicians pay attention to numbers.** Even though I witnessed the difference one well-connected voice could make in terms of influencing a policy decision, in general, the more broad based the pressure that is brought to bear, the more likely a policy maker will respond. Twenty letters or phone calls supporting a particular position can be much more effective than two at capturing the attention of a legislator.

4. **You have to get off the porch to run with the big dogs.** This phrase was often repeated by one of my employers during my tenure on Capitol Hill. It is highly unlikely that a health legislative assistant or policy maker will call an advanced practice nurse and ask whether he or she can meet to discuss issues in which APNs have an interest. It is equally unlikely to find a legislative assistant on Capitol Hill poring through a nursing journal to get new ideas about health problems and solutions from nursing's perspective. If APNs want to be sought out as resources and have their views reflected in health-policy debates and decisions, they must deliberately set out to build the foundation for involvement in public policy.

5. **Occasionally other people really do know what's better for you than you know yourself.** Early on in my work on Capitol Hill, I was encouraged to participate in political activities outside of the office. Initially, I resisted the offer, believing that I could accomplish what I needed to and expand my knowledge base by focusing just on health legislation—a policy purist, if you

will. Very quickly I recognized that broader experiences would enhance the quality of work in which I was engaged and have application in other arenas. For example, after involvement with two congressional campaigns, I amassed significant knowledge about polling, the media, working with different national organizations, communicating messages, and even marketing a product—in these cases, U.S. senators. Virtually everything learned has been transferable and useful in other facets of my professional career.

6. **Knowledge helps to build bridges. We need to continue to expand both our depth and breadth.** In the world of health care and health policy, I learned that one cannot just engage in "nurse speak." Parochial concerns often appear self-serving. In order to help others view a nursing issue as important, I needed to be able to articulate how nursing was part of a solution to an important health-policy problem. It became clear that nurses need to be aware of what is going on in health care, well beyond the environment and the practice in which they work. Being well-informed across a range of health-related issues allowed me to converse more readily with policy makers, business leaders, and consumer advocates; that is, others did not have to engage me on nursing's turf regarding nursing issues. Rather, I had a knowledge base from which I could reach out and find common concerns and interests as points of departure for discussion.

7. **Wear your profession like a badge of honor.** Of the hundreds of individuals with whom I interacted while I was on Capitol Hill, very few were unaware that I was a nurse. In fact, when introducing me as his chief of staff, the last senator for whom I worked always pointed out that I had a doctorate in nursing. I firmly believe that it was important to me and to the profession that my nurse identity—and the associated education and expertise—was recognized as part and parcel of my policy work. At the same time most of my peers were lawyers or political science majors, "being different" helped me establish a separate identity that, because of its uniqueness in the policy arena, helped people to remember the profession from which I hailed. It is important to me that people know that nurses are capable of functioning in many different roles and making substantial contributions. Ultimately, my nursing experience turned out to be a strength, not a handicap. Though I had to learn the policy-making process, confidence came from knowing the health issues for which policy was being developed.

8. **Blow up a bridge only if you're sure you'll never need to cross there again.** Although partisan politics have fueled highly publicized gridlock and hostility, more frequently than not, at the end of the day policy makers typically sit down and negotiate compromises. Congress is a prime example of a group of people with very different views who must work together to accomplish agreed-upon objectives. Initial inflexibility generally gives way to negotiate agreements on issues. Throughout the process of working on contentious issues, it became clear that if an organization or another member of Congress would not join in on one issue of importance, he or

she may be the critical player on another. Consequently, the bridge burned behind you may have provided, on another occasion, the only route to getting you where you want to go.

9. **There is no advantage to being a wallflower.** Initially, I often had to resist the primordial "flight" response at receptions, meetings with international dignitaries, and experts across a range of fields or black-tie events. I eventually convinced myself that most individuals were friendly and all of them were interesting. What was most helpful was finding a standard "ice-breaker" to use. Mine was simply "Hello, I don't believe that we've met. My name is . . . and I work for. . . ." The worst that could come of this opener is a response such as "Well, in fact, we have met."

10. **If you have expertise—share it.** As a neophyte in the policy arena, I cast a wide net in search of nurses and others who were willing to take a few minutes to answer my questions and provide counsel. Lending a hand to nurses coming up after us benefits all of us—and, although these willing mentors may never have thought that I could someday provide assistance in return, they were nevertheless generous with both their time and assistance.

11. **If you need expertise—seek it out.** For nurses new to the policy arena in local communities, state capitols, or the nation's capitol, guidance and support can come from many people of diverse backgrounds. Accomplished people, nurses and nonnurses alike, are often the same individuals who value mentoring others. In the process of seeking or providing support, using strategies to nurture relationships leave lasting impressions. A quick note of congratulations or a well-timed phone call were efforts made by some of the busiest people with whom I came in contact.

Discussion Points

1. Describe the role of legislative assistants for health. Indicate how relationships between APNs and LAs can be developed and why such relationships are important.
2. Explain the significance of media to public-health policy and the nursing profession.
3. Contrast appropriations committees with authorizing committees and describe their roles in the formulation of health policy.
4. Explain the following statement: APNs can enhance the likelihood of influencing health legislation when they advocate a specific concern couched within a broad health-policy context.

References

DeVries, C. and Vanderbilt, M. (1992). *The Grassroots Lobbying Handbook.* Washington, DC: American Nurses Association.

Gingrich, N. (2003). *Saving Lives and Saving Money.* Washington, DC: The Alexis de Tocqueville Institution, p. 35.

Gray, B. H., Gusmano, M. K., and Collins, S. R. (2003). AHCPR and the changing politics of health services research: Lessons from the falling and rising political fortunes of the nation's leading health services, *Health Affairs,* Health Services Research: AHCPR Politics Web Exclusive. http://www.healthaffairs.org/WebExclusives/Gray 062503.

Longest, B. B., Jr., (1998). *Health Policymaking in the United States* (2nd ed.). Chicago, IL: Health Administration Press.

Rundquist, P., Schneider, J., and Pauls, F. (1992, Jan. 24). Congressional staff: An analysis of their roles, functions, and impacts. *Congressional Research Service Report for Congress.* Washington, DC: The Congressional Research Service, The Library of Congress.

Weissert, C. and Weissert, W. (1996). *Governing Health.* Baltimore, MD: The Johns Hopkins University Press.

What is ANA-PAC? (information sheet). Washington, DC: American Nurses Association Political Action Committee.

Government Regulation: Parallel and Powerful

4

Renatta S. Loquist, RN, FAAN, MN

Key Terms

Board of nursing   A state government administrative agency charged with the power and duty to enforce the laws and regulations governing the practice of nursing in the interest of public protection.

Certification   A form of voluntary credentialing that denotes validation of competency in a specialty area with permission to use a title.

Ethical dilemma   A situation that requires an individual to make a choice between two equally unfavorable alternatives.

Ethical principle   Declaration of what is right or wrong based on a set of widely held human beliefs.

Federal Register   A daily publication of the federal government that contains current executive orders, presidential proclamations, rules and regulations, proposed rules, notices, and sunshine act meetings.

Interstate compact   The legal agreement between states to recognize the license of another state to allow for practice between states. The compact must be passed by the state legislature and implemented by the board of nursing.

Licensure   A form of credentialing whereby permission is granted by a legal authority to do an act that would without such permission be illegal, a trespass, a tort, or otherwise not allowable.

Lobbying   The act of influencing a governmental entity to achieve a specific legislative or regulatory outcome.

Multistate regulation   The provision that allows a profession to be practiced in more than one state based on a single license.

Mutual recognition   A method of multistate regulation in which boards of nursing voluntarily agree to enter into an interstate compact allowing the state to recognize and honor the license issued by the other state.

Professional self-regulation   Voluntary process of compliance to a set of moral, ethical, and professional standards agreed to by a profession.

Public hearings   Meetings held by state or federal administrative agencies for the purpose of receiving testimony from witnesses who support or oppose regulations or to receive expert testimony.

Recognition (official recognition)   A form of credentialing that denotes a government authority has ratified or confirmed credentials of an individual.

Registration   A form of credentialing that denotes enrolling or recording the name of a qualified individual on an official roster by an agency of government.

Regulation   Governing or directing according to a rule, or bringing under the control of a constituted authority, such as the state or federal government.

Rules/Regulations   Orders that outline methods of procedure issued by government to operationalize a law.

Introduction

Regulation of the United States health care delivery system and the health care providers who practice within the system is complex. Much of the complexity is attributable to the vastness of the industry, the manner of financing health care, and the proliferation of laws and regulations that govern practice and reimbursement in the interest of public welfare.

This chapter focuses on the major concepts of the regulation of health professionals with emphasis on advanced practice nurses. Understanding the process of licensure and credentialing and its impact on the practice of advanced practice nursing is fundamental to practicing as a competent practitioner. Understanding the regulation of the health care system empowers the APN to advocate on behalf of the profession and consumers of health care.

Regulation versus Legislation

The legislative process is one approach to governance. A parallel, yet equally powerful, approach is the regulatory process. Together, laws and regulations shape the way public policy is implemented. It is important for the APN to understand both processes and know how to influence each process. Major differences between the two processes are described here.

Laws are promulgated and passed by the legislative branch of government (Congress at the federal level or the state legislature for state laws) and establish the framework and authority base for the regulatory process. Once passed, laws must be implemented by administrative agencies (the executive branch) of government. The administrative agency promulgates regulations that outline or define the process of implementing the law.

Laws are written using broad language to provide for flexibility and adaptability in application of the law over time. To assure uniform and consistent application of the law, regulations and/or rules (terms used interchangeably with the same meaning) are written using more specific language that describes how the administrative agency that has jurisdictional authority will implement the law. Regulations are interpretive in nature and dictate "how" the law will be implemented.

> Example: One provision in the nurse practice act provides that a duty of the board of nursing is to examine, license, and renew the license of duly qualified individuals. The regulations to implement that provision of law specify the criteria for eligibility, application procedures, and how and when examinations are conducted. The regulations may change as the board develops new policies and procedures regarding licensure and examination, but the law (statute) continues to provide the board with the broad authority to examine, license, and renew licenses.

The first step in promulgating a law begins with the introduction of a bill by a legislator or group of legislators (sponsor) during a legislative session. The sponsor may introduce legislation to address an issue or concern of his or her constituents. The bill must be passed during the legislative session in which it is introduced or it "dies" and must then be reintroduced in a subsequent session.

Regulations, on the other hand, can be promulgated at any time during the year by an administrative agency. The time frame for implementation of the regulation varies according to the administrative procedures act (APA) of the state, but generally can become effective within 30 days of publication of the final regulation. The APA governs the manner by which an administrative agency accomplishes its functions, conducts meetings, and manages records and information. The APA also specifies the procedure for rule making (the process of promulgating regulations). Each state has an administrative procedures act codified in the laws of the state.

Legislators may amend bills at any time during the legislative process. Amendments may be made to a bill during several points of review: during a subcommittee hearing, a full committee hearing, on the floor of the House or Senate, or in a conference committee. Amendments may be favorable to the sponsor and constituency, or they may be unfavorable as a result of political maneuvering. Some amendments may change the intent of the original bill. There is always risk involved when bills are up for discussion and debate. It is important for the APN to monitor a bill throughout the legislative process and exert influence for positive outcomes.

Regulations may be amended by the issuing agency based on public input prior to the publication of the final regulation. The administrative agency promulgating the regulation has discretion in determining what amendments, if any, are made.

Health Professions Regulation and Licensing

Definitions and Purpose of Regulation

Regulation, as defined in *Black's Law Dictionary*, means "to govern or direct according to rule, or to bring under control of a constituted authority" (Black et al., 1992, p. 1286). Health-professions regulation provides for an ongoing monitoring and maintenance of an acceptable standard of practice for the professions in the interest of public welfare. Regulation is needed to protect the public because of the technical complexity of the health care system. The complexity of educational credentialing, proliferation of types of providers, lack of public information about competency of health care providers, and outcomes of care make it difficult for the public to understand and evaluate options. The bundling of health care services also makes it difficult for consumers to make choices about providers of care. The public trusts that every health care provider is competent to perform the duties assigned, particularly those who are licensed or registered by a state authority. Because the secondary harm that can come to an individual by an incompetent provider may be life threatening, a major role of the regulatory agency is competency assessment and evaluation. In addition, the regulatory process provides the public a forum to resolve complaints against health care providers (Sheets, 1996).

> Example: Ms. Smith is admitted to an acute care facility for major surgery. Upon admission, a registered nurse obtains a patient history and conducts a physical examination. The laboratory technician arrives to obtain blood samples for testing. The certified registered nurse anesthetist meets with the patient to obtain a brief history from the patient and conducts a routine preoperative examination. A nursing technician arrives to prepare the patient for surgery. After surgery the patient in taken to postanesthesia care where another nurse monitors the patient. The respiratory therapist checks the airway and administers treatments. The patient is then transferred to a room where yet another nurse is assigned to administer care. The patient has been a participant in a series of well-rehearsed and routine events, trusting that each provider is making decisions and providing care to produce positive outcomes.

The laws (statutes) and regulations promulgated to credential and govern a profession are called the *practice act*. The practice act includes the laws governing the practice and the accompanying regulations that specify the entry-into-practice requirements, standards for acceptable practice, disciplinary procedures, and standards for continuing competence.

The regulatory process is used to clarify and interpret enabling statutes and to define the methods that the governing authority will use to enforce an existing law. Specifically, regulations set forth standards, criteria for enforcing standards, definitions of terms, procedures, and eligibility requirements for various programs or processes. Regulations cannot be promulgated by an administrative agency without the expressed intent of a law. Silence of the law on an issue cannot be presumed to be the will of the legislature. When there is no prior statutory authority or legislative precedent to address an issue, the legislative process must be enacted.

> Example: An APN petitions the board of nursing to clarify whether or not prescriptive authority is within the scope of practice for the APN. The board staff review the NPA and find a provision in the statute that allows the APN to "diagnose and treat" common, well-defined health problems under approved written protocols. The staff conclude that "treatment" may include prescriptive authority as an "additional act" if permitted in the approved written protocols of the nurse and physician preceptor. No specific language is found in the statute that authorizes writing prescriptions by the APN. When the medical board receives the board of nursing opinion, an attorney general's opinion is requested. The attorney general concludes that the board of nursing may not extend the scope of practice of the APN through regulation. The expressed will of the legislature in regard to the scope of practice for the APN must be sought using the legislative process.

History of Health Professions Regulation

At the end of the 19th century, physicians were the first health care providers to gain legislative recognition for their practice. The definitions of the practice of medicine are all-encompassing of any act to diagnose or treat, or attempt to diagnose or treat, any individual with a physical injury or deformity. Herein lies the problem faced by APNs and other health care providers who are not physicians: to define a scope of practice that does not overlap with this broad definition. The history of nursing regulation is characterized by efforts to accommodate this medical preemption (Safriet, 1992).

The early regulation of nurses was permissive (voluntary), providing for nurses to register with the governing board, hence the title "registered nurse." In some states, nurses were "registered" by the medical board prior to the establishment of a separate board of nursing. During this period, there was no competency assessment. Nurses seeking registration provided evidence of graduation from an approved nursing-education program, and "good moral character" was evaluated by requiring references or endorsements from nurses registered by the board.

The first board of nursing and nurse practice act was passed in 1903 by North Carolina, followed by New York, New Jersey, and Virginia (Sheets, 1996). Boards of nursing began to establish written and practice examinations to measure competency; however, the practice acts were still permissive. Graduates of nursing-education programs not registered with the board were permitted to practice nursing, but they were not permitted to use the title "RN." The first mandatory licensure law was enacted by New York in 1938 (Weisenbeck and Calico, 1995). By the 1950s, mandatory licensure laws for the practice of nursing became widespread, requiring anyone who practiced nursing to be licensed by the state board of nursing. These mandatory licensure laws protected not only the title but also the scope of practice for nurses, resulting in greater public protection.

History of Advanced Practice Nursing Regulation

The 1960s set the stage for the expansion of nursing practice and the practice and regulation of APNs. The birth of the federal entitlement programs, Medicare and Medicaid, increased the number of individuals entitled to government-subsidized health care. With a predicted shortage of primary care physicians, the first formal nurse practitioner programs were opened (Safriet, 1992).

In 1971, Idaho became the first state to legally recognize diagnosis and treatment as part of the scope of practice for the advanced practice nurse. The regulation of APNs was accomplished through joint agreement of the state board of nursing and the state board of medicine for each permissible act of diagnosis and treatment. The model of regulation established in Idaho set a precedent for subsequent models for the regulation of APNs, that is, some form of joint regulation by the board of nursing and board of medicine. The joint regulation was designed to compensate for the broad definition of the practice of medicine and based on the determination that advanced practice nursing was a "delegated medical practice" that required some oversight by physicians. Today the struggle continues between nursing and medicine to define the scope of practice of the APN as nursing practice, regulated solely by state boards of nursing.

Since 1971, virtually every state has developed some form of legal recognition of the APN. Both the American Nurses Association (ANA) and the National Council of State Boards of Nursing (NCSBN) have proposed model rules and regulations for the regulation of advanced practice nursing. However, because the battles for regulation of APNs are fought in highly political state-by-state environments, there is a patchwork of titles, definitions, criteria for practice, scopes of practice, reimbursement policies, and models of regulation that are difficult for policy makers to navigate and understand in today's rapidly changing health care delivery system.

Since 1988, *The Nurse Practitioner: The American Journal of Primary Health Care* has provided an annual survey of each state board of nursing and nursing organizations to gather information on the legislative status of advanced practice nursing. Significant strides have been made by many states in regard to APNs gaining sole authority for scope of practice with no requirements for direct physician supervision. As of 2002, 21 states had indicated that APNs had sole authority for practice with no requirement for physician supervision. Five of the 21 states required physician collaboration only if prescriptive authority was requested. Thirty states require the APN to have some form of collaboration or written protocols, but none require direct supervision by a physician. Thirteen states allow APNs to prescribe without physician involvement, 31 states allow the APN to prescribe controlled substances with physician involvement, and 6 states do not allow APNS to prescribe controlled substances. All states allow some form of prescriptive authority (Pearson, 2002).

Methods of Professional Credentialing

Regulation of the health professions is achieved through various methods of credentialing. The method selected is determined by the state government based on at least two variables: (1) the potential for harm to the public if safe and acceptable standards of practice are not met, and (2) the degree of autonomy and accountability for decision making by the professional. The least restrictive form of regulation to accomplish the goal of public protection should be selected (Gross, 1984; Pew Health Professions Commission, 1994). The term *restrictive* as used in this context means the degree to which the model restricts an individual who has not met the prescribed criteria in the law and the explicit authority of the administrative agency from practicing within the scope of practice of the profession. There are four methods of credentialing used in the United States. Each of the methods is based on the regulation of the individual provider. The methods are described separately, moving from the most restrictive to the least restrictive method of credentialing.

Licensure

Licensure is "granting permission by a competent authority to do an act which, without such permission, would be illegal, a trespass, a tort, or otherwise not allowable" (Black et al., 1992, p. 920). Licensure is the most restrictive method of credentialing and requires anyone who practices within the defined scope of practice to obtain the legal authority to do so from the appropriate administrative agency of the state. Licensure implies competency assessment of the professional at the point of entry into the profession. A licensing examination is administered and ongoing competency assessment by the legal authority is conducted to ascertain that acceptable standards of practice are met. Licensure offers the public the greatest level of protection by protecting the title and the scope of practice of the profession. Unlicensed persons cannot call themselves by the title identified in the law, and they cannot practice lawfully within any part of the scope of practice. The administrative agency holds the licensee accountable for practicing according to the legal, ethical, and professional standards of care defined for the profession. Disciplinary action may be taken on the license of incompetent or unethical licensees, sometimes removing them from practice through an administrative disciplinary procedure. Most of the health professions are regulated by licensure due to the potential for harm to the public by individuals who are not qualified to practice the profession.

Registration

Registration is the "act of enrolling or recording on an official roster" (Black et al., 1992, p. 1283). Registration provides for a review of credentials to determine compliance with the criteria for entry to the profession and permits the individual to use the title "registered." Registration serves as title protection, but does not preclude individuals who are not registered from practicing within the scope of practice, as long as they do not use the title. Registration does not necessarily imply that any competency assessment has been conducted prior to the registration. Some state laws may have provisions for removing incompetent or unethical providers from the registry or marking the registry when a complaint is lodged against a provider. Removing the person from the registry may not necessarily provide public protection, because the individual may continue to practice as long as the title is not used. States are required to maintain a registry of unlicensed assistive personnel who practice in long-term care facilities as a result of the Omnibus Budget Reconciliation Act of 1987.

The title "registered nurse" was formulated in the early days of nursing regulation when the state boards registered nurses. Though nurses have been subject to licensure requirements for many years, the term "registered" has historical significance and has never been changed.

Certification

Certification is the "formal assertion in writing of some fact" (Black et al., 1992, p. 227), that is, providing a certificate. As applied to nursing regulation, certification is a voluntary process of competency assessment conducted by proprietary professional or specialty nursing organizations denoting that the individual has achieved a level of competence in nursing practice beyond the entry-level competence measured by licensure. Certification, like registration, is a means of title protection. Certification, however, is not a governmental process and, therefore, has no force or effect of law. Astute consumers may inquire as to whether or not a provider is certified as a means of determining competency when choosing a provider. Employers also use certification as a means of determining eligibility for certain jobs or as a requirement for promotions within the agency. Some states have promulgated regulations that require an APN to be certified by a specialty nursing organization in order to be eligible to practice in the advanced role.

Recognition

Recognition is a process of "ratification or confirmation" (Black et al., 1992, p. 1271). As applied to nursing regulation, "official recognition" is a method of regulating APNs used by several boards of nursing that implies the board has validated and accepted credentials for the specialty area of practice. Criteria for recognition are defined in the practice act and may include requirements for certification. Official recognition is the least restrictive method of credentialing.

Professional Self-Regulation

Self-regulation occurs within a profession through the desire of members of the profession to set standards, values, ethical frameworks, and safe-practice guidelines beyond the minimum standards defined by law. This voluntary process plays an equally significant role in the regulation of the profession, as does legal regulation. The definition of professional standards of practice and the code of ethics for the profession are examples of professional self-regulation. The members of national professional organizations set standards of practice for specialty practice and determine who can use selected titles by administering certification examinations. Continuing education requirements as well as documentation of practice competency are often required for periodic recertification. The standards are periodically reviewed and revised to reflect current practice. Legal regulation recognizes professional standards as the acceptable standard of practice when making decisions regarding what constitutes safe and competent care.

Even though professional organizations can develop standards, they lack the ability to ensure compliance with the standards. Legal regulation provides a mechanism for monitoring and enforcing compliance with standards of practice. Legal regulation and professional regulation are two sides of the same coin, working together to fulfill the profession's contract with society.

Regulation of Advanced Practice Nurses

Advanced practice nursing regulation has been the focus of the Advanced Practice Task Force of the National Council of State Board of Nursing (NCSBN) for two decades. The evolution of APN practice across the United States has resulted in a patchwork of titles, scopes of practice, and regulatory methods. In order to bring some uniformity to the regulation of APNs, the NCSBN convened the Advanced Practice Task Force. Through the years the task force has developed position papers for consideration by state boards of nursing in a quest for greater standardization and to strengthen the public protection mandate held by boards.

National nursing certifying agencies play an important role in the professional regulation of APNs. Specialty nursing organizations develop certification examinations to measure the competency of nurses in a clinical specialty area. Most boards of nursing require the APN to be certified in the clinical specialty area appropriate to the educational preparation in order to legally practice in the role. The regulatory body has the authority to accept certification examinations if the examination meets the criteria predetermined by the board. The board may not "surrender regulatory authority by passive acceptance without evaluation of the examination content, procedures and scoring process" (NCSBN, 2002). To be legally defensible for licensure purposes, the certification examination must meet certain psychometric standards. The foundational basis for regulatory sufficiency is the examination's ability to measure entry-level practice; be based on a job analysis that defines the job-related knowledge, skills, and abilities; and be developed on psychometrically sound principles of test development.

The NCSBN and the national nursing specialty organizations collaborated to establish criteria that boards of nursing could use in the evaluation of certification examinations (Canavan, 1996). The *Requirements for Accrediting Agencies and Criteria for APRN Certification Programs* were developed in 1995 and updated in 2002 (NCSBN, 2002). The criteria can be located on the NCSBN Web site at http://www.ncsbn.org.

The national organizations that prepare certification examinations for APNs include:

- American Academy of Nurse Practitioners
- American Association of Nurse Anesthetists Council on Certification
- American College of Nurse-Midwives Certification Council
- American Nurses Credentialing Center
- National Certification Board of Pediatric Nurse Practitioners
- National Certification Corporation for the Obstetric, Gynecologic, and Neonatal Nursing Specialties

In addition to the standards of practice set by professional organizations, there are additional standards for practice that govern professional behavior to include policies and procedures of the employing institution, standards and criteria imposed by accrediting agencies such as the state health licensing authority, and the Joint Commission on the Accreditation of Healthcare Organizations (JCAHO).

The NCSBN Advanced Practice Nursing Task Force has also sought to bring greater standardization to APN regulation in an effort to increase mobility of APNs. In 2000, the NCSBN Delegate Assembly passed the *Uniform Advanced Practice Registered Nurse Licensure/Authority to Practice Requirements*. These requirements included:

- unencumbered RN license;
- graduation from a graduate level advanced practice program accredited by a national accrediting body;
- current certification by a national certifying body in the advanced practice specialty appropriate to educational preparation; and
- maintenance of certification or evidence of maintenance of competence (NCSBN, 2002).

Adoption of these uniform requirements by boards of nursing will facilitate APNs becoming a part of the multistate regulation model.

The State Regulatory Process

The Tenth Amendment of the U.S. Constitution reserves for the states all powers not specifically vested in the federal government. The duty to protect its citizens (police powers) is provided to the states. The power to regulate the professions is one way the state exercises its responsibility to protect the health, safety, and welfare of its citizens. State law provides for administrative agencies to assume the responsibility for regulation of the professions. These agencies have administrative, legislative, and judicial powers to make and enforce the laws.

Administrative agencies have sometimes been called the fourth branch of government because of their significant power in the daily execution and enforcement of the law. They are given referent authority by state and federal governments to promulgate rules and regulations, develop policies and procedures, and interpret laws to implement the agency mission.

Boards of Nursing

Each state legislature designates a board or similar authority to administer the practice act for the profession. The board's composition is defined by the law, as are the duties and powers of the board. Traditionally, there are three major duties for licensing boards: (1) control entry into the profession through examination and licensure; (2) monitor and discipline licensees who violate the scope and standards of practice; and (3) monitor continuing competency of licensees to protect the public from unsafe or poor quality practice. Boards of nursing have the additional duty in most states to establish criteria for review and approval of nursing education programs that lead to licensure as a registered nurse (RN) or licensed practical nurse (LPN).

There are 61 boards of nursing in the United States and its territories. Each board of nursing is a member of the National Council of State Boards of Nursing. Some states have separate boards for licensing RNs and LPNs. As members of the NCSBN, the boards have the privilege of using the national licensure examination and meeting together to discuss matters of common interest (NCSBN, 1997).

Composition of the Board of Nursing

Generally, the board is composed predominately of licensed nurses and consumer members. In most states, the governor appoints the members. One state, North Carolina, conducts elections for the board vacancies. Some state laws designate that nurses from specific educational and practice settings, as well as APNs, must be represented on the board of nursing. In other states, the criteria for appointment only require licensure in the profession and a residency requirement. Information on vacancies on the board of nursing can be obtained from the board office or the governor's office. Knowing the composition of the board and when vacancies occur is important to allow the profession to exercise political influence in gaining the desired representation on the board.

Board Meetings

All state government agencies function within open meeting or "sunshine" laws that permit the public to observe or participate in the discussions of the board. Executive sessions and the purpose of the executive session will be announced, when necessary. Rules for executive sessions are specified in the

APA and must be adhered to by the agency. Generally, there are only limited reasons that the board may meet in executive session. Some examples include matters of personnel, obtaining legal advice, contract negotiation, and disciplinary matters. In general, no votes may be taken in executive session. All voting is a matter of public record.

Board meetings may vary in the degree of formality. Most states' APA requires the board to post notice of meetings and the agenda in a public place usually 30 days prior to the meeting. Sometimes the notice of meeting is published in major state newspapers. The agenda is posted in the board of nursing office and can be obtained by calling the board office.

Participants in the board meeting include the board members, the staff of the board, and legal counsel for the board. Legal counsel advises the board in matters of law and jurisdiction. There may be reports during the meeting from staff or other invited guests. Individuals may provide testimony to the board on matters of interest. In making decisions, board members must consider several factors, including implications for the public welfare, national standards of care, impact of the decision on the state as a whole, and the legal defensibility of the decision. All actions of the board must be recorded for the public. Most boards of nursing publish newsletters that summarize the major actions of the board during each meeting. Licensees may request to be placed on the mailing list for the newsletter if one is not automatically received.

Attending meetings of the board of nursing when issues concerning advanced practice nursing are discussed may be the first step in the formulation of policy on APN regulation. Input can be provided to the board during discussion, and information can be obtained on the rationale for decisions by the board.

Monitoring Competency of Nurses

The most critical role of the board of nursing is assuring public protection by monitoring the competency of licensees. Most nurse practice acts have mandatory reporting provisions that require employers to report violations of the NPA. Licensed nurses also have a moral and ethical duty to report unsafe and incompetent practice to the board of nursing. The NPA defines those acts that are considered misconduct and provides for a system of due process to investigate complaints against licensees. Procedures for filing complaints, conducting investigations, and issuing sanctions for violations are enumerated in rules and regulations of the NPA.

The licensed nurse is accountable for knowing the laws and regulations that govern the practice of nursing in the state of licensure and adhering to the legal, ethical, and professional standards of care. Some NPAs include standards of practice in the regulations. Other states may refer to professional standards established by professional associations. The employing agency also defines standards of practice through policy and procedures that must be followed by each nurse employee.

A nurse who holds a multistate license (one license that permits a nurse to practice in more than one state as long as the state is entered into a multistate compact) is held accountable for knowing and abiding by the laws of the state in which the practice occurs in addition to the home state of licensure. Multistate regulation is discussed in more detail later in this chapter. Ignorance of the law is not an excuse for misconduct. Most boards of nursing now have the complete NPA online on their Web sites, as does the National Council of State Boards of Nursing (see http://www.ncsbn.org).

Ethical Principles

In addition to maintaining professional standards of care, the nurse is required to practice according to ethical principles. The *American Nurses Association (ANA) Code of Ethics for Nurses with Interpretive Statements* (ANA, 2001) guides the practice of the registered nurse and is recognized by the regulatory community as a standard for ethical decision making (Exhibit 4–1). The ANA describes the code of ethics for nurses as a document that is "a succinct statement of the ethical obligations and duties of every individual who enters the nursing profession; the profession's non-negotiable ethical standard; and an expression of nursing's own understanding of its commitment to society (ANA, 2001).

Increasingly, nurses are facing ethical dilemmas as advances in technology and scientific discovery coupled with a move toward a market-driven, for-profit health care system create situations where decisions about approaches to care are more difficult to make. The nurse can make sound decisions based on established ethical principles. The study of ethics is gaining prominence in nursing curricula. A more detailed exploration of ethical principles is encouraged. This chapter briefly describes the principles most commonly applied in biomedical ethics.

Autonomy, or *patient self-determination,* provides the individual with the right to choose and implement one's own decisions free from coercion or duress (Aiken, 1994). There are some limits imposed on autonomy when the decision negatively impacts society, such as in refusing treatment for a communicable disease. The concept of informed consent is derived from the ethical principle of autonomy as are the policies regarding advanced directives and health care power of attorney.

Justice (distributive justice) is the obligation to be fair to all people, treating people without regard for race, gender, status, religion, or medical diagnosis (Aiken, 1994). This principle is particularly relevant in the light of cost-containment strategies and access to health care by the uninsured.

Beneficence is directed toward promoting good and preventing evil or harm. The term suggests acts of mercy and charity (Edge and Groves, 1994). Ethical conflicts surrounding the duty of beneficence are more common today with advanced life-support techniques that may postpone death, but leave the patient with a poor quality of life. Also, some treatments meant for good often also cause harmful side effects, i.e., chemotherapy. In general, doing good for the patient implies caring for the patient with a holistic approach.

EXHIBIT 4–1 **Major Provisions of the ANA Code of Ethics for Nurses**

- *Provision 1.* The nurse, in all professional relationships, practices with compassion and respect for the inherent dignity, worth, and uniqueness of every individual, unrestricted by considerations of social or economic status, personal attributes, or the nature of health problems.
- *Provision 2.* The nurse's primary commitment is to the patient, whether an individual, family, group, or community.
- *Provision 3.* The nurse promotes, advocates for, and strives to protect the health, safety, and rights of the patient.
- *Provision 4.* The nurse is responsible and accountable for individual nursing practice and determines the appropriate delegation of tasks consistent with the nurse's obligation to provide optimum patient care.
- *Provision 5.* The nurse owes the same duties to self as to others, including the responsibility to preserve integrity and safety, to maintain competence, and to continue personal and professional growth.
- *Provision 6.* The nurse participates in establishing, maintaining, and improving health care environments and conditions of employment conducive to the provision of quality health care and consistent with the values of the profession through individual and collective action.
- *Provision 7.* The nurse participates in the advancement of the profession through contributions to practice, education, administration, and knowledge development.
- *Provision 8.* The nurse collaborates with other health professionals and the public in promoting community, national, and international efforts to meet health needs.
- *Provision 9.* The profession of nursing, as represented by associations and their members, is responsible for articulating nursing values, for maintaining the integrity of the profession and its practice, and for shaping social policy.

Source: Reprinted with permission from American Nurses Association. *Code of Ethics for Nurses with Interpretive Statements.* © 2001 Nursesbooks.org, American Nurses Association, Washington, DC.

Nonmaleficence is the principle directed toward doing no harm, either intentionally or unintentionally. In addition, the principle implies protection of patients from harm, particularly vulnerable populations who cannot protect themselves, i.e., children, frail elderly, mentally incompetent, and unconscious (Aiken, 1994). This principle is foundational to the role of the nurse as a patient advocate and is embodied in the Nightingale Pledge, which is recited in ceremonies and convocations for nursing graduates.

Veracity is the obligation to tell the truth and not to mislead or deceive. This principle is foundational to documentation and charting as well as conveying information to other care providers.

Confidentiality is the obligation to maintain a patient's right to privacy, to treat records and communications as confidential. This principle will have increasing importance in the emerging health care system where automated patient records and universal patient tracking systems become routine. Enactment of the Health Insurance Portability and Accountability Act (HIPAA) has placed increased emphasis on patient privacy rights making violations of the regulations punishable by fines and imprisonment or both. The HIPAA provisions are further discussed later in this chapter.

Ethical dilemmas occur when the nurse must make a decision that violates one principle in order to adhere to another, creating a conflict. Ethical dilemmas by their very nature require the nurse to make choices between two equally unfavorable alternatives. Areas where ethical dilemmas may be raised in the evolving practice of nursing include:

- Right-to-die situations
- Assisted suicide
- Genetic testing/genetic alteration
- Human cloning/asexual reproduction
- Health care rationing

Boards of nursing will be forging new territory in regulating ethical professional practice as the rapid growth in science and technology provides society with new choices about how human life is created and maintained and how health care policy is viewed. Ethical practice debates will largely be held in the state legislatures, but could also be influenced by federal policy in the interest of protecting the growing numbers of uninsured. The APN must be aware of new legislation and regulations, as well as develop a sound ethical framework for decision making prior to being confronted with complex ethical dilemmas.

Promulgating State Regulations

Government agencies promulgate regulations out of the agency's general administrative duties and jurisdiction in response to a particular issue or concern or as required by specific legislation. The APA of each state specifies the process for the promulgating regulations that includes how the public is notified of proposed regulations and the opportunity for public comment. It is important that the APN becomes familiar with the APA to know when and how to provide comment. States differ in the structural units that review a regulation as it proceeds through the approval process. Some states have designated commissions or committees responsible for review and approval of regulations; other states submit regulations to the general assembly or the committees of the legislature. Whatever procedure is defined, there are certain common elements to promulgating regulations:

- notice to the public that a regulation has been proposed
- opportunity to submit written comment or testimony
- publication of the final regulation in a register or state bulletin

EXHIBIT 4–2   Questions to Ask When Analyzing Regulations

1. Which agency promulgated the regulation?
2. What is the source of authority (the statute that provides authority for the regulation to be promulgated)?
3. What is the intent or rationale of the regulation? Is it clearly stated by the promulgating agency?
4. Is the language in the regulation clear or ambiguous? Can the regulation be interpreted in different ways by different individuals?
5. Are there definitions to clarify terms?
6. Are there important points that are not addressed, i.e., omissions?
7. How does the regulation impact the practice of nursing? Does it constrain or limit the practice of nursing in any way?
8. Is there sufficient lead time to comply with the regulation?
9. What is the fiscal impact of the regulation?

In some states, a requirement for a fiscal impact statement is added. This statement estimates the cost of compliance with the regulation. In this time of cost constraints, the fiscal impact of regulation is a very important concern to businesses and professionals.

Monitoring State Regulations

There are hundreds of regulations promulgated by administrative agencies each year. Regulations that impact advanced nursing practice could be promulgated from a variety of agencies. Knowing which agencies are most likely to have the authority to put forth regulations that impact health care and professional practice, as well as monitoring the legislation and regulations proposed by those agencies, is important to protect the scope of practice of APNs.

The most obvious agencies the APN should consider tracking are the licensing boards of other health professions, such as medicine, pharmacy, counselors and therapists, and other health professionals. In the reforming health care environment, there are numerous conflicts over scope of practice issues, definitions of practice, right to reimbursement, and requirements for supervision and collaboration.

When reviewing regulations, there are several points that are important to consider. Exhibit 4–2 provides some key questions to consider when analyzing a regulation for its impact on nursing practice.

Consider the following situations and how the proposed regulations would affect the practice of the APN.

Example: Assume the board of pharmacy has offered the following definition of the practice of pharmacy. *The practice of pharmacy includes, but is not limited to, the interpretation, evaluation, and implementation of medical orders; the dispensing of prescription drug orders; initiating or modifying the drug therapy in accordance with written guidelines or protocols previously established and approved by a practitioner authorized to independently prescribe drugs; provision of patient counseling as a primary health care provider of pharmacy care.*

If this definition was included in the pharmacy practice act requiring that anyone who "initiated or modified a drug therapy in accordance with written guidelines or protocols" must be licensed as a pharmacist by the board of pharmacy, how would this impact the practice of nursing and, especially, the APN? This is but one example of numerous definitions of scope of practice that are promulgated that has significant overlap with the practice of nursing. It is very important to assure there are provisions within the pharmacy practice act to recognize the practice of nursing as being exempt from the regulation.

Example: Assume the board of medicine has offered the following regulation to clarify the practice of medicine. *Any person who treats, or renders a written or otherwise documented medical opinion concerning the diagnosis or treatment of a patient within the state, as a result of transmission of individual patient data by electronic or other means from within the state to a person or his agent located inside or outside of this state, or renders a determination of medical necessity, appropriateness of proposed treatment, or appropriateness of a patient's length of stay in a hospital, clinic, or other medical treatment facility shall be regarded as practicing medicine within the meaning of the law.*

How does this definition impact the practice of nursing? Knowing that insurance companies use licensed nurses to assist in making a determination of medical necessity regarding payment of claims, what would your response be to this regulation?

Example: Assume the banking and insurance subcommittee of the state House of Representatives is considering a provision to require employers who subscribe to a closed-panel health plan to offer employees an option to dis-enroll and immediately enroll in an open-panel plan, with certain provisions. The provision states that: "Any open- or closed-panel plan offered pursuant to this article may not discriminate against a physician, podiatrist, optometrist, oral surgeon, or chiropractor from practicing as a provider in the plan by excluding the provider on the basis of the profession."

What implications can you see for APNs who may want to provide services to patients in an open-panel plan if this provision passes as written? Note that language missing from a proposed regulation may be just as critical to the practice of the APN as language that is written into the regulation.

In a growing managed-care market, it is critical for APNs to be aware of regulations that mandate benefits or reimbursement policies and to lobby for inclusion of APNs. Several states have promulgated open-panel legislation known as "any willing provider" and "freedom of choice" laws. These bills mandate that any provider who is authorized to provide the services covered in an insurance plan must be recognized and reimbursed by the plan. Insurance company lobbyists as well as business lobbyists oppose this type of legislation. As managed-care contracts are negotiated, APNs must assure that services of the APN are given fair and equitable consideration. Other important areas include worker's compensation participation and reimbursement provisions and liability insurance laws.

The federal government entitlement programs, Medicare and Medicaid, are administered at the state level. The state has the responsibility for complying with the federal mandates on reimbursement, while being given a certain amount of discretion in program implementation. It is important for the APN to be knowledgeable about the state reimbursement policies and procedures and to understand how to influence the decision-making process.

APNs achieved landmark success in 1997, with grassroots lobbying efforts, to gain Medicare reimbursement for all nurse practitioners, regardless of location of practice. Prior to 1997, Medicare reimbursement for nurse practitioners was restricted to those nurse practitioners who provided services in specific geographic locations and who practiced with physician supervision.

In summary, state agencies that govern licensing and certification of health care facilities, administer public health services (public health, mental health, alcohol and drug abuse), govern reimbursement, as well as the health professions licensing boards, are all agencies that could promulgate regulations that would have implications for the practice of the APN.

Serving on Boards and Commissions

One way to actively participate in the regulatory process is to seek an appointment to the state board of nursing or other board or commission that impacts health policy. Active participation in the political process, especially during times of rapid change and reform, will ensure the voice of APNs is heard in setting the public-policy agenda.

When seeking appointments to boards and commissions, consider selecting an agency whose mission and purposes are consistent with your interest and expertise. Because most board appointments are gubernatorial or political appointments, it is important for the APN to obtain endorsements from legislators, influential community leaders, and employers who are willing to write letters of support to the governor.

A personal letter to the governor expressing interest in serving on the board should include a statement of qualifications and rationale for why the APN is interested in serving. Explain the contributions that can be made and willingness to commit the time and effort to accomplish the terms of the appointment. Include previous volunteer work to demonstrate interest in the community and the ability to serve effectively. Attach a resume of educational and work experiences and provide a means of communication to follow up on any missing information.

The letters of support should document the contributions made in employment and community service. Delineate involvement in local, state, and national organizations. The letter from the employer should indicate a willingness to provide the time to fulfill the responsibilities of the position during the term of office. There will be a significant time commitment required in service, and it is very important that the APN be able to fulfill the responsibilities in a competent manner. To obtain information regarding the time commitment, speak to other members of the board or call the executive director or administrator of the agency.

The Federal Regulatory Process

There are many forces that have contributed to the federal government becoming a more central figure in the regulation of the health professions. The most significant factor is the advent of the Medicare and Medicaid programs. The federal initiatives that have grown out of these programs are largely focused on cost containment (prospective payment) and consumer protection (combating fraud and abuse) (Jost, 1997; Roberts and Clyde, 1993).

With the "graying" of Americans, the cost of administering the Medicare program is skyrocketing, with predictions of bankruptcy if substantive changes are not made in either the criteria for eligibility, the methods of reimbursement, or both. There are expected to be numerous changes to the system over the next several years.

One of the most significant changes occurred in July 2001 when the Center for Medicare and Medicaid Services (CMS) was created to replace the former Health Care Financing Administration (HCFA). The reformed agency provides an increased emphasis on responsiveness to beneficiaries and providers, and quality improvement. Three new business centers have been established as part of the reform: Center for Beneficiary Choices, Center for Medicare Management, and Center for Medicaid and State Operations (CMS, 2001).

APNs have also been impacted by changes in the Medicare reimbursement policy. Legislation was passed in Congress in 1997 calling for Medicare reimbursement of APNs regardless of setting and went into effect in January 1998. These regulations provide direct reimbursement to APNs for providing Medicare Part B services that would normally be provided by a physician. These services are not restricted by site of geographic location as services have been in the past. Under this legislation, APNs can see both new and continuing patients without restriction. Reimbursement rates are set at 80 percent of the lesser of the actual charge or 85 percent of the fee schedule amount for the physician (AANP, 2003). APNs must secure a Medicare provider number to be eligible for reimbursement. In order to obtain a Medicare PIN number, the APN must have a masters degree in nursing, be nationally certified, and recognized in his or her state as practicing at an advanced level.

The devolution of government has changed the relationship between the state and federal regulatory systems. Responsibilities once assumed by the federal government have been shifted down to the state level, such as administration of the Medicaid programs and management of the welfare program. The philosophy that states are better equipped to make decisions about how best to assist their citizens and the sentiment against creating federal bureaucracy and increasing the tax burden have been the impetus to this devolution.

Even though states have primary authority over regulation of the health professions, federal policies also have an enormous effect on health care workforce regulation. All the policies related to reimbursement and quality control over the Medicare and Medicaid programs are promulgated by the U.S. Department of Health and Human Services (HHS) and administered through its financing agency, the CMS. Other federal statutes that have a regulatory impact on health care providers and should be familiar to the APN include:

- Clinical Laboratory Improvement Amendments of 1988 (CLIA 88)
- Occupational Safety and Health Act of 1970 (OSHA)
- Mammography Quality Standards Act of 1987 (MQSA)
- Omnibus Budget Reconciliation Act of 1987 and 1990 (OBRA 87 and 90)
- Americans with Disabilities Act of 1990 (ADA)
- North American Free Trade Agreement of 1993 (NAFTA)
- Telecommunications Act of 1996
- Health Insurance Portability and Accountability Act of 1996 (HIPAA)

The veterans administration hospitals and the Indian Health Services both are regulated by the federal government, as are the uniformed armed services. Individuals who are employed in these services must be licensed in at least one state and are subject to the laws of the state in which he or she is licensed and the standards of care and policies established in the federal system. This license may or may not be in the state in which the individual is practicing or residing. If the individual decides to practice in the civilian sector, the individual must become licensed by the state where the practice is occurring.

The Supremacy Clause of the U.S. Constitution gives legal superiority to federal laws (Braunstein, 1995). When a federal law or regulation is promulgated, it takes precedence over any state law. State laws in conflict with federal laws cannot be enforced. At times, the courts may be asked to determine the constitutionality of a law or regulation to resolve jurisdictional disputes.

The Commerce Clause of the U.S. Constitution limits the ability of states to erect barriers to interstate trade (Gobis, 1997). Courts have found that the provision of health care is interstate trade under antitrust laws. This finding sets the stage for the federal government to preempt state licensing laws in the practice of professions across state boundaries, if it chooses to do so.

The impact of technology on the delivery of health care, such as "telehealthcare," allows providers to care for patients in remote environments and across the geopolitical boundaries defined by traditional state-by-state licensure. This raises the question as to whether or not the federal government will intercede in standardizing licensing requirements across state lines to facilitate interstate commerce, usurping the state's authority. Licensing boards are beginning to identify ways to facilitate the practice of telehealthcare, at the

---

EXHIBIT 4–3 **Federal Rule-Making Process**

Congress Authorizes Law That Provides
Authority for Rule Promulgation
↓

Advance Notice of Proposed Rule-Making
(Optional)
↓

Proposed Rule Published in the *Federal Register*
(Comment Period Specified, Informal Hearings Optional)
↓

Final Rule Published in the *Federal Register*
↓

Rule Becomes Effective in 30 Days after Publication
↓

Final Rule Updated in Code of Federal Regulations
(Update Done on a Quarterly Cycle by Agency Title)

Source: Goehlert, R. U. and Martin, F. S. (1989). Federal administrative law. *Congress and Law Making: Researching the Legislative Process* (2nd ed.). San Francisco, CA: ABC-CLIO, pp. 82–83.

---

same time preserving the power and right of the state to protect its citizens by regulating the professions at the state level. One innovative approach to nursing regulation, multistate regulation, is discussed later in this chapter.

Promulgating Federal Regulations

The federal regulatory process is a two-step process established by the federal Administrative Procedures Act. A notice of proposed rule-making (NPR) is published in the proposed rule section of the *Federal Register* that informs the public of the substance of the intended regulation and provides information on how the public may participate in providing comment, attend meetings, or otherwise participate in the regulatory process. The second step involves careful consideration of public comment by the agency and amendment to the regulation, if warranted. The final regulations are issued by the agency through publication in the rules and regulations section of the *Federal Register* and become effective 30 days after publication (Exhibit 4–3).

Emergency Regulations

Provisions for promulgating emergency regulations are defined at both the state and federal levels. Emergency regulations are promulgated if an agency determines that the public welfare is immediately adversely affected. Emergency regulations may take effect immediately upon publication. They are usually temporary measures that are effective for a limited time (usually

90 days, with an option to renew) and must be followed with permanent regulations that are promulgated in accordance with the APA process.

Locating Information

The *Federal Register* is the bulletin board or newspaper of the federal government. It is published daily, Monday through Friday, except for federal holidays. It contains executive orders and presidential proclamations, rules and regulations, proposed rules, notices, sunshine act meetings, as well as corrections to previous copies of the *Federal Register*. Each document in the *Federal Register* begins with a heading that includes the name of the issuing agency, the *Code of Federal Regulations* title, and a brief synopsis of the contents. After the heading, a preamble is published that contains the type of action, summary of action, deadline for comments, address to which the comments may be sent, a contact person, and other supplementary information (Goehlert and Martin, 1989). The *Federal Register* may be accessed online via the Governmental Printing Office at http://www.gpoaccess.gov/fr/index.html.

The *Code of Federal Regulations* (CFR) is a compilation of all final regulations issued by the executive branch agencies of the federal government. The CFR consists of 50 titles that represent broad subject areas. Each executive agency has jurisdiction over a topic area that is identified in the chapter heading. The CFR is updated annually in sections. Each quarter, one section of the CFR is updated according to a schedule that includes all regulations that have been passed since the prior printing. Consequently, there is never a publication that has all the regulations passed in it for the year. An index is published and revised semi-annually that helps in locating rules by agency name and subject headings (Goehlert and Martin, 1989). The *Code of Federal Regulations* is online via the Government Printing Office (GPO) at http://www.gpoaccess.gov/cfr/index.html.

Each state government publishes similar documents that identify the proposed regulations, notices, final regulations, and emergency regulations. The publication is usually called the *State Register* or the *State Bulletin*. The publication cycle can be obtained by calling the state legislative printing office or the state legislative information system office. Copies of these documents are usually available in the local libraries and may be available online on the state's governmental Web site.

The APN has a daunting task to read the myriad of proposed regulations promulgated by agencies at the state and federal levels. There are several aids that can be employed to assist in the monitoring process, such as legislative services, monitoring services, bulletins that summarize proposed regulations, and specialty organization newsletters and journals.

Lobbyists are employed by organizations to monitor and track legislative and regulatory activities of interest to an organization. Subscription services are available that will track legislation for an agency or organization and will provide an abstract of the substance of bills and regulations as well as the progress through the legislative or regulatory process. Both free and subscription legislative information services are available online. Examples of online services include:

- State Net: information and intelligence for the 50 states and Congress, located at http://www.statenet.com.
- Thomas Legislative Information: sponsored by the U.S. Library of Congress, located at http://thomas.loc.gov.
- GPO Access: located at http://www.gpoaccess.gov.

In addition there are numerous private services available by searching the Internet. Several nursing and health care associations also feature relevant updates and information on current legislative and public policy issues (see Exhibit 4–4).

EXHIBIT 4–4   **Selected Web Sites of Interest**

URL	Summary of Content
http://www.statenet.com	Legislative and regulatory reporting services from all 50 states and Congress. A subscription service that provides comprehensive and timely information on legislation.
http://thomas.loc.gov	Thomas Legislative Information System. Sponsored by the U.S. Library of Congress. Summarizes bills, provides full text of bills and the *Congressional Record,* information on the legislative process and U.S. government Internet resources.
http://www.ahrq.gov	Agency for Healthcare Research and Quality. Information on health care research, evidence reports, clinical practice guidelines, consumer health information, hyperlinked to U.S. Dept. of Health and Human Services (HHS).
http://www.ctl.org	Center for Telemedicine Law. Information on the latest findings in the regulation of telemedicine, proceedings of national telemedicine task force, state-by-state updates on telemedicine legislation.
http://www.nursingworld.org	American Nurses Association. Access to all ANA services; access to *Online Journal of Issues in Nursing,* jointly prepared with Kent State Univ.
http://www.ncsbn.org	National Council of State Boards of Nursing. Information on all National Council services and committee activities, access to state nurse practice acts, information on progress of multistate regulation.

Continued

EXHIBIT 4-4 **(Continued)**

URL	Summary of Content
http://www.hhs.gov	U.S. Dept. of Health and Human Services. Access to all agencies within the department, i.e., ACHPR, CDC, CMS, HRSA, NIH, etc. Consumer information and policy information.
http://www.hschange.com	The Center for Studying Health Systems Change. A Washington DC based research organization dedicated to studying the nation's health care systems and the impact on the public.
http://www.nurse.org	State-by-state display of advanced practice nursing organizations, links to related sites that contain legislative and regulatory information, NP Central (a comprehensive site for APN CE offerings, salary information, job opportunities).
http://www.nursingethicsnetwork.org	Nursing Ethics Network. A nonprofit organization committed to the advancement of nursing ethics. Site contains ethics research findings and online inquiry.
http://www.acnp.org	American College of Nurse Practitioners. Comprehensive site featuring latest trends and issues impacting APN practice and regulation.
http://www.aanp.org	American Academy of Nurse Practitioners. Comprehensive site featuring latest trends and issues impacting APN practice and regulation.
http://www.cms.hhs.gov/hipaa	Center for Medicare and Medicaid Services. Latest legislative and regulatory information on reimbursement, HIPAA implementation.
http://www.hhs.gov/ocr/hipaa	Office of Civil Rights. Fact sheets, sample forms, FAQs on HIPAA implementation along with related links and educational materials.
http://www.iom.edu	Institute of Medicine. Provides objective information to further science and health policy. A leading and respected authority on health issues. Access to published reports.

Providing Public Comment

There is a small window of opportunity for public input into the development of regulations. Most comment periods are a minimum of 30 days from the date of the publication of the proposed rule. Sometimes an NPR will provide for a longer period of time to submit comments if the agency anticipates the issue will be one of strong public interest or will be controversial in nature. It is very important that the APN is vigilant as to when the comment periods are set.

Public hearings may be held by an agency on a proposed rule, but are not required unless the APA establishes criteria for when a public hearing must be held by the agency. Generally the agency is required to hold a hearing when a request is made by a specified number of individuals or agencies. Written comments received by the agency are made a part of the permanent record and must be considered by the agency's board or commission members prior to the publication of the final rule. A final rule can be challenged in the courts if the judge determines that the agency did not comply with the APA or ignored public comments.

The *Register* names the individual in the agency who can be contacted to submit comments. It is best to place the comments in writing to assure inclusion in the public record. It is permissible to call the agency and provide comments orally, if time is of the essence. Faxing comments may also be an option if the comment period is near expiration. It is of utmost importance that the deadline that is posted in the *Register* is met, because agencies can rightfully disregard comments received after the deadline.

When providing public comment in writing, or testimony at a hearing, it is important for the APN to:

- Be specific regarding whether the regulation is supported or opposed. Give examples using brief scenarios or experiences when possible.
- Have credible data to back the position, such as statistics. Utilize research findings that can be explained in common language; avoid medical jargon.
- Know what the opposition is saying and respond to these concerns.
- Convey a willingness to negotiate or compromise toward mutually acceptable resolutions.
- Demonstrate concern for the public good, rather than self-interest.
- Be brief and succinct. Limit remarks to one or two pages or 5 minutes for oral testimony.

Regulatory agencies charged with public protection are more likely to address concerns that are focused on how the public may be harmed or benefited rather than concerns that seem like turf protection and professional jealousy. Demonstrate support for your position by having colleagues that represent a variety of organizations and interests submit comments. It is important to demonstrate the degree of concern, because the number of comments received is one way the agency measures support or nonsupport for the regulation.

Often APNs believe that their voice or points of view will be ignored or that the perceived power of the medical profession will override nursing's concerns. APNs may be surprised to find that there is a strong sentiment toward consumer welfare in government and that nurses are seen as expert clinicians and consumer advocates, making them a powerful voice in the regulatory process.

Lobbying and Political Decision Making

Lobbying is the act of influencing a governmental entity to achieve a specific legislative or regulatory outcome. Anyone can lobby, and it has been demonstrated that the grassroots lobbyists can achieve the most effective lobbying efforts. Grassroots lobbyists are the local constituents who have the power to elect officials through their vote. Grassroots lobbying efforts take organization and a commitment on the part of the constituent to be well-informed on the issue being considered and to respond when called. Professional nursing organizations have become increasingly more aware of the strength in grassroots lobbying efforts and have made concerted efforts toward educating their members regarding ways to communicate with legislators and regulatory agencies. The "Aunt Mary Network," a method of linking legislators with a nurse who is a relative or friend has proven very successful (Pruitt et al., 2002). Legislative workshops are excellent forums to teach nurses how to exert their political influence to shape public policy in the interest of consumer welfare.

It is important to be aware of state ethics laws as they relate to lobbying. There are strict reporting requirements in most ethics laws in a state along with restrictions that apply to the use of funds and gifts.

Participating in organized lobbying efforts is critical to successful outcomes. There is no substitute for visibility in the legislative and regulatory process. Building trusting relationships, demonstrating interest and concern for the public good, and providing information on issues important to the profession are all things that can be done on a regular basis through regular participation in the legislative and regulatory process. It is best not to wait until there is an important bill or regulation pending to begin developing relationships with legislators and staff of administrative agencies. A brief contact to convey interest in the activities and issues of the agency will help to develop name recognition. Leave a business card and offer to serve as a resource in the future. Volunteer to serve on committees and task forces to build your credibility and trust.

Legislators are most commonly the targets of lobbying efforts. However, it is equally important and often most effective to cultivate a relationship with the legislative staff. Legislators rely heavily on the advice of their staffs. Provide information to the staff and have them keep you informed of progress on a particular issue.

There are several key points to include in developing a successful lobbying plan.

• *The importance of unity within the profession.*   Divisiveness within the ranks of the profession is a sure road to defeat. There will be plenty of opposition to a controversial issue outside the profession, so make sure nurses understand and support the cause. At a minimum, if a group cannot agree to support the initiative, work toward a compromise so that the group will not openly oppose the cause.

> Example: When APNs were seeking prescriptive authority in South Carolina, the certified registered nurse anesthetists (CRNAs) chose not to be included in the regulation so they would not be subject to protocols and supervision of a physician. Rather than oppose the APNs in their quest for prescriptive authority, the CRNAs supported the APNs by presenting testimony and remaining an active part of the advanced practice coalition.

• *Seek and define a base of support external to the profession.*   Identify groups and individuals who have something to gain if your cause is successful, i.e., consumers and other licensed professionals.

> Example: A major initiative of rural counties in South Carolina is to attract new business and industry. One very important aspect of attracting new businesses to an area is the quality of life. Adequate health care services, education, and infrastructure are critical components to a prospective client. APNs met with the state department of commerce to share how using APNs to increase access to primary health care could improve the ability of rural counties to recruit new businesses. The department of commerce, along with local mayors, began to join the APN coalition to support regulations to provide prescriptive authority to APNs.

• *Timing is everything.*   There are times and windows of opportunity for a political agenda to be moved forward. Sometimes it is just as important to wait for a favorable climate. At the same time, be vigilant of the environment and know when the time is right to avoid missing a critical window of opportunity. During periods of reform, unfreezing occurs and there is a stronger propensity for changes to be made.

• *The regulatory process is an evolving process.*   Do not be discouraged if regulations do not include all the aspects supported by the nursing community. Amendments to regulations can be made at a later time. Sometimes success comes one step at a time.

Identify who the proponents and the opponents are on a particular issue, and realize that all have the same goal—to influence the governmental entity in their favor. Reason and rationality are not always the basis for political decision making. There are, however, effective strategies such as bargaining, compromise, trade-offs, and negotiation that can lead to agreement on controversial issues.

Understanding that there are many tactics that can be employed to influence the regulatory and legislative process will enhance success in the process. The American Nurses Association has published the *Grassroots Lobbying Handbook* to provide information to nurses on to how to influence the legislative and political process (DeVries and Vanderbilt, 1992).

Another effective strategy in influencing legislative and regulatory outcomes is attendance at board and committee meetings. Listening to the dialogue and understanding the issues and concerns of the regulators can provide invaluable insight into what strategies need to be employed. Through observing and participating in the meeting, the APN will gain recognition and begin to build a relationship with the regulators that may pay significant dividends in the future.

Strengths and Weaknesses of the Regulatory Process

The regulatory process is much more ordered than the legislative process in that the administrative procedures act in each state and at the federal level directs the process that must be undertaken. There is guaranteed opportunity for comment and public input. The regulatory process has built-in delays and time constraints that slow down action. On the other hand, the regulatory process also is much more controlled by administrative agencies and can often become tedious and complex in detail of implementation. The regulations may not always be written by individuals who are knowledgeable about the impact of the regulations, making the public input process especially important.

One power provided to administrative agencies is to interpret regulations. It is especially important to be aware that existing regulations may be misinterpreted by the staff or board of an agency, resulting in a new meaning being imposed rather than the original intent of the regulation. One example of how the interpretation of regulations can have significant impact on advanced practice nursing is the 1991 decision of the Drug Enforcement Administration regarding the issuance of DEA numbers to APNs.

> Example: The Federal Controlled Substances Act requires providers who are authorized to prescribe, dispense, administer, or conduct research with controlled substances to obtain a federal DEA number. Prior to 1990, many APNs applied for and received DEA registration numbers. In 1991 the DEA began to question the applications based on the new interpretation that registration was only available to those providers who had "plenary authority" (authority that was not derived from protocol) and who worked without supervision. The DEA determined that because restrictions for the prescription of controlled substances by APNs were imposed by the individual states and within practice settings, the APNs did not meet the standard for receiving a DEA registration number.

This new interpretation had a significant effect on the practice of the APN because many insurance companies use the DEA number as a unique identifier for reimbursement purposes. The message in the DEA interpretation was damaging to APNs because it equated the collaborative and supervisory practice agreements between APNs and physicians as one of control (Safriet, 1992). The proposed rule was not promulgated, but rather a strong lobbying effort by nurses was successful in developing a system for the registration of APNs with a designated prefix that went into effect in 1995. The registration of APNs with the designated prefix allows the APN to apply for a unique number separate and distinct from the physician number and allows the APN to prescribe controlled substances within the parameters established by state law.

With turnover in the composition of administrative agency board members and staff, new interpretations to existing statutes and regulations may occur. For this reason, it is especially important to review opinions and/or declaratory rulings of the board, attorney general opinions, and opinions of the court. These opinions carry the force and effect of law even though they are not promulgated according to the APA. There is a fine line between the duty to interpret existing laws and regulations and establishing new laws or standards without complying with the APA. The courts have revoked several board rulings requiring boards to promulgate new regulations according to the APA.

Current Issues in Regulation and Licensure

Regulation in a Transforming Health Care Delivery System

The current system of regulation of health care professionals is based on the regulation of the individual provider and the employment setting. Questions have been raised as to whether this system is the best means of public protection or whether the system has become a means of protecting the profession and creating monopolies for services (Gross, 1984; Pew Health Professions Commission, 1994). As new health care occupations and professions have emerged, there has been increasing professional debate about what tasks can be accomplished by what professions. Overlapping scopes of practice have naturally emerged among nursing, medicine, pharmacy, social work, physical therapy, occupational therapy, and other licensed health professions. Overlapping scopes of practice are appropriate when competency and education to perform the acts are substantially equivalent. However, restrictive practice acts have made overlapping scopes of practice a battlefield for debate, a debate with which APNs are very familiar.

The Pew Health Professions Commission (1995) has suggested that the current century-old regulatory system is out of sync with the nation's health care delivery and financing structures and in need of major reform. The web of laws and regulations created by bureaus, agencies, boards, and legal departments makes it difficult for the public and those regulated to participate in what Dower and Finocchio call an "exclusionary scheme" (Dower and Finocchio, 1995, p. 2). The Pew Health Professions Commission suggests that states review the regulatory process in light of the following criteria:

- Does regulation promote effective health outcomes and protect the public from harm?

- Are regulatory bodies truly accountable to the public?
- Does regulation respect consumers' right to choose their own health care providers from a range of safe options?
- Does regulation encourage a flexible, rational, and cost-effective health care system?
- Does regulation allow effective working relationships among health care providers?
- Does regulation promote equity among providers of equal skill?
- Does regulation facilitate professional and geographic mobility of competent providers? (Dower and Finocchio, 1995, p. 1)

Workforce regulation has a tremendous impact on the access, cost, and accessibility of health care. Restrictive scopes of practice limit the ability of comparably prepared providers to provide care. Concurrently, employers have expanded the use of unlicensed assistive personnel (UAP) who infringe on the scope of practice defined for the licensed nurse. Boundary disputes within and across disciplines flourish—between nursing and other allied health providers, allied health providers and medicine, nursing and medicine, dental hygienists and dentists, and nurses and UAPs.

The Pew Task Force on Health Care Workforce Regulation has challenged the state and federal government to respond to the complex issues regarding the education and regulation of the health professions. The task force has offered 10 recommendations to make the state regulatory system more responsive to the evolving health care system (Exhibit 4–5).

The creation of super boards with a majority of consumer representatives is one suggestion the Pew Health Professions Commission has advocated. Gross (1984) advocates for increasing competition among providers and giving the consumer more choice. Gross suggests one alternative to individual licensure of professionals would be to regulate dangerous procedures, or those procedures that, when inadequately performed, would cause irremediable consequences. This system of regulation has been implemented in Ontario, Canada. The Ontario model of regulation regulates 13 dangerous procedures and determines which professionals may engage in these procedures based on demonstrated competency and education. This model is under study by those groups interested in alternatives to the current regulatory system and could be the next frontier of debate in reforming health care regulation.

There is a window of opportunity to achieve significant reform in the regulation of the health professions in the 21st century. Advanced practice nurses must be open to the concept of new regulatory models that may emerge. Regulation will determine who will have access to the patient, who will serve as the gatekeeper in a managed-care environment, who will get reimbursed, and who will have autonomy to practice. APNs must be visible participants throughout the political process to shape a dynamic and evolving system that is responsive to the health care environment and ensures consumer choice and protection.

EXHIBIT 4-5   Ten Recommendations for Reforming Health Care Workforce Regulation

1. Use standardized and understandable language for health professions regulation and its functions to clearly describe them for consumers, provider organizations, business, and the professions.

2. Standardize entry-to-practice requirements and limit them to competence assessments for health professions to facilitate the physical and professional mobility of the health professions.

3. Base practice acts on demonstrated initial and continuing competence. Allow and expect different professions to share overlapping scopes of practice. Explore pathways to allow all professionals to provide services to the full extent of their current knowledge, training, experience, and skills.

4. Redesign health professions boards and their functions to reflect the interdisciplinary and public accountability demands of the changing health care delivery system.

5. Educate consumers to assist them in obtaining the information necessary to make decisions about practitioners and to improve the board's accountability.

6. Cooperate with other public and private organizations in collecting data on regulated health professions to support effective workforce planning.

7. Require each board to develop, implement, and evaluate continuing competency requirements to assure the continuing competence of regulated health care professionals.

8. Maintain a fair, cost-effective, and uniform disciplinary process to exclude incompetent practitioners to protect and promote the public's health.

9. Develop evaluation tools that assess the objectives, successes, and shortcomings of their regulatory systems and bodies to best protect and promote the public's health.

10. Understand the links, overlaps, and conflicts between their health care workforce regulatory systems and other systems that affect the education, regulation, and practice of health care practitioners and work to develop partnerships to streamline regulatory structures and processes.

Source: Pew Health Professions Commission (1995). *Task Force on Health Care Workforce Regulation: Policy Considerations for the 21st century.* San Francisco, CA: UCSF Center for the Health Professions, pp. 3–8.

Multistate Regulation

Technology has transformed the health care delivery system and is challenging the state-by-state regulatory and licensing system. Mergers, acquisitions, and buyouts of health care systems have produced giant conglomerates that operate across state lines. Care is coordinated by case managers who may be located in distant states. Nurses staff telephone hot lines across state boundaries to provide advice and consultation to patients on health care issues. The Internet and e-mail afford patients hundreds of disease specialty home pages on the World Wide Web sponsored by institutions and voluntary associations. The Cyberspace Telemedicine Office is a Web site that collects and stores basic medical information provided by patients. Individuals can access the information on diseases and medicines tailored to their clinical status and receive online consultation from a physician (Braunstein, 1995). United HealthCare's Web site, called Optum Online, offers nursing online services. Individuals submit questions, and then nurses research answers and provide personalized information within 48 to 72 hours (Gobis, 1997). Current law mandates that a nurse must be licensed in each state where he or she practices. There are nurses who currently hold up to 50 licenses that are expensive and unduly cumbersome to maintain. These scenarios raise many questions as to how the current state-by-state regulatory system can be adapted to fit the new health care environment. Boards of nursing must continue to minimize barriers to health care imposed by unnecessarily restrictive regulations, particularly in light of the nursing shortages that are projected over the next several years. Access to nursing care by the public is critical to maintaining the quality of health care in the United States.

Although states have done much over the years to facilitate interstate mobility of nurses, there are still cumbersome licensure processes that produce difficulty for seamless transitions across geopolitical boundaries. The confusion is prominent especially in the regulation of APNs. Not only are there a variety of methods used to regulate APNs, ranging from second licensure to official recognition, titles vary from state to state, as do the scopes of practice and even the jurisdiction for regulation (i.e., nursing, medical, or joint boards). The NCSBN's definition of *Uniform Advanced Practice Registered Nurse Licensure/Authority to Practice Requirements* will promote standardization of APN regulation to allow APNs to participate in multistate regulation as well as compete in a global market.

Moving to a multistate regulatory system has advantages for the profession and must be carefully executed state by state to assure that the mission of the boards to protect the public is achieved. Central databases for reporting disciplinary actions and procedures for investigating complaints on licensees who are not located in the state where the patient resides have been developed. Boards must strengthen their roles in assuring continuing competence of licensees and making information available to the public so that the public can make informed choices about providers.

The concept of a "national" license is not very difficult to conceive. Boards of nursing have used a national licensure examination to measure competency for entry into practice since 1951. General and specialty professional nursing organizations develop national standards of care and standards for professional practice. The courts have held that a national standard of care is expected and should be received by the patient. Patients should be able to expect the same level of care from nurses regardless of where the patient lives. Model practice acts have been developed by the NCSBN and ANA to promote national standards of care and regulatory models. In spite of all these efforts, the politics of state-by-state regulation have resulted in variance and confusion. The NCSBN's Nursing Practice and Education Committee has developed

Uniform Core Licensure Requirements that will assist in the implementation of the mutual recognition compact by diminishing concerns over disparate qualifications for licensure in compact states. These core licensure requirements for initial entry into the nursing profession are considered *minimum* requirements that are essential to promote public protection (NCSBN, 1999).

The NCSBN delegate assembly adopted the "mutual recognition" model of multistate regulation in 1997. Mutual recognition is a method of licensure in which boards voluntarily enter into an interstate compact to legally recognize the policies and processes of a licensee's home state to permit practice in the remote state without obtaining an additional license. This model is similar to the driver's license model of regulation that permits an individual who is licensed to drive in one state to drive in any state, as long as the individual obeys the laws of the state in which he or she is driving. Suspension of the driver's license by the home state invalidates the individual's privilege of driving in any state. If a violation of law occurs, the state in which the violation occurs is responsible for disciplinary action (NCSBN, 1998).

The mutual recognition form of regulation is common in the European Union and Australia (Winn, 1995). Mutual recognition preserves the sovereignty of the state while fostering collaboration and cooperation among the states. When applied to nursing licensure, the nurse is licensed in the state of residency, and the nurse is required to practice according to the laws of the state where the patient resides. Although national criteria for licensure and regulation are not required to operationalize this model, such criteria would facilitate multistate practice.

The NCSBN and its member boards made an historic decision in 1998 to adopt the mutual recognition concept. To implement the mutual recognition model of nursing regulation, each state legislature must sign the interstate compact into law. Since 1999, there have been 20 states to pass compact legislation (NCSBN, 2003). Advanced practice nurses initially were not a part of the interstate compact agreement. With the move toward adoption of the Uniform Requirements for Licensure/Authority to Practice, APNs will be able to participate in the multistate regulation process. The APN must reside in a state that has already joined the interstate compact and subscribed to the uniform requirements. The multistate license does not, however, include prescriptive authority. Prescriptive authority must be sought independently in the state of practice.

Given the climate in the federal government related to the business of health care and the concept that this business is interstate commerce, it would seem that states will begin to move quickly to preserve state regulation of the professions while facilitating interstate practice.

The Future of Advanced Practice Nurse Regulation

Much has been written in this chapter on the problems and issues related to the regulation of APNs. However, not all of the problems associated with the full utilization and practice of the APN are external to the profession; some of the problems have been created within the profession. The proliferation of APN educational programs with numerous specialty areas that have limited scopes of practice has created much of the public confusion regarding the role and scope of practice of the APN. Multiple educational pathways to achieve APN certification and legal credentialing have complicated the regulatory process further (O'Malley et al., 1996). The numerous titles used for APN practice are confusing not only to the public but to regulatory agencies such as the Center for Medicare and Medicaid Services that establishes national reimbursement policies. Clear definitions of APN role and title, educational requirements, and scope of practice must become a regulatory priority.

Credentialing APNs has been a major source of debate at the national level. Should this level of provider be licensed rather than officially recognized? Should there be a core competency examination developed at the national level for APN credentialing? Do certification examinations developed by the specialty nursing organizations meet the legal defensibility of an entry-level licensure examination? Who is an APN? Should there be a minimum education requirement for use of the title? These are all questions that continue to be raised in forums between specialty nursing organizations and licensing agencies. Until the role of the APN is clearly understood by consumers and policy makers, APNs will continue to be underutilized and undervalued.

O'Malley and colleagues (1996, p. 67) state that "success in the future will be contingent on nursing's ability to figure out how national health care priorities have been reordered and on the ability to create and implement a preferred future for nursing that supports health care delivery needs for individuals and populations within the framework of building healthier communities." Nurses must align themselves with community leaders, look for opportunities to educate the community about the valuable services that APNs provide, and become visible participants in the decision-making processes of government.

Reimbursement Issues

Significant breakthroughs are being made in reimbursement policy for APNs, largely due to the formation of grassroots lobbying efforts and coalitions of APN specialty nursing organizations. With the passage of federal legislation in 1997 allowing APNs to bill Medicare directly for services, APNs will have the opportunity to increase consumers' access to care. The managed-care markets value efficiency and effectiveness in providers. APNs are learning how to cost out services in the competitive market to win contracts and demonstrate cost-effective, quality-care outcomes to patients. In managed-care contracts where reimbursement is capitated, the amount of reimbursement is not as important as knowing whether the services can be provided for the capitated fee. Research studies are needed to document the cost of care and demonstrate nursing interventions that reduce the use of costly health care services over time. Studies that demonstrate the value-added activities of nursing intervention, cost-benefit analysis of interventions, and patient satisfaction with care are emerging in the literature and can be very useful in negotiating contracts for patient populations. Understanding the business aspects of health care financing and creating successful practices are new roles for entrepreneurial APNs who are managing the health care for a group of clients. It is a role in which APNs are gaining more comfort and experience.

Medicare and Medicaid programs saw significant reform in 2001. The Health Care Financing Agency (HCFA) has been renamed the Centers for Medicare and Medicaid Services (CMS). The agency has been restructured to focus more clearly on direct service lines of business to include the Center for Medicare Management, Center for Beneficiary Choices, and Center for Medicaid and State Operations (HHS, 2001).

Health Insurance Portability and Accountability Act

Congress passed a major regulatory reform initiative in 1996 during the Clinton administration. The Health Insurance Portability and Accountability Act (HIPAA) has four major objectives:

1. Guarantee health insurance access portability and renewal by eliminating preexisting condition exclusions and prohibiting discrimination based on health status
2. Reduce health care fraud and abuse by simplifying administrative processes and promoting electronic filing of claims
3. Enforce standards for health information
4. Guarantee security and privacy of health information

The sections of the act that are the responsibility of the CMS include Title 1 (health insurance reform) that guarantees portability of health insurance from one employer to another and Title 2 (administrative simplification provisions) that requires national standards for electronic health care transactions and national provider identifiers. The Office of Civil Rights is empowered to enforce the privacy rules associated with HIPAA. All health care providers who have a direct treatment relationship with patients in a practice setting that conducts electronic payment transactions must comply with the rules. The major components of the rules include to

1. establish policies and procedures for protecting patient information
2. provide training to employees on the rules
3. designate an employee who will be responsible for implementation and compliance with the rules
4. provide patients with notice that states how the provider will use their health information
5. obtain written consent for using or disclosing information in providing treatment, obtaining payment, or operating the practice
6. obtaining written authorization for using patient information for purposes other than treatment, payment, or operations
7. provide patient security (Buppert, 2002)

The rules cover all medical records and other identifiable information held at the practice site. Fines of up to $100 per violation or a maximum of $100,000 and 5 years imprisonment can be levied for failure to comply.

Impact of the Nursing Shortage on Regulation and Licensure

Supply-and-demand projections substantiate that the shortage of nurses and other health care providers will continue well into 2015. The factors driving the shortage include a growing aging population who will consume more health care services, the aging of the nursing workforce resulting in a large cohort of nurses retiring from the profession, and the inability of nursing to attract men, minorities, and young people into the profession. Even though there have been numerous initiatives at the state and federal level to reverse this trend, the nursing shortage continues to fuel policy on work environment issues across the nation.

There are several issues that bear monitoring during this period of a declining nursing workforce. They include:

1. Delegation and supervision of unlicensed assistive personnel (UAP). Practice for UAPs will continue to be debated and expanded as the shortage of licensed staff make it difficult to meet all the care demands of the public. Providing safe and effective care while delegating care to UAPs will place additional responsibilities on the licensed nurse.

2. Mandatory overtime legislation. When there are insufficient numbers of staff to meet care requirements, employers have often initiated policies to require staff to work additional shifts. Research has shown that fatigue impacts the mental acuity of an individual, leading to more errors in judgment and in medical errors that could result in harm to the patient. The Institute of Medicine (IOM) has published findings that link medical errors to the number and educational level of nurses employed as well as to fatigue of the staff (IOM, 1999). Employers have used the concept of "patient abandonment" to force employees to remain on duty against their will, threatening staff who leave the employment setting with patient abandonment that would result in a report to the licensing board. Laws have been passed in several states that preclude an employer from requiring staff to work beyond their scheduled assignment against their will.

3. Staffing ratios. In some states the nurses have organized to pass legislation to implement staffing ratios that guarantee a nurse-to-patient ratio dependent on the acuity of the patient. Staffing ratios have both positive and negative implications. Although the regulations for staffing ratios may require a set number of nurses to be employed, the minimum ratios imposed by law may be seen by the employer as the maximum number that must be employed, thereby placing a cap on hiring and negatively impacting the quality of care.

4. Foreign nurse recruitment. There is often an attempt to increase the recruitment of foreign-educated nurses when there is an acute nursing

shortage in the United States. Legislation is often introduced during these periods of time to relax the standards for licensure and to accept competency examinations that are not equivalent to the National Council Licensure Examination (NCLEX). The nursing community must be vigilant to these attempts to lower the standards for licensure and thus prevent discrimination against U.S.-educated graduates.

Other trends and issues will surface over the next several years that may impact the regulation of nurses and APNs. It will be increasingly more important to stay abreast of legislative and regulatory initiatives and to affiliate with professional organizations to preserve and protect professional standards.

Conclusion

Today is an era of rapid transformation in almost every aspect of life. Change is constant, and it rapidly forces adaptability and flexibility on the part of all individuals. Changes in the delivery of health care are transforming the practice and regulation of the APN. Today the APN must develop skills to capitalize on the chaos in the health care system and create opportunities for the advantage of the profession rather than fear the future. One way to capitalize on the times is to become politically astute and learn to shape public policy through working with coalitions of nurses, other providers, and consumers to advocate for quality health care at an affordable cost.

Knowing how to navigate the regulatory process will give the APN the tools needed to become a confidant spokesperson. Seeking and finding information on the status of issues critical to the APN, such as reimbursement, scopes of practice, and licensure issues, keeps the APN knowledgeable about how best to influence outcomes. Participating in professional nursing organizations provides a forum for building strong coalitions and gaining power in the political process. Each APN has the ability to make a difference.

Discussion Points

1. Contrast the major differences in the legislative and regulatory processes.
2. Describe the major methods of credentialing. List the benefits and weaknesses of each method from the standpoint of public protection and protection of the professional scope of practice.
3. Discuss the role of professional organizations in regulating professional practice.
4. Review the American Nurses Association *Code of Ethics for Nurses with Interpretive Statements*. Select the ethical principle on which each provision of the code of ethics for nurses is based. Explain why you made that selection.
5. Describe an ethical dilemma that you have recently experienced. What principles were in conflict with each other? Which principle ruled in your decision? Why?
6. Obtain a copy of a proposed or recently promulgated regulation. Using Exhibit 4–2, analyze the regulation for its impact on nursing practice.
7. Assume the board of nursing has promulgated a regulation requiring all APNs to have 20 contact hours of continuing-education credit in pharmacotherapeutics

each year to maintain prescriptive authority. Write a brief (no more than two pages) testimony supporting or opposing this proposed regulation.

8. Describe the federal government's role in the regulation of health professions. Do you believe the role will increase or decrease over time? Explain your rationale.

9. Discuss the pros and cons of multistate regulation. Based on your analysis, defend a position either for or against multistate regulation.

10. Prepare written testimony for a public hearing defending or opposing the need for a second license for APNs.

11. Contrast the board of nursing and the national or state nurses association vis-á-vis mission, membership, authority, functions, and source of funding.

12. Identify a proposed regulation. Discuss the current phase of the process, identify methods of offering comments, and submit written comments to the administrative agency.

13. Download at least one resource from each Web site listed in Exhibit 4–4 and evaluate them according to reliability of the author, last update, and appropriateness of data. Share the resources with colleagues.

14. Evaluate the board of nursing in your state using the criteria for review of regulatory agencies developed by the Pew Health Professions Commission (1995).

15. Identify the states that have implemented nurse staffing ratios. List some of the obstacles the state has encountered in the implementation phase.

References

Aiken, T. D. (1994). *Legal, Ethical and Political Issues in Nursing.* Philadelphia: F. A. Davis Co., pp. 20–26.

American Academy of Nurse Practitioners (AANP) (2003). Medicare reimbursement fact sheet. Retrieved from http://www.aanp.org.

American Nurses Association (ANA) (2001). Code of ethics for nurses with interpretive statements. Kansas City, MO. Retrieved from http://www.nursingworld.org.

Black, H. L., Nolan, J. R., and Nolan-Haley, J. M. (1992). *Black's Law Dictionary* (6th ed.). St. Paul, MN: West Publishing Company.

Braunstein, M. (1995). Homecare in cyberspace. *Computer Talk for Homecare Providers,* pp. 5–12.

Buppert, C. (2002). Complying with patient privacy requirements. *The Nurse Practitioner: The American Journal of Primary Healthcare* 27(5), 12–32.

Canavan, K. (1996). Credentialing agencies agree on outside review. *The American Nurse* 28(5), 6.

Center for Medicare and Medicaid Services (CMS). (June 14, 2001). Fact Sheet: The New Center for Medicare and Medicaid Services (CMS). Retrieved from http://www.hhs.gov/news/press/2001pres/20010614a.html.

DeVries, C. M. and Vanderbilt, M. W. (1992). *The Grassroots Lobbying Handbook.* Washington, DC: American Nurses Association.

Dower, C. and. Finocchio, L. (1995). Health care workforce regulation: Making the necessary changes for a transforming health care system. *State Health Workforce Reforms* 4, 1–2.

Edge, R. S. and Groves, J. R. (1994). *The ethics of health care.* Albany, NY: Delmar Publishers, Inc., pp. 28–45.

Gobis, L.J. (1997). Licensing and liability: Crossing the borders with telemedicine. *Caring 16*(7),18–24.

Goehlert, R.U. and Martin, F.S. (1989). Federal Administrative Law. *Congress and law making: Researching the legislative process* (2nd ed.). Santa Barbara, CA: ABC-CLIO.

Gross, S. (1984). *Of Foxes and Hen Houses*. Westport, CT: Quorum.

Health Care Financing Administration. (1995). *Health Care Financing Review 16*(4), 237–238.

Institute of Medicine (IOM) (1999). To err is human: Building a safer health system. (report of the IOM). Retrieved from http://www.iom.edu.

Jost, T.S. (1997). *Regulation of the Health Professions*. Chicago: Health Administration Press.

National Council of State Boards of Nursing (NCSBN). (1997). Using nurse practitioners certification for state nursing regulation: An update. *Issues 18*(1).

National Council of State Boards of Nursing. (1998). Multi State Regulation Task Force Communique. NCSBN, Chicago, IL. April 1998.

National Council of State Boards of Nursing (NCSBN). (1999). Uniform Core Licensing Requirements: a supporting paper. July 1999. Retrieved from http://www.ncsbn.org/ public/regulation/nursing_practice_licensing.htm.

National Council of State Boards of Nursing (NCSBN). (2002). Regulation of advanced nursing practice position paper. Retrieved from http://www.ncsbn.org.

National Council of State Boards of Nursing (NCSBN). (2003). Compact implementation. Retrieved from http://www.ncsbn.org.

O'Malley, J., Cummings, S., and King, C.S. (1996). The politics of advanced practice. *Nursing Administration Quarterly 20*(3), 62–69.

Pearson, L.J. (2002). Fourteenth annual legislative update. *The Nurse Practitioner: The American Journal of Primary Health Care 27*(1), 10–52.

Pew Health Professions Commission. (1994). *State Strategies for Health Care Workforce Reform*. San Francisco, CA: UCSF Center for the Health Professions.

Pew Health Professions Commission. (1995). Report of task force on health care workforce regulation (executive summary). San Francisco, CA: UCSF Center for the Health Professions.

Pruitt, R., Wetsel, M., Smith, K., and Spitler, H. (2002). How do we pass NP Autonomy Legislation? *The Nurse Practitioner: The American Journal of Primary Health Care 27*(3), 56–65.

Roberts, M.J. and Clyde, A.T. (1993). *Your Money or Your Life: The Health Care Crisis Explained*. New York: Doubleday.

Safriet, B.J. (1992). Health care dollars and regulatory sense: The role of advanced practice nursing. *Yale Journal of Regulation 9*, p. 2.

Sheets, V. (1996). Public protection or professional self-preservation. *NCSBN Monograph*, p. 3.

U.S. Department of Health & Human Services. (2001). The New Centers for Medicare and Medicaid Services (CMS). Fact sheet retrieved from http://www.hhs.gov/news/press/2001pres/20010614a.html.

Weisenbeck, S.M. and Calico, P.A. (1995). *Issues and Trends in Nursing* (2nd ed.). St. Louis, MO: Mosby.

Winn, J.R. (1995). Endorsement: State vs. national licensure. *Federation Bulletin 82*(1), 9–15.

Policy Design

Patricia Smart, PhD, RN, FNP

5

Key Terms

Fire alarms   Signals built into a policy that alerts policy makers that the design, implementation, or evaluation phase is in danger of failing.

Fuzzy/crisp charges   Degree of clarity of objectives and directions for implementation in a mandate or law.

Participation   Extent to which individuals in the target population join in government programs.

Policy link   Connection between policy ideas and their implementation.

Introduction

The scope of government's involvement in social issues in the United States has increased rapidly during the last 75 years. Federally funded health care programs such as Medicare and Medicaid have made a major impact on how health care is implemented by providers and perceived by the public. As noted by Comer (2002), government involvement in health care has occurred at the state and local levels through program administration, educational preparation, licensing, and regulation of practice.

The United States has one of the most sophisticated health care systems (although challengers call it a "sick care system") in the world in terms of technology and preparation of health care professionals. Yet in many of the health indices designed to evaluate the overall health of the citizens of a country, state, or county, the United States rates comparatively low. For example, as found in Healthy People 2010 Goals (USHHS), life expectancy in the United States for females is 78.9 years, while in many other developed countries such as Japan, France, Canada, and England a female's life expectancy is 82.9 years, 82.6 years, 81.2 years, and 79.6 years, respectively. Infant mortality also is an important measure of a nation's health. Healthy People 2010 notes that in 1995, the United States ranked 25th among industrialized countries in infant mortality. Furthermore, new cases of low birth weight and very low birth weight, both of which contribute to infant mortality, have increased in the United States. (USHHS, 2002)

Frequent failure of solutions to many social problems and tactics to restrict government spending have combined to raise questions about the effectiveness of social programs. Efforts to restrict spending continue to be in the process of debate with no resolution in sight. Ulbrich (2003) comments on American ambivalence regarding expanding the role of government, particularly in the area of health care. She notes that an underlying basis from which all discussions and arguments regarding the role of government in health care are formed is based in the belief that personal financial risks should be individually assumed. These risks are associated with earning a living and managing one's income and assets wisely as opposed to shared responsibility through government.

Policies are usually designed to influence behavior and get people to do what they ordinarily might not do. As noted by Longest (2002), health policies address health concerns through laws, regulations, or programs that focus on health determinants including behavioral choices, physical environment within which people live and work, and social factors. Although many studies regarding the policy process have been conducted, few have examined the process of policy design in issues of health care, particularly prenatal health care and infant mortality. The focus of most policy studies has been on the implementation of effective programs, and data have been gathered on statistical outcomes. This author argues that design considerations should be a component to be considered during all phases of the policy process to promote policy success. For example, in the agenda-setting phase, the social issue must be stated in such a way that it will capture the attention of lawmakers and framed so that government response will be feasible and adaptable. During the implementation phase, the design of the policy provides guidance and also provides an overall picture of the plan by specifying the intended outcomes. During the evaluation phase (included in the design), the program objectives are clearly identified and measurable.

The Policy Process

The policy process is the act of addressing or ignoring a publicly perceived problem. Leichter (1979) notes that policy is contained in legislative enactments including budgets, court mandates, and executive orders. According to Thompson, the policy process "involves a complicated interaction among government institutions, actors, and the particular characteristics of substantive policy areas" (Thompson, 1981, ix). This scholar agrees with Heclo's notion that "a policy, like a decision, can consist of what is not being done" (Heclo, 1978, p. 134).

Policies that address social problems in the United States usually are formulated by a combination of legislators and aides, the executive branch, courts, and special-interest groups. Professional experts are often asked to serve as panel members or consultants or to serve on committees that provide input to policy makers. Advanced practice nurses (APNs) are asked to serve on committees that relate to health care. For example, nurse leaders were invited to sit at the table during the early 1990s when Hillary Clinton was proposing a national plan to change existing health care policies. The proliferation of participants in policy formation makes systematic program design focused on outcomes difficult to achieve. Social problems are usually intractable and difficult to solve. As noted by Safriet (2002), most social issues are not brought to the attention of policy makers until there is a crisis with multiple causative factors. Decision making with regard to relevant factors that relate to or have an impact on perceived social problems often is conducted hastily due to lack of information, constituency impatience, and lack of expertise (Dryzek, 1983).

Review of Policy Research

Much of the research contributing to an understanding of the policy process is found in implementation literature. Although the design of a policy affects the implementation phase, many studies have ignored environmental factors existing in the design phase that would have impact on policy implementation. For example, attitudes and expectations of policy makers are often different from the attitudes and expectations of policy participants. Policy success or failure is seen by many policy scholars as occurring only within the implementation phase of policy making. The study of implementation has been described as falling into three "generations" of works. Each generation of implementation scholars is marked by specific pitfalls and contributions. It is important to understand how the pitfalls can produce a negative impact upon policies and programs. APNs are in a position to play a key role in the design of health policies and must have knowledge of ways to improve the probability of success.

Pressman and Wildavsky (1973) note the complexity of implementation and difficulty in achieving policy success when many branches and divisions of government attempt to work together. They attribute this to the many "veto points" that occur within a "seamless web" of interaction among policy players. Veto points are those areas of vulnerability in the policy process where decisions might be made that could undermine the original intent of the policy makers. For example, in the process of obtaining a state's recognition for prescriptive authority for APNs, the proposal (beginning of the policy) was examined critically by many interested groups, including physicians, pharmacists, and health insurance agencies. At any point, members of these groups could recommend amendments that could alter, at best, or, at worst, "shoot down" the proposal.

Pressman and Wildavsky also identify the use of time as a tool among players. For example, delay tactics have been used to improvise original plans and objectives for the benefit of the players. Pressman and Wildavsky's seminal research contributes to the policy process because it points out many areas of failure in a large government program.

Bardach (1977), another first-generation policy scholar, moves away from the litany of "nothing works" and identifies several factors required for sound implementation. He looks at relationships among implementation actors and labels the activity process among policy players as "game playing." He identifies activities, such as bargaining and negotiating among players, that make a tremendous impact on policy success and failure. For example, in some states, APNs have to be willing to allow a representative from the board of pharmacy or the board of medicine to be on the governing board that regulates nursing at the advanced level.

Bardach (1977) notes that to incorporate such concerns as policy success through bargaining and negotiating in strategic planning of policy, one must begin with a design that incorporates scenarios, which will anticipate games and "fire alarms." For example, if a sex-education program is being considered as a means of reducing teen pregnancy, an interest group may use a fire-alarm technique of trying to sabotage the program because the education material is at odds with the group's beliefs. The group also may try to control the curriculum or move to have local government determine the content, thus restricting the material.

Second-generation policy scholars tended to criticize the work of first-generation researchers as being pessimistic about program success. Early scholars emphasized identification of key variables, but the emphasis was placed not on how variables affect implementation itself, but how variables impede the implementation planning or structural process of implementation.

As second-generation scholars noted weaknesses of previous work, they began to build models from which to analyze implementation. The structural process of implementation was studied from a top-down, bottom-up, and backward-forward mapping approach (Elmore, 1979–1980; Mazmanian and Sabatier, 1983; Van Meter and Van Horn, 1975). The top-down approach is used when describing traditional hospital governance. The policies are derived at the top bureaucratic layer and flow downward. In the bottom-up design, the ideas and concerns come from the lower echelons or the "street-level bureaucrats" (Lipsky, 1980), the implementers who work with policy-target populations. An example of street-level bureaucrat is the public health nurse who is concerned about the current policy that addresses drug-addicted pregnant teens. These concerns are then brought forward to the administrators. The backward-forward mapping concept is described as a flow of information that travels up and down channels between bureaucrats and the target population as programs develop.

Through the work of second-generation implementation scholars, several variables were identified, including policy form and content and organizations and their resources and people. A major contribution produced by these scholars is the development of frameworks from which to conduct scientific inquiry and theory building.

A third generation of implementation scholars worked to build a solid theoretical framework. Goggin and colleagues (1990) combine the major concerns and variables of the top-down and bottom-up models into an analytical framework that provides a mechanism to address questions of conceptualization and measurement. Durant and Legge (1993) tested the effects of alternative implementation strategies at different time periods. In a longitudinal analysis, they determined that initial implementation choices exerted a more favorable impact than those strategies that were chosen later in the policy process and that produced no impact.

Agenda Setting

Many scholars focus on how a perceived problem reaches the government agenda within the process of policy making. For example, Kingdon utilizes the Cohen and colleagues' description of the decision process (Cohen et al., 1972) as a loose collection of ideas that emerge from "organized anarchies." Kingdon, speaking about the public decision-making system in the United States, adds the notion of independent streams that he labels the policy stream, the political stream, and the problem stream. He contends that a choice opportunity occurs when the person with a problem and the person with a solution come together. He describes this rather cavalier, fluid activity as decision making within the realm of policy making, and the outcomes as a function of how the streams happen to combine.

On the other hand, Dryzek (1983) argues that a modicum of reasoning should be introduced into the policy process. He asserts that haphazard, loose coupling of ill-defined streams will not produce policies with the properties of adaptation, homeostatic capability, and feedback that are necessary to withstand policy analysis and revision. Dryzek further argues that the type of policy designed for specific problems depends on the complexity and uncertainty of the policy and the lack of feedback to the policymakers.

Ingraham (1987) also rejects the notion that policy making takes place in a "garbage can." The garbage can metaphor refers to a process of decision making that consists of separate streams of problems, solutions, participants, and choices that couple and uncouple to produce alternative solutions to problems (Kingdon, 1995). Ingraham states that more rigorous studies should be conducted to examine the critical components of the policy process. She says that the most notable omission has been the effort to "determine the exact nature of the problem and its causes, the potential range of solutions and the most appropriate strategy for achieving desired outcomes" (p. 613). Ingraham also notes that the problem-solving nature of public-policy design has rarely been examined. Instead, she states that "design activities have been viewed simply as a product of political compromise as an ad hoc effort to determine legislative or executive intent."

Policy Links

During the 1980s, political scientists studied the content of policy with the intention of providing a clearer understanding of the link between policy design and policy outcome. Their efforts hold importance for APNs whose roles often require interpretation and implementation of policies. To improve the likelihood of policy success, APNs must be able to critically analyze policy content; that is, what is the original intent of the policy, and is the policy designed in such a way to assure the intended outcome? Dryzek (1983) argues that efforts to analyze the policy process should place more emphasis on the study and utilization of policy design. Schneider and Ingram (1990) also argue for a closer look at design and proposed a framework to examine behavioral assumptions and attributes of policy content that can be employed by APNs to conduct the work of government.

Government policies are subject to a wide scope of interpretation that depends on who brings problems to national attention and which legislative group attaches itself to problems and solutions. Jones (1984) maintains that often a policy is not the direct result of a perceived public problem because the problem itself is not stated clearly. He insists that it is fairly standard for policies to be vague in order to allow flexibility in implementation and administrative discretion at the program level. Jones notes further that policy formulation often follows a haphazard path that may proceed without a clear problem definition. This author agrees that policy formulation is often haphazard and argues that policy formulation rarely includes a clear, well-thought-out design. An opportunity exists for APNs who recognize the value of vagueness. Rather than waiting for clear directives, the nurse must learn and become comfortable with vagueness, because it allows discretion and flexibility in decision making and action, thereby enhancing the ability to individualize management.

The Design Issue

Until the 1990s, most policy-process research focused on policy implementation and evaluation. Both areas of policy research have contributed to the study of the policy process. These studies have isolated factors that may impact upon policy success. Some of these factors are the tools by which government addresses social issues. Since the 1980s, however, scholars have begun to analyze the link between policy design and implementation. Mandates that often are not clear in intent or purpose, or that are unclear regarding implementation, often are handed down by legislators and are difficult to conceptualize and operationalize. The result of unclear mandates often results in a mismatch between congressional intent and bureaucratic behavior. For example, federal money that is allocated to states for harm-reduction programs, such as smoking cessation during pregnancy, may reach a segment of the target group that may not need it. Many college-educated women will not smoke during pregnancy, yet the private health care providers have access to as much federal money to develop an antismoking program as their public agency counterparts.

There has been concern among some scholars that the historically strong focus on implementation has not contributed significantly to a theoretical understanding of policy making. They argue that whereas policy making and implementation design individually have been taken seriously and neither has been taken for granted, each should be viewed as a complex process involving multiple actors in a political arena (Linder and Peters, 1987). Scholars argue that when the focus is only on the fundamental idea of the policy making or implementation design as separate entities without action on the relationship between design and implementation, the focus may have normative implications for analyzing policy that may be highly undesirable. For example, placing a focus only on implementation may lead to subjective input from policy makers who may not be responsive to the needs of the target population. These scholars disagree with the belief that implementation determines policy and that policy formulation should revolve around implementation, and they argue for a closer look at policy design and content.

Linder and Peters (1987) state that attention should shift to the phase of the policy-making process where original intent and design are spelled out, rather than focusing research on policy implementation as the determining factor of success or failure. In their study, policy design is listed as a reason for policy failure. Describing some programs as "crippled at birth," these scholars note that the best bureaucracies in the world may not be able to achieve desired goals successfully using a particular policy that may be excessively ambitious (the problem is too complex for single policy) or where there is a misunderstanding of the nature of the problem. Linder and Peters propose that implementation should be examined, but only as one of the conditions that must be satisfied for successful policy making. They maintain that by shifting the focus of study to policy design, a more reliable and explicit answer can be found regarding policy success.

This author proposed that by examining the assumptions made by policy makers regarding participation of the target population, the process of development of policy, the tools used to develop a definition of the problem, and the match between policy development and outcome, policies relating to infant mortality and low birth weight can avoid some of the factors that may contribute to the policies being "crippled at birth."

Policy Design

Policy design can be conceptualized as a process that can occur at both the policy formulation and implementation phases or as a blueprint approach that shapes policy (Linder and Peters, 1990). Scholars agree that policy design is an integral component of implementation, yet design has been the subject of few studies. Some scholars have discussed policy formulation, design, and legitimation as important links between problem identification and policy implementation, and they argue that formulation functions (research, review, projection, and selection) may occur either systematically or haphazardly. Thus, design is a critical and vulnerable factor in the overall policy process.

In their proposal, which supports shifting of research focus from implementation to policy design, Linder and Peters (1987) argue that goal determination should be a priority in order to choose the appropriate matching policy instruments. Their proposal emphasizes a general approach to design of policy instruments and implementation structures, which facilitates a more positive approach to policy making.

Other scholars concur with Linder and Peters. During the 1970s and 1980s, studies regarding the policy process began to focus on policy design, instruments chosen by policy makers, and policy content. Ingraham (1987) argues that a systematic analysis of program design, rather than analysis via the garbage can model, could enhance policy success by allowing the option of considering alternative strategies and providing causal links culminating in theory building. She focuses her work on two areas of policy design.

The first area is related to the level of design; that is, the extent to which a program has been structured consciously and systematically and the extent to which several elements of design content and process are examined. For example, what is the range of solutions that was considered, how is strategy chosen, and is the match between strategy and available resources examined? She argues that the lowest level of design activity is the simplistic two-step process involving direct transference of political rhetoric to a program with absence of design considerations. Ingraham (1987) notes that Lowi (1960) suggests that many liberal policies of the past suffered from this translation and notes further that more conservative rhetoric and policies suffer due to lack of design considerations as well.

Ingraham (1987) also examines the location of design activities as her second focus on policy design. Her posture is that policy formulation and design no longer take place exclusively in the legislative arena. Instead, activity is seen more often in many different locations within the policy system. She notes that input from experts outside the legislative body require a greater effort toward clarifying goals and objectives and require negotiation and bargaining. Ingraham identifies several variables that may influence both level and focus of policy design including problem intractability, goal consensus, commitment to solution, and alternatives. She maintains that continued identification and elaboration of factors influencing policy design is necessary to understand the policy process further. Advanced practice nurses should heed Ingraham's advice by staying abreast of societal and environmental changes that could impact health policy. For example, the recurrence of tuberculosis has become a major public health concern. With earlier detection, many individuals could have been protected against the recent recurrence, and the national economic impact would have been less.

Often there are mismatches between legislative intent and bureaucratic outcomes. Bureaucrats often receive "fuzzy" (as opposed to "crisp") charges with vague marching orders (Lerner and Wanat, 1983, p. 500). Fuzzy charges can be a problem with a program in general or may refer to more micro factors such as determining which clients are eligible for services. One major consequence when executing fuzzy mandates is the need to interpolate a workable mandate from the vague charge. This results in "conceptual satisficing" (p. 505) because of lack of time to explore all alternatives fully. These scholars contend that a continuous line of fuzzy mandates often requires extensive organizational shifts with subsequent changes in bureaucratic outcomes. For example, many contend that the *Roe v. Wade* decision by the U.S. Supreme Court in which the court contended that a woman has the right to decide what happens to her body has been abused by a society that has used the decision to support broader issues of contraception.

In his thesis regarding the complexity and uncertainty in social policy, Dryzek (1983) contends that more, not less, cogitation is needed. He argues that critique must be appropriate and discerning to the issue and contends that greater use should be made of policy design through analysis of substantive content of policy choices.

Upon reviewing the current policy literature, it is apparent that the design phase of the policy process continues to be an area where few policy scholars choose to focus their efforts. However, there are a few policy studies that are looking at design when examining social policy. For example, in a study conducted to examine policy-instrument utilization to promote electricity-efficient household appliances and office equipment, Varone and Aebischer (2001) determine that the political climate within which a policy was implemented is a critical factor to be considered when choosing instruments.

In summary, policy design is an integral component of implementation. An understanding of policy tools or instruments chosen for policy design and the underlying assumptions of policy makers during the design process is critical to an understanding of the overall policy process.

Policy Instruments

Some policy scholars have directed their attention to instruments chosen by policy makers in developing policy, the process by which strategy is chosen, and have identified factors, which influence policy design. Sardell (1990) notes that the definition or framing of an issue is critical to the nature of activity on the issue, the type of groups that become involved, and the development of specific policies. Thus, the study of instruments or tools by which the government achieves desired policy goals has allowed researchers to examine policies in relation to their intent and to begin to infer predictive capabilities of tools. Originally, many scholars argued that this method of analysis eliminated or reduced significantly the aspect of political practice and political community. The idea has become somewhat modified and acceptable to most scholars. Linder and Peters (1990) note that most instrument research efforts focus on the presumed merits of tools, as opposed to the heuristics and decision-making routines employed by those who choose the instruments or tools.

Other scholars have noted the dearth of information regarding the decision-making process and policy content within the design phase. Dryzek (1983) contends that the fit of policies to their environments usually is related directly to the complexity of the problem and that complex and uncertain circumstances often lead to avoidance of policy analysis. In other words, the more complex the problem and subsequent policy, the less likely that analysis will occur. He notes that most policy-design analysis focuses on methods of alternative selection or how the selections should be made. Design quality would be improved with the shift of analytical focus toward the generation of alternatives. That is, by exploring the various alternatives and the potential for success, greater enlightenment of the intricacies of the problem would be experienced. He examines what factors lead to decisions reached by policy makers toward instrument choice (i.e., the content of the decision-making process).

Dryzek also argues that strategic thinking should be conducted that involves the consideration of the cultural, institutional, physical, and biological environments. By encompassing these components, a tendency toward following standard operating procedures is avoided. Such considerations lay the groundwork to enhance the decision-making abilities of future generations. Advanced practice nurses can exert great influence in helping policy makers understand the components. For example, a nurse can provide information on health beliefs and practices of diverse cultural groups that can assist a legislator in designing an appropriate program or policy.

Several scholars have proposed ways to examine the tools of government. For example, Hood (1986) also ascribes to the notion of using tools as a way of simplifying analytical examination of government behavior. He describes governments' tool kits as containing both detecting and effecting tools. Detecting tools bring information to the attention of government and effecting tools influence consumer behavior. Hood identifies several resources that can serve as tools available to government, such as modality (the centralized position held by government), treasure (fungible properties or common money), authority (possession of legal power), and organizations (the possession of people with various talents and capabilities).

Two other scholars proposed a framework for studying policy based on tools. Schneider and Ingram (1990) offer a framework to analyze implicit or explicit behavioral theories found in laws, regulations, and programs. Their analysis uses government tools or instruments and underlying behavioral assumptions as variables, which guide policy decisions and choices. Their contention is that target group compliance and utilization is an important form of political behavior that should be examined closely. Combined with process variables such as competition, partisanship, and public opinion, Schneider and Ingram argue that the tools approach moves policy beyond considering the standard analysis and improved frameworks. They note that policy tools are substitutable and often states use a variety of tools to address a single problem. To understand which tools are most productive, emphasis should be placed on using them in conjunction with a particular policy design. APNs use their knowledge of policy tools to make suggestions and recommendations to government leaders who are designing policies and programs.

Policy Design Model

Schneider and Ingram (1990) state that public policy almost always attempts to get people or enable people to do things they would not have done otherwise. These scholars describe policy tools as those methods chosen by policy makers to overcome barriers to policy-relevant actions. Large numbers of people in different situations are involved in policy making. Actions required by these players include compliance with policy rules, utilization of policy opportunities, and self-initiated actions, which promote policy goals. Schneider and Ingram list several reasons they suggest may impact the failure to take actions needed to ameliorate social, economic, or political problems: (1) lack of incentives or capacity; (2) disagreement with the values implicit in the means or ends; or (3) the existence of high levels of uncertainty about the situation that make it unclear what people should do or how to motivate them. Schneider and Ingram describe five specific policy tools used by governments in designing policy. They identify five broad categories of tools, which include authority, incentives, capacity building, symbolic, and hortatory and learning.

The Tools

Authority tools are used most frequently by governments to guide behavior of agents and officials at lower levels. Authority tools are statements backed by the legitimate power of government that grant permission and prohibit or require action under designated circumstances. An example of an authority tool is a law, regulation, or mandate that requires women to qualify under regulated criteria for prenatal services.

Incentive tools assume individuals are utility maximizers and will not be motivated positively to take action without encouragement or coercion. These tools rely on tangible payoffs (positive or negative) as motivating factors. Incentive-policy tools manipulate tangible benefits, costs, and probabilities that policy designers assume are relevant to the situation. Incentive tools assume individuals have the "opportunity to make choices, recognize the opportunity, and have adequate information and decision-making skills to select from among alternatives that are in the best interests" (Schneider and Ingram, 1990, p. 516). An incentive tool, for example, may be an offering of coupons for free public transportation to prenatal clinics to encourage pregnant women to seek care. If the APN assumes that lack of transportation is a barrier to access prenatal care, the outcome from an attempt to use of this particular incentive may fail.

Capacity tools provide information, training, education, and resources to enable individuals, groups, or agencies to make decisions or carry out activities. These tools assume that incentives are not an issue, and target populations will be motivated adequately. For capacity-building tools to work, populations must be aware of what risk factors the tools possess and how these tools can help. Capacity tools focus on education. For example, information may point out the risks of smoking and drugs on a fetus, and information on such risk factors is distributed to the target population. The underlying assumption is that information about the cessation of smoking is considered valuable, and that pregnant women will stop smoking if they have correct information.

Symbolic and hortatory tools assume that people are motivated from within and decide whether to take policy-related actions on the basis of their beliefs and values. An example of this type of tool is a poster directed at adolescents that uses an adolescent model to issue advice or a warning. Such tools seek to gain the attention of the target population (adolescents) through use of peer imagery.

Learning tools are used when the basis upon which target populations might be moved to take problem-solving action is unknown or uncertain. Policies that utilize learning tools often are open-ended in purposes and objectives and have broad goals. A needs assessment of the target population may be conducted by a task force. This type of survey provides knowledge and insight for policy makers and is an example of a learning tool.

Policy tools are important resources for the APN, because they can enhance efforts to provide accurate information so that the patient can make informed decisions. For example, educational pamphlets relating to health promotion behaviors such as dietary considerations for the diabetic can be sent home with the patient. This will reinforce information received from the care provider and help the patient adhere to a fairly complicated change in lifestyle.

Behavioral Dimensions

In addition to understanding the types and the roles of tools in developing policy, the nurse in advanced practice must understand behavioral assumptions and the political context within which tools exist. The political climate in which social problems are addressed often prescribes the choice of tools to be implemented. Various tools are used when addressing similar social problems. Often these tools are interchanged and many times result in differing outcomes when used by different agencies, states, or countries. In the United States, for example, liberal policy makers are inclined to use capacity-building tools when developing policy for the poor and minority groups, whereas conservative policy makers might use the same types of tools in developing policy applicable to businesses.

Schneider and Ingram (1990) report that a shift in focus to the behavioral dimensions of policy tools permits comparative analysis across policy types, which yields information about the effectiveness of alternative tools when particular circumstances of the policy arena are held constant. The two researchers propose that the concept of policy-tool choice in policy making can be used to compare the behavioral assumptions of policy from different states and countries, particularly on like issues that have shown contrasting results.

Health care is fraught with a multitude of factors that are difficult to identify and control. One of the most elusive factors inhibiting policy success is the ability to predict consumer behavior and participation in a program. Another factor that exacerbates the problem of control is the introduction of policies designed to control health care costs. Recently, the main shift in the health policy agenda has been from access to cost containment. For 25 years after World War II, the priority was to ensure access to advanced medical care for all citizens. Health insurance schemes were extended, new hospitals were built, old ones modernized, and numbers of physicians grew. However, when escalating costs coincided with the recession of the 1970s, efforts to cap health expenditures occurred.

Cost-containment policies threaten to jeopardize access to health care and its quality. For example, health care staff power has decreased, and the most sophisticated technology is available to only a few. Not only are the poor at risk for not receiving adequate health care, but the crisis affects the middle-income sector also.

Child health is an area in which the paradoxes of health policy are seen very clearly. Industrialized nations provide high technology and specialized services to those with acute conditions, while often misdirecting the focus away from primary care and the social factors that increase medical risks. The United States ranks first in the world in its ability to save the lives of premature and very small infants, yet ranks fifteenth in the proportion of babies born at low birth weight (Sardell, 1990) and, currently, ranks twenty-fifth in infant mortality (USHHS, 2002). In spite of this country's ability to save these special-care infants initially, neonatal mortality (death up to 27 days after birth) and postneonatal mortality (death from 28 days to 1 year) impact the United States profoundly. Although the infant mortality rate has declined over the past 20 years, the overall rate in the United States for infant mortality is still 7.2 percent. In addition, one can anticipate that with budget crises and the lack of resolution regarding access, the infant mortality rate will not improve and may, in fact, increase due to less-than-adequate prenatal visits. Rather than expanding national health insurance coverage as most liberal-democratic countries, the United States, with its bias against public solutions, allowed employment-based insurance to expand to the point where the state could merely fill main gaps with welfare-oriented safety nets. According to Sardell (1990), studies conducted at local levels in the 1960s and 1970s found that reductions in neonatal mortality were related to the introduction of neonatal intensive care services, the availability of family planning services, Medicaid services, and the legalization of abortion.

Miller (1988) was commissioned by the U.S. Institute of Medicine to study outreach for prenatal care. He compared rates of low birth weight and infant mortality in 10 European countries with the United States. All of the nine European nations whose rates of low birth weight were lower than that of the

United States had national standards for prenatal care with organized community services at the local level and national financing and monitoring of these services. In all 10 countries, services were provided to all women, regardless of income with minimal financial barriers to care. Incentives were offered for women to seek prenatal care, such as paid leave for prenatal classes or visits, transportation to services, early reservations for delivery, and children's allowances. Furthermore, home visits were routinely made after delivery in every cited European country. Although most states and counties in the United States have begun to offer home visits, it is due to an insurance-driven mandate of 24-hour stays in the hospital for uncomplicated vaginal deliveries and 72-hour stays for women who have delivered by cesarean.

Infant Mortality: Comparative Issues

One of the most important issues facing nations today involves pregnant women and their infants. The problem of infant mortality has been on the government agenda of the United States for decades, and policies have been designed and implemented to relieve this problem. However, infant mortality and its causes and consequences in the United States remains a critical social issue, and the country lags behind most industrialized nations in solving the problem. A major cause of infant death is low birth weight (2,500 grams or less). Even though the infant mortality rate is improving, the problem of low birth weight is becoming more prevalent.

A major contributor to low birth weight and subsequent death is unplanned pregnancy. At particular risk for unplanned pregnancy is the adolescent. In a report published in the *Journal of the South Carolina Medical Association,* Blackhurst and colleagues reported that in 1993 more that 404,000 adolescents gave birth in that state. Of these adolescents, 10,135 were less than 15 years of age and 149,751 were between the ages of 15 and 17. The researchers also noted that estimated pregnancy rates among women between the ages of 14 and 17 in South Carolina increased from 47.0 per 1,000 in 1983 to a high of 56.9 per 1,000 in 1988. Since that time, there has been a steady decline to a low of 44.8 per 1,000 in 1993. However, this rate still translates into slightly under 5,000 pregnancies in 1993 (Blackhurst et al., 1996).

Low birth weight costs both lives and money. According to the former federal Office of Technology Assessment, the U.S. health care system spends between $14,000 and $30,000 per low birth-weight child, mainly in intensive care costs during the infant's first year. Life-long costs for the low birth-weight infant have been estimated at $250,000 per child (Singh, 1990).

Prenatal Care

Experts recognize that early and adequate prenatal care is one of the most important factors in preventing low birth weight; however, more than 24 percent of American women do not receive adequate prenatal care (Lee and Estes, 1990). The question emerges as to why a significant portion of American women living in a country with a highly developed and sophisticated health care system are not receiving prenatal care needed to prevent low birth weight and potential death of their infants.

Political Culture: South Carolina

Consideration for political environments must be taken into account in comparing social indicators because structure and function of governing bodies include differences that could affect policy decisions. Government action in South Carolina is often partisan as each administration opts to target its own social issues. Subsequent action on health care reflects partisanship.

Unlike the centralized states of Europe, the Constitution of the United States does not provide for a single, decisive locus of political power or will. The United States pluralist system of checks and balances has led to a federal legislature that, even when dominated by the same party as the executive, has considerable autonomy but may be divided strongly on a given issue. Interest groups may veto or modify programs and policies at many points in the legislative process, as well as through executive agencies. The executive branch is relatively weak and has been likened to one interest group among many others. This diffusion of power in the United States makes it difficult to enact and implement policies. State policies often replicate this diffusion of power and its constraint upon substantive change. Finally, in the prevailing two-party system, both parties tend to advance centrist policies and avoid the risk of bolder positions.

The structure of federalism (a system of government that allows each state considerable room for decentralized development in terms of adapting to unique human and environmental circumstances) offers opportunities for bolder programs in states than at a national level. The role of elected governor is weak constitutionally. The state is governed by a strong bicameral legislature and an appointed cabinet. South Carolina is a predominately Republican state with politically conservative views.

Due to the explicit separation of powers between the federal government and the states, states and counties, and counties and municipalities, policy making in states is often considered uncoordinated overall, although particular sectors called subgovernments may be well organized. Each subgovernment deals with a relatively narrow facet of government, such as health or education. Slow-paced or incremental policy making occurs frequently. Due to the growth of regulatory activities, policy making has become even more complex with more interdependency and conflict. Complex issues and limited resources have begun to blur boundaries between subgovernments.

APNs often work in settings where even small policy changes involve multiple disciplines or departments and actors. For example, in a primary-care setting, such as a family-planning center, a policy change relating to Medicaid payment would affect patient recordkeeping for the social worker, dietitian, physician, and business manager as well as the nurse. The APN must be prepared to assume a leadership role in the collaboration of the various disciplines in providing comprehensive care to the patient.

Political Culture: The Netherlands

The Netherlands is a pluralistic nation that has a homogeneous and secular political structure with a highly differential role structure. The Netherlands has a constitutional monarchy that is vested with symbolical rather than actual power. The centralized nature of the Dutch government is reflected by a monarch-appointed representative who resides within each province and municipality. An example of the centrally controlled nature of Dutch government is the method of disbursement of government funds. Historically, in contrast to the United States and South Carolina, there was very little discretion allowed to lower-level administrators in municipalities. This was a result of clear, specifically stated policies that limit administrative and management flexibility. Since 1985, however, the Dutch government has become more decentralized with more political discretion and power being assumed at the local levels.

As noted by Lijphart (1977), the Netherlands has managed to overcome potential problems caused by cleavages through exceptional cooperation and coordination among elite members of each segment in the policy-making process. Elite members are those who have the greatest influence in policy making. For example, popular legislators, intellectuals, and business leaders are often considered elites. Political changes have occurred in the Netherlands, however, that have brought more average citizens into positions of political power. This factor will have an impact upon the decision-making process of policy making as well as the various tools used to address social problems.

The South Carolina policy-making system, on the other hand, is fraught with cleavages and turf issues that have affected policy making in critical areas. An excellent example of this is seen in the problem of infant mortality. This study suggests that the polarization over the issue of infant mortality before it becomes a problem (preventing unplanned pregnancies) has kept South Carolina in the top ratings in ratios of infant mortality per one thousand live births.

Economies

The gap between equality and distribution of income is greater in the United States than in the Netherlands. Income in the Netherlands falls within a closer range. Sardell (1990) notes that access to health care among the poor and unemployed is a long-standing concern of proponents of maternal and infant care. However, despite an unemployment rate that exceeds that of South Carolina, prenatal services are provided to all Dutch women, regardless of income, with minimal financial barriers to care.

Health Care: South Carolina

Dery (1984) notes that the definition of a social problem often determines how difficult it will be to address and resolve. The problem of infant mortality in South Carolina is perceived to be an intractable problem, according to key informants. The result is the lack of an overall policy. In its place is an ill-defined, fragmented approach that focuses on small components of the problem. For example, inadequate prenatal care was perceived to be a major problem and access was considered the critical component. Medicaid eligibility was expanded to 185 percent of poverty, making more pregnant women eligible for prenatal care. Incentives such as coupons for free food, medication, and infant care were provided. In order to receive the coupons, the pregnant woman must apply through the local health department. Eligibility is determined through a qualification process, including a thorough history relating to sexual activity, marital status, and educational level. Initially, the process took approximately 6 weeks. Currently, the process takes only 3 weeks; however, the woman has to make many trips to several different government agencies for her eligibility to be processed.

Health Care: The Netherlands

The health care system in the Netherlands is based on a combination of elaborate government regulation on one hand and mainly private provision of health care facilities on the other. The government provides funds to privately administered health care service providers. The present government's policy places greater emphasis than in the past on development of preventive measures, health promotion, and health protection. The Netherlands appears to hold a broader vision of maternal and infant care than does the United States. Along with medical care, Holland places considerable emphasis on social and environmental indicators as determinants of health status. The *Health 2000 Memorandum,* published by the Dutch Government in 1986, and the subsequent volume, *Keydocument Health Care: 1989,* clearly identify the shift toward a more comprehensive health policy. According to Sardell (1990), an aspect of the consensus on maternal and infant services is that infant mortality will be reduced only if these services address the social as well as the medical needs of high-risk mothers and infants.

The Dutch system of health care for mothers and infants contrasts to that of South Carolina in both its focus on prevention and promotion and through its provision of universal access to health care. Access is achieved through "sickness funds" which constitute basic health insurance for 62 percent of the Dutch population. According to several informants, workers in 1993 who made up to 55,000 guilders annually (about $30,000) paid 3.15 percent of gross wages to the fund and employers paid an additional 4.95 percent. In 2003, the Dutch system still is not a pure form of socialized medicine. There is no national health system but there is a national health insurance system. Both private and public funding is available to all citizens in the Netherlands and every resident has access from birth to death. Funding for programs is provided through mandatory taxation of all working people and their employers. In 2003, all those 65 years and older who have worked have paid premiums into an AOW (national) insurance system and now receive the full amount allocated plus 2 percent of a fixed amount each year. In effect, those who earn approximately 27,000 euros annually contribute to this system, although those who earn more may choose a private insurance system (Roode, personal communication, July 24, 2004).

Few policy studies have focused on prenatal health care outcomes or programs. Those that have are oriented mainly toward components of the program implementation phase. Scholars have yet to study designs of policies relating to the problem of infant mortality, and, more specifically, have not determined whether there are gaps between assumptions of policy makers when choosing tools for policies and actual outcomes of policies. In addition, there are few studies that compare similar policies and programs, their uses of tools, and their successes with tools. This study examined which program-design factors may have contributed to the difference in infant mortality rates between babies born in South Carolina and the Netherlands.

Policy Design Factors Related to Prenatal Care in South Carolina and the Netherlands

The purpose of this study was to determine which policy design factors, if any, produce desired outcomes in the area of prenatal health care. This study examined and compared policy-making instruments related to infant mortality and low birth weight in South Carolina and the Netherlands. South Carolina's infant mortality rate of 10.5 percent is significantly higher than the 8 percent infant mortality rate in the Netherlands. If factors related to policy design addressing infant mortality are found to impact design outcome, these factors may be isolated to determine degree of impact. Exhibit 5–1 provides an overview of the findings.

General Characteristics

The research component in South Carolina was conducted through the Division of Maternal and Child Health located within the state-level Department of Health and Environmental Control (DHEC). Data were gathered in an urban setting. The program in the Netherlands was under the aegis of the Ministry of Welfare, Health, and Cultural Affairs located in the Amsterdam area. Research was conducted in Amsterdam, Leiden, Nordwijk, den Haag, and Utrecht—all urban settings.

The Netherlands was chosen for the comparative analysis for several reasons. The focus of the program regarding the health of infants is similar to the program in South Carolina. Prenatal care in the Netherlands is part of a comprehensive health care plan. Paradoxically, this aspect is also different from

EXHIBIT 5-1 **Findings: Policy Design Factors**

South Carolina	*The Netherlands*
Infant mortality perceived as a problem. Anecdotal and discretionary approach to policy design.	Infant mortality perceived as a problem. Universal approach to policy design.
Individual, independent initiatives. Abortion policy, family planning, and sex-education programs restricted, limited, and conservative. Policy making slow and incremental.	Overall policy. Abortion policy, family planning, and sex-education programs easily accessible, available to all, and liberal. Policy making slow and incremental.
Reactionary response. Addresses infant mortality as a medical issue, rather than a social problem with medical consequences.	Preventative response. Addresses infant mortality from a holistic approach, which includes social and environmental factors.
Narrow focus on issue of infant mortality as well as family planning, sex education, and abortion. Have leaders who consider these topics politically risky.	Broad, sweeping changes 10 to 12 years ago on family planning, sex education, and abortion. Has political leaders who support and endorse these topics.
Process variables: Factional political and public environments. Strong partisanship exists. Cleavages and gaps exist among players and target population. Public opinion is fragile. Interest group strength is minimal. Policy analysis and evaluation is not a priority. Political support is apathetic with few exceptions.	Process variables: Homogeneous and consociational political and public environments. Harmonious relationships exist among political elites. Public support policies are in place. Strong special-interest lobbyists at work. Statistical data gathered and communicated. Political support consistent and proactive.
Assumptions regarding target group behavior: Co. production is uncoordinated, not encouraged, and there is no joint tenancy; compliance is minimal; utilization is below expectations and political support is apathetic with a few exceptions.	Assumptions regarding target group behavior: Co. production is organized and joint tenancy is encouraged; compliance is responsive; utilization is sought and maximized and political support is strong and proactive.
Tools: Findings support that Schneider and Ingram's defined policy-making tools (1990) are comparable to those used in the Netherlands. Focus of tools is retrospective.	Tools: Findings support that Schneider and Ingram's (1990) defined policy-making tools are utilized and are consistent with those used in the South Carolina. Focus of tools is prospective.
Social indicators and demographics appear to have minimal impact.	Social indicators and demographics appear to have minimal impact.

South Carolina. South Carolina participates in a relatively free market system while the Netherlands has a national health care program. Another reason the Netherlands was chosen as a comparative site is that both South Carolina and the Netherlands are governed by a bicameral legislature and an appointed cabinet. In both sites, an elected leader holds actual power, but the two legislative bodies (Senate and House in the United States, First and Second Chambers in the Netherlands) exert a strong measure of control on the leadership activities. The population of South Carolina is 3,487,000, with 69 percent of the population white, 29.8 percent African American, and the remaining 1.1 percent from other racial and ethnic origins.

The Netherlands is one of the most densely populated countries in the world with 14.6 million inhabitants in 1988, including 570,000 foreigners. Since the 1960s, Western European countries such as the Netherlands have experienced a major influx of migrants from former colonies such as the Dutch Antilles and some Mediterranean countries. The most numerous immigrant groups in the Netherlands are from Surinam, the Dutch Antilles, Morocco, and Turkey. These ethnic minorities are concentrated in larger urban centers. In Amsterdam in 1981, 44.5 percent of all children age 5 and under were born to non-Dutch families, primarily from Surinam and Morocco (Miller, 1988).

A qualitative approach was used to address two questions that emerged regarding design of policy toward prenatal care. The first question sought the content of the policy itself. What policy-design factors are crucial to program strategists to ensure an effective program? Several questions evolved from the first. Which tools were being used to attain program success, and why did policy makers choose these tools? Were there other alternatives? What were the assumptions underlying decisions regarding tool and instrument choice? Were these assumptions correct? Were the tools accomplishing what policy makers assumed they would? Were the tools bringing pregnant women into a health care setting? Did the attendance of the prenatal women seeking prenatal care foster the expected outcome of higher birth weight in infants?

In responding to the first question, several types of tools were examined as described by Schneider and Ingram (1990). For example, they describe incentive tools as ways to induce compliance or encourage utilization. Incentive tools are used to manipulate tangible benefits, costs and probabilities policy designers assume are important to the target population. As an incentive, a policy might offer free infant diapers with a certain number of visits to a prenatal care center with the assumption that the pregnant women would value this gift and, thereby, encourage visits to a prenatal health care center. However, if the assumptions are incorrect and the target group values factors other than those considered by policy makers, the policy is doomed. For example, the incentive may be useless if the patient does not want to spend time going to the clinic in the first place or if free diapers are not perceived by the pregnant women as something they will need.

In relation to the first group of questions, the decision-making process was examined when tool selection occurred. Dryzek (1983) argues that strategic thinking, including a balance of creation and criticism, is needed. He contends that incremental thinking lends itself to a return to the mode of standard operating procedures without consideration of new ideas. One question to be asked relative to policy revision or change is the causality and degree of change. Each time policy is revised or changed, what is the cause and degree of change? Does tool selection reflect dominant ideologies or interest group strength? How mature is the current design? Schneider and Ingram (1990) argue that newer policies begin with relatively benign strategies, such as inducements or capacity building, and then shift toward more coercive policy tools, such as authority tools, learning tools, and symbolic and hortatory tools.

In researching the group of questions, this author determined that the aspect of design is impacted by the key figures formulating it. For this reason, the values of the key figures formulating the policy design were of paramount importance. It was necessary to determine whether the policy-making experts recognized their own biases and to what extent these perspectives and beliefs were included in policy formation. Motivating factors of the policy makers to assume responsibility for the process and the outcome needed to be identified.

A second group of questions emerged regarding the discrepancy in outcomes between South Carolina and the Netherlands. How were the tools and assumptions of a developed country (the Netherlands) with a lower rate of infant mortality and significantly less expenditure different from those used by South Carolina? The second group of questions also explored causality. Is the discrepancy in infant mortality due to poor design, or is it due to environmental factors such as cultural or ethnic behaviors or values? What is the cultural or ethnic composition of each program? Do environmental factors contribute to the outcome? Schneider and Ingram (1990) note that there is a dearth of information about comparative effects of different policy tools on consumer utilization, compliance, coproduction, and political support for the policy.

The study was conducted in Greenville and Columbia, South Carolina, and Amsterdam, Leiden, and Nordwijk, the Netherlands. Subjects were selected on the basis of expertise in areas of legislative process and health policy. Key informants from South Carolina and the Netherlands were interviewed. The researcher chose a semistructured interview guide using general, but directed, open-ended questions. Data were compiled and analyzed to establish commonalties among concepts, which produced patterns or themes allowing comparisons among programs. Following the framework of Guba and Lincoln (1989), the process of data analysis was employed immediately and compared continuously with each subsequent interviewing session until category saturation was achieved (Glaser and Strauss, 1967). Coding of responses into categories and subsequent saturation occurred after responses were analyzed. When a satisfactory number of interviewees offered the same responses to the guided interview, the categories became saturated.

Key informants from South Carolina and the Netherlands included bureaucrats, legislators, elected officials, nurses, physicians, and consumers. Informants from both sites were interviewed on areas of legislative process and health policy. Informant input was analyzed for patterns and themes of information. Informants were asked specifically to provide knowledge of the impact of the political philosophy and political process guiding policy decisions. These areas were chosen as being indicative of the assumptions about the target population when making decisions regarding choice of policy tools. Analysis of the concepts derived from the study was organized within the Schneider and Ingram (1990) framework. Using their conceptual basis of tool choice and their underlying assumptions, themes emerged that were proposed as a basis for further study of policy content.

The policy-making tools developed by Schneider and Ingram (1990) are described as instruments that can be substituted for one another and are often used in conjunction and cooperation with one another. Policy-making tools may conflict with one another. For example, the law in South Carolina requires that health care must be provided for pregnant women who are within 185 percent of the poverty level. Yet, incentive tools such as funding are limited, and the reimbursement process is cumbersome and not prompt. Thus, most private physicians providing prenatal care are not willing to serve this population. Each of the tools has the capacity to allow institutions to achieve the same policy purpose, yet this utopian outcome does not often occur. Policy variables, policy players, demographics of the target population, and policy influence were shown to play a significant role in outcome differences.

The findings from both sites were described under four headings:

1. policy background, which relates to the way each government perceives the problem and describes the approach taken by each site in problem resolution

2. government responses, which describe the direction taken by each government in addressing prenatal care as a deterrent to infant mortality and the effectiveness of governmental response (this section also discusses policies and initiatives of each site with applicable policy tools used for decision making and implementation)

3. policy-process variables, which relate to the components that impact the policy makers' decision making

4. policy participation, which discusses policy participation. Policy background examined aspects of problem identification.

Policy Background

In South Carolina, Dery's (1984) description of problem identification was found to be applicable. Dery notes that the way a problem is defined determines how difficult it appears to policy makers to address and to discover solutions. If information relating to causative factors impacting upon a problem is not identified, available, communicated to, or understood by policy decision makers, the problem usually appears to be so complex and insurmountable that problem solving is ignored or attention is focused on smaller components of the problem that are more easily addressed. Current approaches to the problem of infant mortality in South Carolina are described by a majority of respondents in this state as fragmented, undefined, and lacking a specific plan.

Most subjects described the issue of infant mortality as a problem that encompasses a multitude of social and economic factors rather than merely a singular, unique problem. Interviewees related that the causes of infant mortality are intertwined with many socioeconomic factors such as poverty, lack of education, and poor self-esteem. Each of these factors alone encompasses many seemingly unsolvable issues that impact upon the others.

The data obtained through interviews with key informants in South Carolina provide rich descriptions of how poorly informed key policy makers are about the nature of infant mortality and the impact of prenatal care as a major determinant to infant mortality. Yet, the study showed that, on average, 12 percent of pregnant women in South Carolina were known to visit a prenatal health care provider no more than five times during their pregnancies and, therefore, received less than adequate prenatal care. Seven percent of white women did not receive adequate care and more than 18 percent of "black and others" received less-than-adequate care.

Most notable, key policy makers commented about the lack of a cohesive, comprehensive policy addressing infant mortality. This lack was noted by most informants to be a result of policy makers' unwillingness to make broad sweeping changes in the way they historically have addressed this issue. Most informants described change in policy as being slow and incremental.

Most informants described the communication infrastructure between researchers and decision makers as poor, and direct communication of information regarding problem factors as being transmitted rarely. In addition, the many layers of bureaucracy proved to be a formidable barrier to clarity of facts regarding issues and problems.

Data providers in South Carolina expressed that they lacked clarity regarding what information decision makers were requesting. Furthermore, data providers did not believe that decision makers were always clear on what information they needed. On the other hand, informants in the Netherlands perceived that they were able to resolve communication problems effectively. For example, when studies were conducted to examine factors impacting pregnancy outcome, Dutch decision makers communicated effectively the areas that they wanted included in the study and data providers designed the study to those specifications. When the study revealed that unwanted pregnancy impacted pregnancy outcomes, the information was communicated directly and explained to decision makers who developed policy immediately to address unwanted pregnancy. The policy designed and implemented by Dutch policy makers was a nationwide effort at reducing unwanted pregnancies. This effort included the introduction of formal sex-education classes to begin in the fifth and sixth grades and to continue throughout the high school program. Church leaders and the media became committed to providing accurate, objective information regarding reproductive anatomy, birth control, and prevention of sexually transmitted diseases. There is no teen pregnancy "problem" in the Netherlands.

In South Carolina, problem identification and communication of the perceived problem of high infant-mortality rates is made complex by multiple political actors involved in addressing the concern. Again, most informants agreed that the actors often are uninformed about factors affecting infant mortality and, thus, have difficulty addressing the problem. Complicating the issue is the political environment surrounding policy making. Reflecting the general political condition of the United States, South Carolina is a pluralist state with political factions and cleavages among factions. This often results in stagnation of progress on social issues.

Most informants noted the lack of a "bold thinker" within the policy-making body with a special interest in infant mortality. Kingdon (1995) notes that bold thinkers and charismatic leaders provide the energy and direction to address problems through methods and plans not tried before. As noted by Schneider and Ingram (1990), the presence of a bold thinker provides the impetus to explore different ways to address problems. APNs can provide the bold thinking to explore innovative ways of addressing many of the health problems existing today.

In contrast to South Carolina, respondents from the Netherlands reported that infant mortality was not perceived as a social problem. When asked how the issue of infant mortality is addressed by government programs, most respondents noted immediately that it was no longer a unique problem because it has been addressed effectively by the Dutch government. The majority of respondents stated that the factors surrounding the issue of infant mortality, which in the past may have been defined as problematic, had been identified and, for the most part, resolved. Because infant mortality is no longer considered an intractable problem with unsolvable factors, informants were interviewed to determine how factors that might have impacted problem identification were resolved in order to make such a definitive and conclusive statement.

Informants in the Netherlands agreed that the issue of infant mortality was recognized to be a multifaceted arena, as in South Carolina, and was not perceived to be a singular, isolated issue. However, the Dutch related that when the issue became a part of managed health care, fragmentation of services, access to care, participation, and utilization of care ceased to become relevant issues. They noted that open dialogue and communication also impacted the perception that the problem of infant mortality was a manageable one in the Netherlands. Dutch informants stated that sex education was taught in all schools during the fifth and sixth grades. In addition, issues relating to reproduction, birth control, and prevention of sexually transmitted disease were openly discussed by the parents, churches, and the media. The same, factual information was consistently provided to young people. Key informants in the Netherlands noted that sex is discussed as a knowledge issue rather than a moral one.

Most informants (those who initiate and conduct research and those in decision-making capacities) agreed that the infrastructure between the two groups involved consistent and direct communication of problem factors as they occurred. A preventive approach to problematic areas is utilized. Though not described as perfect, the infrastructure is viewed as making regular efforts to enhance communication and coordinate services. Competition for scarce resources was described as a concern in the Netherlands. However, the target population was described as important to policy formulators, and the government saw that funds were available for this care.

In the Netherlands, as in South Carolina, there are multiple political actors who were involved in addressing infant mortality. As a pluralist country, many political factions exist with cleavages between factions. However, as described by Lijphart (1984), Dutch politics have the unique characteristic of being able to overcome major disputes because political elites from each faction work together to reach a consensus regarding programs. For example, policy-making actors were able to overcome factional cleavages regarding moral issues surrounding unwanted births to consider the overall good for society by the prevention of unwanted births.

The solution process in South Carolina was noted to be an anecdotal approach to finding solutions for social problems. For example, an infant, who spent the first 3 weeks of life in a neonatal intensive care unit due to premature birth and subsequent problems related to low birth weight, was described as unable to go home on the scheduled date because the home was without heat. Financial support had to be obtained from a social agency to enable the mother to take the infant home. Although this method of solving an immediate problem is recognized by policy makers and providers as a less-than-desirable way to handle a crisis, all respondents stated that it was the feasible thing to do at the time. Subjects noted consistently that crossing financial boundary zones occurs frequently and exacerbates the original problem of murky functional areas. This appears to intensify the difficulty in clearly identifying and subsequently addressing the problem of infant mortality.

Solutions to problems in South Carolina often are localized and are not communicated to other areas within the state that may be attempting to address the same issue. This results in a "reinvention of the wheel" approach to resolution and likely assures that solutions chosen will continue to be case specific. This anecdotal approach to problem solving is very different from the universal approach to problem solving utilized by the Dutch.

Interviewees in the Netherlands related that solutions chosen are universally applied. All Dutch women have access to prenatal health care, counseling, and information about pregnancy alternatives. All pregnant women who use the health care system are assessed uniformly and consistently using identical criteria and are referred to appropriate services on an equal basis. Those with risk factors are provided care consistent with the risk. All Dutch women have access to the same social services. There are no eligibility criteria to be met in order to gain access. Specific problems, such as lack of resources to pay for health services, do not arise because basic health care insurance is available to all.

When questioned about what policies in South Carolina address infant mortality, subjects responded that there are no clear policies. Instead, there are many "initiatives." Each initiative has its own set of objectives and goals that are described as rather vague and which have not been evaluated to determine effectiveness. According to the Department of Health and Environmental Control (2003), although the 5-year trend in infant mortality has shown steady improvement (12.9 percent in 1987 to 10.7 percent in 1992), respondents were not able to determine which initiatives were instrumental in the improvement rate. They felt that clarification of the issue was needed in order to establish a policy with overall encompassing objectives that could be evaluated. This lack of action on studying causation of improvement rates kept the state focused on addressing most social problems, including infant mortality and lack of prenatal care. These problems appeared easier to address anecdotally than through an overall policy. In contrast, the Netherlands used policy types that were described as effective and consistent.

Government Response

This research found that governments in both countries used tools similar to those described in Schneider and Ingram's framework (1990), although the policy environments differed a great deal. Policies and initiatives developed and implemented by policy makers were analyzed by applying policy tools used in the conceptualization and implementation of the policy. As noted by Schneider and Ingram, "policy tools are used to overcome impediments to policy relevant actions" (1990, p. 510). Successful realization of policy goals requires active participation by the target population. However, if policy makers are not cognizant of motivating and deterring factors impacting upon the decision-making process of the target group, incorrect assumptions regarding participative behavior can result in an ineffective policy.

Although data relating to government responses to the problem of infant mortality revealed that policy makers are informed regarding beliefs and values of the target population, government-designed policies to address infant mortality have not been successful in reducing the rate of infant mortality. Although key informants in South Carolina were unable to identify a specific policy that addresses infant mortality, several initiatives established by the executive branch were discussed. The initiatives are implemented by the Department of Health and Environmental Control and are available only to those pregnant women who qualify on the basis of financial status. These initiatives employ tools such as providing free bus passes for prenatal patients to the prenatal clinic, which may help in achieving initiative goals, although specific goals relating to specific tools are not clearly stated or specified.

One of the more encompassing initiatives is a federally funded grant project that places an emphasis on identifying barriers to prenatal care and posing solutions to remove the barriers. Various tools were chosen by policy makers to aid in accomplishing the goal of improving access for pregnant women to prenatal health care. An example is a program in which private physicians agree to provide prenatal care for a certain number of patients who qualify for nationally funded prenatal care. This program is entitled Partnership for a Healthy Generation.

Although total compliance for participation in the Partnership for a Healthy Generation is not mandated by law for the target population or for localities, access to federal and state financial support for prenatal health care is accompanied by certain expectations of the state. An example of an authority tool used by South Carolina is found in the requirements stipulated by this policy. In order to receive government-funded coupons that provide free food, medication, infant care (including immunizations), and free maternal care, the pregnant woman must apply through the local health department. Eligibility is determined through a qualification process, including a thorough history relating to sexual activity, marital status, and educational status. Initially, the process took approximately 6 weeks. The initiative's goals were to decrease the process to 2 to 3 weeks. If the patient has been identified as being at high risk (through past obstetric history, family history, or current disease), the process is often hastened further.

In the Netherlands, there is only one system of health care. All patients, wealthy and those on welfare, seek prenatal care from the same health care providers. There is no qualifying process to receive prenatal care.

Another initiative in South Carolina is the High Risk Channeling Project that channels high-risk pregnant women into appropriate levels of care. This regulatory project determines which health care provider and which hospital setting a pregnant woman uses during her pregnancy. The Netherlands also has a high-risk channeling policy in which pregnant women, who are considered at high risk, are referred to an obstetrician. The pregnant women who are not considered at risk are seen by family practitioners and midwives.

The area of family planning reflected the widest gap in the choice of tools. Several initiatives exist in South Carolina that address family planning. All initiatives are activated through local and individualized programs with no single program providing a clear and consistent framework to be followed by other programs. Family-planning health professionals are not allowed to enter the schools to provide counseling. Students are encouraged to visit health departments in order to receive family-planning advice and are urged to inform their parents of their visits. Although sex education is taught in the state-funded schools, each county may present the package in any form it chooses. Most key policy makers, who are informed about the content of the sex-education curriculum practices around the state, report that it is often a very brief (15 minute) discussion each semester that covers broad concepts. In contrast, Dutch schools mandate a comprehensive sex education to all students beginning in the fifth grade. In addition, a government-funded family-planning service is available through all general practitioners and midwives.

The government is supported in these efforts by the majority of the Dutch citizens and most of the clergy.

Policy-Process Variables

Policy-process variables may make a major impact on the success or failure of a policy or program. Process variables include partisanship, public opinion, interest-group strength, homogeneity between policy makers and the target population, and influence of policy analysis.

In South Carolina, partisanship affected decisions on policies addressing maternal and infant health. Schneider and Ingram (1990) note that Democrats are disposed more favorably than Republicans toward capacity-building tools or positive inducements for populations such as the poor. However, Democrats in South Carolina have traditionally been politically conservative. Therefore, most policies relating to family planning, unwanted pregnancies, and infant mortality have been conservative in nature. The Netherlands, in contrast, is noted for its ability to provide an arching relationship among political elites to provide harmony and stability. Lijphart notes that the Netherlands is "a dramatic example of the survival of a nation state as a stable democracy despite extreme social pluralism" (1977, p. 103).

Public opinion regarding policies that address unwanted pregnancies in South Carolina is polarized. The divisions between those who favor open, factual, and consistent information regarding sexuality and sex education and those who feel that such an environment would foster more promiscuity and unwanted pregnancies are also reflected in the legislature.

In the Netherlands, public opinion is strongly and cohesively in favor of open communication between adolescents and the community at large regarding unwanted pregnancies. Statistics show that the results of unwanted pregnancies—infant mortality and elective abortions—are at a much higher rate in South Carolina than in the Netherlands. A gap also exists in South Carolina between policy makers and the target population. Most informants state that this gap attributes to relative lack of public support and the weakness of special-interest groups lobbying for prenatal care. Quite the opposite exists in the Netherlands. Political support is apathetic and inconsistent in South Carolina, yet is supportive, consistent, and proactive in the Netherlands.

Policy Participation

The success of a policy or program is highly dependent upon whether the target population perceives the services provided by the program to be valuable enough to warrant participation. Policy participation in this study revealed that coproduction (assumption of the values and involvement of establishment of goals) of a policy is not coordinated in South Carolina, but that Dutch citizens are very involved with policy design and formulation. All Dutch citizens use the same health care system and, therefore, have more interest. Utilization of services in South Carolina is poor, which informants suggest is the result of very little input regarding policy formulation from the target population. Dutch women fully participate in family planning and prenatal health care programs.

CHIP Project

In a 2000 unpublished study called the Community Health Interagency Project (CHIP), a collaborative multidisciplinary team studied the incidence of diabetes II and the incidence of limb amputation in a rural area in South Carolina. As part of the team, this author conducted an analysis of the health care system in that region to (1) identify key players in the health care policy realm in that county and (2) identify patterns of health care utilization in that county. An additional purpose of the study was to identify those health care policies and/or programs that specifically addressed the issue of increased incidence of diabetes and related morbidity and mortality rates. In addition, factors impacting upon the success or failure of the program were examined including the tools utilized and the behavioral assumptions made by the policy designers and implementers.

Similar to the previously described study, data were obtained through interviews from health care administrators and providers. The subjects were selected on the basis of expertise in areas of health care and knowledge of the citizenry in the community. Key players in the design and implementation of the program were identified and were interviewed regarding the purpose and objectives of the programs and which tools were chosen to enhance program success. Questions asked included:

- What did you intend to accomplish with this program?
- What tools were included in the design of the program to reach your objectives?
- In general, do you perceive that the program is working?
- What factors outside your control kept you from reaching all objectives?
- How did you think the program would promote the desired objectives?

Multiple initiatives were implemented to improve patient education and access that would, subsequently, improve the rate and morbidity of type II diabetes in that county. The assumption of the policy makers was that once people are educated (capacity tool) and health care programs are made easily accessible (incentive tool), citizens of the county would participate in programs that would identify and provide health care for type II diabetic patients. However, statistics demonstrate that the rate and morbidity of type II diabetes in that county continues to remain high.

In addition to the discussions with health care professionals and policy makers, transcribed reports of discussions with focus groups held by members of the research team with citizens and diabetic patients were reviewed and analyzed. A review of records of type II diabetic patients hospitalized at the regional hospital in 1998 were reviewed to analyze records of frequency of physical assessment checks, appropriate diabetes-related teaching to patient and family, and knowledge of available community resources. Consistent with multiple studies regarding the incidence of diabetes, causative factors, and impact of type II diabetes, discussions with both health care professionals and diabetic patients described the issue of type II diabetes and subsequent morbidity and mortality as a problem that encompasses a multitude of social and economic factors rather than merely a singular, unique problem.

Several community initiatives focused on education and/or care were discussed with policy players and focus group participants; however, they were described by a majority of subjects as fragmented, undefined, and lacking a specific plan. For example, community initiatives, such as exercise classes in local churches and hospital-sponsored services for diabetic patients, were sporadic and usually not well-publicized. Another community initiative involved a mobile unit set up at a health fair to screen for diabetes; however, one participant noted "those people who didn't have transportation or didn't know someone up here to bring them missed that."

Several other initiatives were described that address issues of select groups of type II diabetics. For example, a local college provided a support group for diabetic students. Another community initiative, a children's rehabilitation service with an endocrine clinic, was held every other month with individual meetings with parents and family to provide information and education regarding office visits, desired outcomes, and diet.

A program addressing the provision of education and training to lunchroom staff members in schools to make sure diabetic diets were maintained through school was discussed; however, these services were provided only to those students who met financial guidelines. A program called Smart Shopping was offered for a short period of time in which a dietician would gather a group of people who had preregistered and would go to the grocery store to assist them in food choices. One respondent described this program as very helpful "but we haven't done that in a long time."

Conclusion

The nursing profession is undergoing rapid changes in educational and training programs and in tasks and roles that nurses assume. Beginning as a helping profession with a hospital-based background, nursing education in the United States has moved to university settings that offer bachelors and advanced degrees. Baccalaureate-prepared nurses currently represent 32 percent of the total number of nurses in the country and the number is rising. The number of baccalaureate nurses returning to universities for advanced education in nursing through master's and doctoral degrees also is growing. Nurses in advanced practice are taking their rightful places as providers of quality nursing care in diverse settings.

As a component of advanced practice nursing, active participation in the policy process is essential in the formulation of policies designed to provide quality health care to all individuals. To be effective in the process, APNs must understand how the process works and the points at which the greatest impact might be made. The design phase of the policy process is the point at which the original intent of a solution to a problem is understood. APNs can be extremely effective in this phase as policy tools are considered and selected.

References

Bardach, E. (1977). *The Implementation Game: What Happens after a Bill Becomes a Law.* Cambridge, MA: MIT Press.

Blackhurst, D.W., Gailey, T.A., Bagwell, V.C., Dillow, P.A., McCuen, K., Warner, L., and Crane, M. (1996). Benefits from a teen pregnancy program: Neonatal outcomes and potential cost savings. *The Journal of the South Carolina Medical Association 5*(92), 209–215.

Cohen, M., March, J.G., and Olsen, J.P. (1972). A garbage can model of organizational choice. *Administrative Science Quarterly 17,* pp. 1–25.

Comer, M.E. (2002, May). Factors influencing organized political participation in nursing. *Power, Politics, and Policymaking 3*(2), 97–107.

Dery, D. (1984). *Problem Definition in Policy Analysis.* Lawrence: University Press of Kansas.

Dryzek, J.S. (1983). Don't toss coins in garbage cans: A prologue to policy design. *Journal of Public Policy. 3*(4), 345–368.

Durant, R.F. and Legge, J.S., Jr. (1993). Policy design, social regulations and theory building: Lessons from the traffic safety policy arena. *Political Research Quarterly 46*(3), 641–657.

Department of Health and Environmental Control. (2003).

Elmore, R.F. (1979–1980). Backward mapping: Implementation research and policy decisions. *Political Science Quarterly 94*(4), 601–616.

Glaser, B. and Strauss, A. (1967). *The Discovery of Grounded Theory: Strategies for Qualitative Research.* Chicago: Aldine.

Goggin, M.L., Bowman, A.O'M., Lester, J.P., and O'Toole, L.J., Jr. (1990). *Implementation Theory and Practice: Toward a Third Generation.* Scott, Foresman and Co.

Guba, E.G. and Lincoln, Y.S. (1989). *Fourth Generation Evaluation.* Newbury Park, CA: Sage Publications.

Heclo, H. (1978). Issue networks and the executive establishment. In A. King (Ed.), *American Political System.* Washington, DC: American Enterprise Institute.

Hood, C.C. (1986). *The Tools of Government.* New Jersey: Chatham House.

Ingraham, P.W. (1987). Toward more systematic consideration of policy design. *Policy Studies Journal 15*(4), 611–628.

Ingram, H.M. (1977). Policy implementation through bargaining: The case of federal grants-in-aid. *Public Policy 25,* pp. 499–527.

Institute of Medicine. (1988). *Prenatal Care.* Washington, DC: National Academy Press.

Jones, C.O. (1984). *An Introduction to the Study of Public Policy* (3rd ed.). Monterey, CA: Brooks Cole Publishing Company.

Kingdon, J. W. (1995). *Agendas, Alternatives, and Public Policies.* Boston, MA: Little, Brown and Company.

Lee, P. R. and Estes, C. L. (1990). *The Nations Health.* Boston, MA: Jones and Bartlett.

Leichter, J. M. (1979). *A Comparative Approach to Policy Analysis: Health Care Policy in Four Nations.* Cambridge, MA: Cambridge University Press.

Lerner, A. W. and Wanat, J. (1983). Fuzziness and bureaucracy. *Public Administration Review*, pp. 500–509.

Lijphart, A. (1977). *Democracy in Plural Societies.* New Haven: Yale University Press.

Lijphart, A. (1984). *Democracies.* New Haven, CN: Yale University Press.

Linder, S. H. and Peters, G. B. (1987). Design perspective on policy implementation: The fallacies of misplaced prescriptions. *Policy Studies Review 6*(3), 459–475.

Linder, S. H. and Peters, G. B. (1990). Research perspectives on the design of public policy: Implementation, formulation, and design. In D. Palumbo and D. J. Calista (Eds.), *Implementation and the Public Policy Process: Opening Up the Black Box.* New York: Greenwood Press, pp. 51–66.

Lipsky, M. (1980). *Street-Level Bureaucracy.* New York: Russell Sage Foundation.

Longest, Jr., B. B. (2002). *Health Policymaking in the United States* (3rd ed.). Chicago: Health Administration Press.

Lowi, T. (1960). *The End of Liberalism.* New York: Norton.

Mazmanian, D. A. and Sabatier, P. A. (1983). *Implementation and Public Policy.* Dallas: Scott, Foresman and Co.

Miller, C. A. (1988). Prenatal care outreach: An international perspective. *Prenatal Care: Reaching Mothers, Reaching Infants.* Institute of Medicine, Washington, DC: National Academy Press.

Pressman, J. and Wildavsky, A. B. (1973). *Implementation: How Great Expectations in Washington Are Dashed in Oakland; Or, Why It's Amazing that Federal Programs Work at All.* Berkeley: University of California Press.

Safriet, B. J. (2002). Closing the gap between can and may in health-care providers' scopes of practice: A primer for policymakers. *Yale Journal on Regulation 19*, 301–334.

Sardell, A. (1990). *The U.S. Experiment in Social Medicine: The Community Health Center Program. 1965–1986.* Pittsburgh, PA: University of Pittsburgh Press.

Schneider, A. and Ingram, H. (1990). Behavioral assumptions of policy tools. *Journal of Politics 52*(2), 510–529.

Singh, H. K. D. (1990). STORK reality, Why America's infants are dying. *Policy Review 2*, 391–398.

Thompson, F. J. (1981). *Health Policy and the Bureaucracy: Politics and Implementation* Cambridge, MA: MIT Press.

Ulbrich, H. (2003). *Public Finance: In Theory and Practice.* Mason, OH: Thomson Publishers.

U.S. Department of Health and Human Services (USHHS). (2002). *Healthy People 2010.* Boston, MA: Jones and Bartlett.

Van Meter, D. S. and Van Horn, C. (1975). The policy implementation process: A conceptual framework. *Administration and Society 6*, 455–488.

Varone, F. and Aebischer, B. (2001). Energy efficiency: the challenges of policy design. *Energy Policy 29*, 615–629.

Policy Implementation

Marlene Wilken, PhD, RN

Key Terms

Environmental factors   A broad category of nonstatutory variables in the implementation process that includes socioeconomic conditions, public support, attitudes and resources of constituency groups and commitment, and leadership of implementing officials.

Implementation games   Refers to a variety of strategies and maneuvers used to achieve control by agencies and groups involved in the implementation process.

Policy implementation   The process of putting a policy or program into effect.

Policy structure   The ability of statute to shape policy implementation based on several elements such as clear, consistent objectives; causal linkages between interventions and objectives; funding; hierarchical integration of agencies; behaviors of agency officials; and access by outsiders.

Tractability   A component of policy implementation that addresses the ease or degree of manageability of a problem. Elements include technology, diversity, target groups, and extent of behavioral change.

Implementation is the "shadow land," the neglected dimension of U.S. governance (Nathan, 1993, p. 122 as cited in Weissert and Weissert, 2002).

Introduction

Policy Implementation Defined

Policy implementation is not widely understood. In fact, some researchers suspect that the phenomenon of policy implementation may elude understanding. Others are challenged by trying to answer the question "What comes first, then, the chicken of the goal or the egg of implementation?" (Theoduolou and Cahn, 1995, p. 140). This uneasiness about how to study this seemingly seamless web of relationships between thought and action is understandable. The subject of policy implementation is slippery, and trying to separate policy design from implementation has consequences; however, what happens after a bill becomes a law is an area of study can enlighten those of us who choose to examine the process.

Implementation is the process of putting a policy into effect, the result of fulfilling or executing policy decisions. The process involves mobilizing human and financial resources to comply with the policy. When implementation occurs, there is usually a directed change, a rearrangement of behavior patterns to honor the prescription set forth in the policy decision. The process involves using the resources necessary to address the who, what, when, where, how, and why of policy mandate (Quade, 1989). Implementation may consist of altering objectives to correspond with available resources or mobilizing new resources to accomplish old objectives. The process of implementation can be smooth, bumpy, or may never happen.

Implementation also can be thought of as the government response to the problem phase. Government agencies respond to the law, policy, or program delegated to them by the government. Ideally, the instructions, in the form of statute, executive order, or court decision, clearly identify the problems to be addressed and give some direction as to the objectives to be pursued, both of which help to shape the structure of the implementation process. The agency charged with implementing the program often develops the guidelines and regulations necessary for a functioning and workable program. Implementation ends successfully when the goals sought by the decision are achieved within the reasonable constraints of time, money, and other costs.

The process of implementation goes through a number of stages that can best be thought of as dependent variables or constants. The stages include passage of the basic statutes, policy decisions of the implementing agencies, compliance of target groups with those policy decisions, the actual impact both intended and unintended, and possible revisions or attempted revisions in the basic statute (Mazmanian and Sabatier, 1983).

Policy analysts, those who study various aspects of the policy process, view implementation as an element in the policy design, which involves comparison of the alternatives in response to a policy decision. According to Mazmanian and Sabatier (1983), the crucial role of implementation analysis is the identification of three broad categories: (1) management or control of the problems being addressed, (2) a coherent structure that favors attainment of the policy objectives, and (3) the degree of achievement of the statutory objectives.

Given this process, advanced practice nurses (APNs) and policy analysts who study implementation need to addresses several issues. The first is to determine the degree to which the policy results or outcomes are consistent with the official objectives enunciated in the original statute, court case, or authoritative directive. Another issue is to identify the extent to which the original objectives and basic strategies were modified during the implementation process. Finally, APNs should try to determine the principal factors affecting the degree of change and modification and any other important effects (Mazmanian and Sabatier, 1983).

According to Bardach (1977), the implementation of a policy or program is an assembly process. The assembly involves numerous and diverse program elements. In addition, the process is a political one, in which the already existing policy mandate affects the strategy and tactics of the implementation struggle. Bardach (1977) sees the politics of implementation as highly defensive, with a great deal of energy used to maneuver in order to avoid responsibility, scrutiny, and blame. The result is an approach that integrates the assembly and the politics via the idea of a system of loosely related implementation games.

The Medicare game is one example. The implementation of Medicare involves a diverse collection of individuals and groups who bring a variety of goals and preferences to the Medicare game. These groups include federal administrators, private insurance companies, medical providers, advocacy groups for the elderly, White House and congressional committees, and others. Each player is trying to influence who gets what, when, where, and how from Medicare through bargaining and compromise. The end result is that the program that finally is implemented may not look much like the one initially envisioned (Litman and Robins, 1997)

Implementation Variables

"During implementation there is almost always something that does not go according to plan" (Quade, 1989, p. 343). In the study of the implementation process, one finds that the components identified are consistent but often given different names. Regardless of the label, each aspect of the process affords room for possible deviation from the original intent of the policy mandate. Thus, one way to conceptualize the components of implementation is as independent variables—identifiable elements common to each implementation process but which vary in their degree of significance to the process itself.

Mazmanian and Sabatier (1983) identified three categories of variables: (1) tractability of the problem, (2) ability of statute to structure implementation, and (3) nonstatutory variables affecting implementation. Within each of the three broad variables, there are identified factors that have been conceptually aggregated. The following discussion provides a closer look at the factors included in each of the categories of variables.

Tractability

Tractability, the first category, is described as the degree of difficulty encountered in the management and control of the problem. Inherent in the nature of the tractability problem itself are several factors. One factor is the availability of technical theory and technology, referring to the ease with which the requisite theory and technology are available to meet the objectives within the constraints of funding and feasibility. An example of easily accessible technical theory and technology developed and used by nurses is the Braden Scale for Predicting Pressure Sore Risk. Nurses use the Braden scale to identify at-risk individuals needing prevention and the specific factors placing patients at risk. The Braden scale is one example of research from the former Agency for Health Care Policy and Research (AHCPR). Established as part of the Omnibus Budget Reconciliation Act of 1989, the mission of AHCPR was to conduct and support general health research. One outcome was the development of clinical practice guidelines, including the Braden Scale, which were disseminated to health care providers, policy makers, and the public. Many acute- and long-term care institutions have incorporated the use of the Braden Scale into their patient-care documentation policy. By using the Braden Scale as a clinical practice standard, agencies and accrediting bodies can better determine the quality and effectiveness of patient care.

Another factor relates to diversity of proscribed behavior. The more varieties of behaviors or services being provided by the policy statute, the greater will be the discretion of the persons involved in the implementation. This may result in considerable variation in program performance. One example is the current state-by-state patchwork approach to APN scope of practice. For over 30 years, APN legal authority to practice has expanded, but not without struggles against organized medicine and others who want to require limitations. Many practice barriers still exist, and APN practice is not equal among the states. APNs face barriers of reduced or denied reimbursement. Restrictions or limitations are placed on primary care provider status for state Medicaid or managed care plans, providing care to certain groups such as workman's compensation claims, sports/school physicals, and hospital privileges. Physician supervision or written collaboration documentation is still required in some states (Pearson, 2002).

APNs are up against the broad authority of the legal scope of practice established by physicians over 100 years ago. Physicians are threatened by the loss of control over the health care dollar, so they continue to challenge APN autonomy. The resistance of organized medicine to APN autonomy has intensified due to the continued movement of APNs into primary-care practice, APNs' eligibility to receive direct reimbursement, and fee-for-service patients and insurers seeking APN services. According to Pearson (2002), APNs must focus their efforts toward achieving fair statutes and regulations and work toward achieving a uniform practice act. A uniform practice act would sanction APNs' scope of practice within their professionally credentialed area and close the door to political influences that seek to undermine the APN's autonomy. This involves APNs seeking exclusions from the medical practice act (Pearson, 2002).

The other two factors of tractability are target groups and extent of behavior change required. The sum of behavioral modification required to achieve the policy objectives is a result of both the number of persons in the target group and the amount of change required of them. Behavioral change of target groups is more likely to occur when the group size is small and capable of being isolated (more definable). APNs are considered a target group because of their relatively small number, which makes the regulation of such groups more manageable, and their desire for achieving a uniform practice act. One way for APNs to achieve national standards for health care workforce regulation, education, and credentialing is to support the Pew Health Professions Commission recommendation that Congress establish a policy advisory board. The policy board would develop national scopes of practice for legislature implementation (Pearson, 2001).

Both behavioral interventions and technological change are creating problems for program implementation against the resurgent HIV epidemic among U.S. men who have sex with men. Men are using the Internet to form sexual liaisons making the efficiency of usual outreach methods woefully inadequate. The program depends upon behavioral strategies for its success, but experts recognize that new biomedical approaches are needed that will appeal to the target population (Gross, 2003).

Structure

The second broad category of variables is the ability of policy decisions to structure implementation. Those who have defined the policy are attempting to induce idealized patterns of interaction. To achieve the idealized policy, legal objectives need to be precise and clearly ranked in order of importance. Clear objectives not only serve as a resource to the actors both inside and outside the implementing institution but also help direct the actions necessary to achieve the objectives (Mazmanian and Sabatier, 1983). The importance of precision has been termed a "top-down" perspective. The top-down viewpoint judges implementation by how closely administrators comply with the law. This viewpoint possess appeal because it gives an agency strong control and lessens the possibility that agency officials will dissipate energy by disagreeing with one another over how to interpret the law. The importance of precise statutes holds considerable appeal in the implementation literature, but precision is not always the best remedy (Thompson, 2001).

One example of lack of precision as a barrier to practice is the current situation some APNs are facing related to collaboration. There is a refusal by physicians to collaborate, resulting in APNs leaving their clinical practice clinics (*American Nurse*, 2003). According to Pearson (2002), there is a misinterpretation by some states over the term *collaboration* and APNs must work to more clearly define the legislative language.

Another example is from a study of acute care nurse practitioners (ACNP). The purpose of the descriptive study was to explore the influence of organizational factors on the role implementation of ACNPs. The following factors that were identified as causing a problem with implementation include lack of acceptance of the role by others; role ambiguity; lack of role definition including policy, scope, and standards of practice; and economic and financial issues (Irvine et al., 2000).

In addition to precision, it is important that there is a clear ranking as to the relative priority of the new directive within the totality of the agencies programs. Without such a clear priority ranking, it is likely the new directive will be delayed and given a low priority status. Thus, the clearer the objectives, the more likely the policy outputs of the implementing agencies and ultimate behavior of the target groups will match the intended policy decisions (Theoduolou and Cahn, 1995).

A second factor in this category requires that two elements are present. First, the causal linkages between government interventions and the attainment of program objectives must be understood. Second, the officials responsible for implementing the policy or program must have jurisdiction over a sufficient number of the critical linkages so that the objectives can be attained. The latter factor depends to some degree on the extent to which the statute involves groups or agencies arranged in rank order, such as federal, state, and local entities.

This grouping according to rank is called *hierarchical integration* and can pose problems for implementation. When hierarchical integration is present, the strategy is to minimize the number of opportunities in which a player can interfere with the policy process and block attainment of legal objectives. The more loosely integrated the hierarchy of the agencies, the greater the chance of variation in the degree of compliance by persons participating in the implementation process.

An example of this is demonstrated with the smallpox vaccination plan of December 2002. The Bush administration called for an initial vaccination of military personnel, frontline health care workers, and "first responders." The officials responsible for carrying out the vaccination plan included federal, state, and local agencies. The American Nurses Association (ANA) asked for a delay in the implementation of the smallpox plan. Why? According to ANA President Barbara Blakeney, "Because we didn't believe there were basic protections for nurses, our patients, or our families, and could not fully support the vaccination program at this time" (*American Nurse,* March–April 2003, p. 4). President Bush had called for the vaccination of over 500,000 frontline care workers by Feb 24, 2003. One month into the program, 4,000 volunteers were vaccinated and 3 months later, the CDC reported that 35,903 civilians including health care professionals had been vaccinated (*American Nurse,* March–April, 2003). Four months after the program was implemented, the executive-ordered plan was considered a failure in the eyes of many because the goal of 500,000 vaccinated was closer to 50,000 after 4 months.

Another strategy to minimize problems with hierarchical integration is to provide the players with sufficient incentives for compliance. Sanctions or inducements, if strong enough, can ensure acquiescence among those who have the potential to veto action (Mazmanian and Sabatier, 1983). The incorporation of linkages and sanctions or incentives is demonstrated by the reintroduction in Congress of the Patient Safety Act (PSA) in 1997. The representative who reintroduced the bill stipulated that institutions not meeting specific criteria (of the PSA) would not qualify for Medicare reimbursement. The criteria-linking requirements to Medicare qualification included making staffing and patient outcome information available to the public and providing support for nurses to report unsafe working conditions, known as *whistle-blower protection.* This incorporation of linkage with sanctions or incentives put teeth in the patient protective initiatives (Reed and Vanderbilt, 1997).

The ability to structure successful implementation depends upon funding. The level of funding at the beginning must be enough to assure the possibility of achieving the objectives. The level of funding above the threshold is proportional to the probability of achieving the objectives. Adequate funding can help but is no guarantee that a program will be a success (Mazmanian and Sabatier, 1983); indeed, the opposite may be true. Inadequate funding may doom a program or sufficiently cripple the implementation process. There is also the possibility that a program can be given to an agency in which the program becomes a *phantom,* meaning the program exists on paper or in name but cannot be readily identified by those around it.

The significance of funding policy is noted in the following two examples. First, the Pew Health Professions Commission Task Force (1995) recommendations on health care workforce regulation indicate that states should use standardized language for health-profession regulation. The premise is reasonable, and the National Council of State Boards of Nursing (NCSBN) acknowledged that consistent definitions of such terms as *licensure, certification,* and *registration* would be helpful to consumers. The NCSBN indicated, however, that such a standardization process would introduce problems of funding and territorial battles among APNs. For example, certification in some states requires a master's degree and in other states it does not. The process would be expensive and consumers would bear the cost. Another problem with standard language is that trying to tackle the "crazy-quilt" approach to advanced practice regulation would be daunting. The differences in APN regulation between the states are due to the political climate within which the regulation developed. Professional groups including APNs are resistant to change that can result in loss of identity, position, and opportunity. Given the number of special interests and professional groups in a jurisdiction, one sees the enormity of the task of standardization (NCSBN, 1996).

The second example of funding deals with the current HIV endemic that started in the 1990s. The profile of clients with HIV in the 1990s changed to include more women and children and a greater number of individuals diagnosed with both HIV and mental illness and/or substance abuse. In addition, the treatment protocols changed with the advent of drugs for HIV. According to the National Commission on AIDS, "The HIV epidemic is already adversely affecting the ability to recruit and retain health care students" (p. 141 cited in

Locher and Didion, 2003). Locher and Didion blame the 1993 decrease in enrollment in nursing schools as evidence of this trend. Occupational-exposure infection became a reality, and the cost of postexposure prophylaxis fell directly on the health care agencies. As costs increased due to larger patient volume and more expensive therapies, the funding has decreased. Locher and Didion blame this decrease in financial support on three major factors: (1) the September 11, 2001, terrorist attack; (2) the flat funding by the Bush administration in conjunction with a shift of donated dollars; and (3) the shift of policy makers to financing the pandemic of HIV in developing countries. The result of insufficient funding is that access is being denied to some, other programs are closing to new clients, and there are waiting lists in yet others. The service capacity lost with the closing of HIV services could result in more patients seeking hospital care.

In addition to providing clear and consistent objectives, few veto points, and adequate incentives for compliance, the implementation process can be influenced by a statute stipulating the formal decision rules of the implementing agencies. When multimembered commissions are involved, rules dictate the number of votes required for specific actions. Through this stipulation process, the findings will be fully consistent with legal objectives (Mazmanian and Sabatier, 1983).

Another factor involved in the ability of a statute to structure implementation is the officials' commitment to statutory objectives. Commitment on the part of officials in the implementing agencies is significant to the success of the program. The requisite commitment to the statutory objectives can be achieved in several ways, including assigning responsibility to a new agency specifically created to administer the statute, assigning to existing agencies whose policy orientation is in harmony with the statute, or stipulating in the statute that top implementing officials be selected from specified sectors known to support the legislation's objectives. Sometimes program designers are unable to make the optimum assignments to supportive agencies, and the implementation process is suboptimal at best (Theoduolou and Cahn, 1995).

The continued evolution of managed care has made the expansion of the credentialing process of APNs necessary. *Credentialing* is the process by which professionals provide evidence they are qualified to perform specific clinical skills. National accrediting bodies for health maintenance organizations (HMOs), such as the Joint Commission on Accreditation of Healthcare Organizations and the National Committee for Quality Assurance, are examining the credentialing process. In addition to the usual information regarding credentialing of APNs, the process will require peer review, in some states medical review of credentialing information, and possibly professional references from the directors of educational programs the nurse completed. According to Rustia and Bartek (1997), such comprehensive credentialing will serve as further assurance to the public that APNs are committed to providing optimal results in health care by providing the types of persons and services necessary.

The final factor that affects the ability of a law to direct implementation involves formal access by outsiders. The participation of external actors to the implementing agencies include target groups, potential recipients, and legislative, judicial, and executive figureheads providing oversight of the agencies. Objectives are more likely to be attained if statutes permit citizen participation as both formal interveners in agency proceedings and as petitioners in judicial review. In addition, the placement of oversight in the hands of statutory supports will enhance the implementation process (Mazmanian and Sabatier, 1983).

The Health Insurance Portability and Accountability Act (HIPPA), passed by Congress in 1996, provides an example of this. In 1997, the U.S. Department of Health and Human Services (HHS) offered recommendations to Congress related to aspects of medical privacy protection in HIPPA. Congress was given a deadline of August 1999 to pass legislation protecting the privacy of health information, but Congress failed to meet that deadline. HIPPA indicated that HHS could issue appropriate regulations, and they did, but not without much controversy. There was a wide range of interests affected by the proposed rules. According to Marietti (Charters, 2003), there were 52,000 public comments on the first version of the privacy rule issued in December 2000 under the Clinton administration and 11,000 on the second version that was proposed by the Bush administration before the December 2000 version was reached. The final medical information privacy rule was published on August 14, 2002, and most of the entities covered in HIPPA had to comply with the privacy rule by April 14, 2003. Small health plans had until April 14, 2004, to comply with the rule.

Health care business groups view the final rule as one they can work with because they were successful in getting a requirement removed from the rule. The requirement concerned getting written consent to use protected information. With its removal, all that is needed is a good-faith effort to obtain acknowledgement that patients received information of their privacy rights and practices. On the other hand, privacy protection groups saw the removal of the requirement as a serious setback that undermined patient control of the use of their health care information. Predictions have been made that the changes will weaken patient trust in the health care system (Charters, 2003). Other groups such as the Health Insurance Association of American view the privacy law as unworkable. They claim that the states will create their own variations of the privacy law and this will cause increases in health care costs (Charters, 2003). Researchers feel that the additional regulations will prevent or impede certain types of research. Overall, complying with HIPPA will be a technical challenge and will require cultural change (Charters, 2003).

Nonstatutory Variables

The third broad category of implementation involves nonstatutory variables. The factors include socioeconomic conditions, public support, attitudes and resources of constituency groups, and commitment and leadership skill of implementing officials. Another term for this category could be *environmental factors*.

Variations occur over time and among governmental jurisdictions that affect policy implementation. Social, economic, and technological changes affect the political support for statutory objectives. Socioeconomic conditions impact the perceptions of the relative importance of the problem addressed by the statute. Political support, over time, is likely to diminish due to fading interest. Local variation in socioeconomic conditions can also affect implementation by producing significant pressure for flexible regulations and noticeable administrative discretion for local government units. It was once assumed that NPs would help replace physicians who were leaving rural communities. That did not happen because often nonphysician practices developed enough demand for medical services to allow a physician to come in and take advantage of that developed market. In recent years, the demand for APNs in nonrural settings has grown, and a migration of APNs to the metropolitan areas is evident (Wilken, 1993).

Policies that are linked directly with technology are subject to changes based upon the state of the art in technology. In response to the 1998 IOM report (*To Err is Human: Building a Safer Health Care System*), the veteran's administration (VA) implemented a new technology called The Bar Code Medication Administration (BDMA) system. Nurses at the VA scan a bar code printed on the patient's ID wrist band that opens the patient's medication record on a computer screen and lists the medications to be given at that time. The nurse then scans the bar code on each unit-dose medication before it is given. Initially the system had problems that actually caused medication administration to take more time. The problems, however, were virtually eliminated because of input from nurses and other staff. Bar coding is a natural progression in using technology in health care. The error rate is one error in one hundred characters when entered manually, compared to one error in a million characters when using a scanner in bar coding (Trossman, 2003).

Two other factors include media attention to the problem and public support. Described as episodic or perhaps cyclical in nature, public opinion waxes and wanes. The interaction between the mass media and the public can affect policy implementation. Sufficient evidence exists to indicate that legislators are influenced by public support, especially if public opinion within the legislator's district is relatively uniform. Agencies often employ opinion polls to help support policy positions. Constituency groups vary their attitudes and financial support based, in part, on public support. In addition, constituency groups can affect policy implementation through direct intervention (Mazmanian and Sabatier, 1983).

The passage of California's new safe-staffing law is just such an example. Sponsored by the California Nurses Association and authored by an elected assembly member, the bill grabbed headlines from coast to coast and around the world. Coverage was national and international using such media as TV, radio, newspapers, and Internet Web sites. One coalition of hundreds of nurses, doctors, and health care advocates was reported in the *Boston Globe*. Public opinion polls disseminated to the media and lawmakers indicated that greater than

80 percent of Californians supported the bill. Nurses in other states were calling for enactment of similar legislation (Harrington C. and Estes C., 2001).

An additional factor is change in the resources and attitudes of constituency groups. Proponents of a regulatory program that seeks to change the behavior of one or more target groups are confronted with an essential, but often problematic, challenge. The challenge for constituency groups is to transform the initial public support for their position into viable organizations that are recognized as legitimate players and consequently called upon by implementing officials to play a part in policy decisions. The opponents of the mandated change also have resources and incentives to intervene in the implementation process. Opponents can generally intervene over a longer period of time than proponents, and regulatory agencies recognize this. The survival of regulatory agencies depends upon accommodation with the interests of target groups.

One example is the 1989 payment system for physicians approved by Congress. The new approach to paying physicians who treated Medicare patients was the resource-based relative value scale (RBRVS). The purpose was to establish a national standard payment scale for a variety of physician services. During the implementation of RBRVS, the federal Health Care and Finance Administration proposed changes that included reductions in payment for surgeries and other highly specialized procedures and increases in payment for delivery of primary care. Because notice of proposed changes must appear in the *Federal Register,* various physician groups took notice, and an invitation to bargain and negotiate occurred (Litman and Robins, 1997).

Historically, analysts have concentrated largely on the idealized policy with little attention to the target group and virtually no attention to the implementing organization or environmental factors. An example of this occurred in New York City when municipal outpatient clinics were set up for preventive health. The problem occurred when the clinics were established in areas where the target population had no understanding of the clinic's purpose. In low-income areas, residents only go to a health clinic when they are sick and need help, never when they are well. When these residents did come to the preventive clinic, they were turned away and referred to a hospital for treatment (Quade, 1989). This resulted in confusion as to the value, even the relevance, of the services provided.

This discussion of broad categories and specific factors of policy implementation provides much information about the process. Factors interact with other factors. The implementation process can be explained further by discussing four components of the process that are, in themselves, independent variables.

Independent Variables

One variable is the organization responsible for carrying out the policy mandate. Institutions can determine their own standards and programs while working within the policy. This flexibility of standards and programs helps to explain how a policy can be implemented differently between and among the institutions and governing bodies involved. Administrative agencies frequently use the regulatory process to include program elements they were unable to put into legislation, thereby undermining congressional intent. The use of unlicensed assistive personnel (UAPs) is an example of institutions, such as hospitals and long-term care facilities, including elements that they were unable to put into legislation. In most states, the activities of UAPs are beyond the reach of existing professional regulatory mechanisms; that is, boards of nursing have jurisdiction only over licensed nurses, not unlicensed assistants. Training, supervision, and discipline of UAPs vary from agency to agency.

Policy implementation requires competent personnel who have adequate comprehension, capability, and willingness to carry out the mandate. One aspect related to personnel is the composition of regulatory boards. The issue raised by the Pew Health Professions Commission Task Force (1995) and others is whether professional boards, including boards of nursing, are unduly influenced by the profession they are regulating so that their decisions are more out of self-interest for the profession than out of interest for the consumer. The American Nurses Association (ANA) responded, saying that professional members must be held accountable to the same standards as public members and that nursing's record in working with state regulatory boards speaks to a collaborative relationship with the public to ensure safe and quality health care services (ANA, 1997).

Another variable is pressure by rival agencies that can influence policy implementation in a number of directions. Division of authority among governments at the federal, state, and local levels makes it difficult for one government level to order another government level to do anything. For example, state governments do not want to be told by the federal government how to administer programs that are jointly funded by both. This explains the differences among the state Medicaid programs related to eligibility and services offered. Block grants are another example of how the division of authority plays out in the implementation process. Block grants are authorized and appropriated by the federal government, with each state receiving a lump sum of money to provide programs and services for a particular population, such as mothers and children. The states are to fulfill the federal mandate that speaks to broad categories. The specifics of how to accomplish this are left to the states to decide. The differences noted in the ranking among states related to such areas as morbidity and mortality reflect, in part, the degree of success in the implementation process.

Bureaucracies and bureaucrats are thought to be responsible for many problems of implementation. Individual officials have varying goals, and each uses his or her discretion in translating orders from above into commands further down the hierarchy. The greater the number of players who can act independently on a policy decision, the less the policy will reflect the decisions made by the government on that issue. The common perception is that lower-level bureaucrats do not carry out the instructions and orders of higher-level bureaucrats. According to Lipsky (Vedung, 1997), typical street-level bureaucrats, including nurses, grant access to government programs and provide services with them. These public service workers who interact directly with citizens have substantial discretion in implementing policy as well as actually creating policy through the multitude of decisions they make. Their discretion cannot be completely controlled due to lack of supervisory resources, so policies are formed by the street-level operators who develop routines and shortcuts for coping with their everyday jobs (Vedung, 1997). This leaves the implementation process open to problems of control and accountability.

Sometimes, the constraints placed by the courts limit the alternatives of implementation. The results of court cases involving the 1990 Americans with Disabilities Act (ADA) provide examples of how the judicial system can affect implementation. The ADA provides comprehensive civil rights protection for people with disabilities by legislating rules for business and service providers. The intention of the law was to empower persons with disabilities through knowledge that there were provisions for registering complaints and determining compliance through the courts (Harrison, 2002). Title 1 of the ADA is related to employment of persons with disabilities. At the time the ADA was passed, employment rates of persons with disabilities was low and, although employers expressed support for ADA, they had concerns about how the provisions of the ADA would affect them. In 1995, 5 years after passage of the ADA under Title 1, the employer has fared better than the employee in the courts, and the disability activists were accusing the court of decreasing the effectiveness of the ADA. Reviews of all court cases filed in relation to employment and the ADA indicated that the employer won in over 95 percent of the cases. In addition, the court narrowed the definition of disability under the ADA. Previously, the criteria for disabled was the inability of persons to perform their jobs. An additional criterion was added by the court—inability to perform activities of daily living. Ironically, employees within the health care system have greater barriers to their success in court than employees of other industries (Harrison, 2002). The court tries to ensure that a balance is struck between ADA compliance and meeting patient responsibilities. The court decides whether persons with disabilities pose a threat to recipients of health care, despite accommodations being provided. Edmonds cites two examples. The first is a nurse with a back injury who was fired. She lost her law suit against the ADA because the court determined that lifting was a crucial part of her job, even though she had her sister perform the lifting. The second case was an HIV-positive operating room technician who refused an accommodation of being transferred to another job. He lost his case under the ADA because the court decided his threat to surgical patients was great, despite the low probability of patients contracting HIV. Based on these and other events, there has been discussion about making the ADA definition of disability less vulnerable to interpretation by the courts. This will, however, require legislation to reauthorize the ADA definition (Harrison, 2002).

Another example of the courts and implementation is the Death with Dignity Act that was the result of Oregon's public initiative process. Voters first approved the act on November 8, 1994. One day before the law would have taken effect, a temporary restraining order was issued by the U.S. District

Court for the District of Oregon with a permanent injunction issued in August 1995 (A. Jackson, executive director, Oregon Hospice Association, personal communication, November 4, 1997). In early 1997, the Ninth Circuit Court of Appeals ordered the district court to lift the injunction. The reasoning for lifting the injunction was that the plaintiffs lacked standing to challenge Oregon's law because persons were not harmed by a law that had never taken effect. In November 1997, citizens voted on a referendum proposed by the Oregon legislature. Ballot Measure 51 asked voters whether or not they wished to repeal the Death with Dignity Act. The issue was decided by mail-in ballots with approximately 60 percent of the voters saying they did not wish to repeal the act (A. Jackson, executive director, Oregon Hospice Association, personal communication, November 4, 1997). This issue has been discussed in the U.S. Congress, but at the time of this writing a bill to repeal has not been passed.

The more clear the objectives and concise the statute, the better chance of meeting the policy objectives because both help limit discretionary powers. According to Thompson (2001), there are several circumstances under which vague laws can foster positive and creative program results. The first circumstance is when Congress cannot find a solid underlying theory in drafting legislation and when there is urgency to do something. A specific, detailed law as to how best to allocate funds to decrease the rate of cancer mortality is not feasible. A second circumstance occurs when there is a threat to the validity of statutes that are too specific due to fast-changing norms or accepted conditions in the economic and social climate. For instance, findings occur frequently regarding the identification of substances that are thought to cause cancer and there is usually not conclusive evidence on what is an acceptable level of exposure. A third circumstance centers on when consensus in the implementing agency as to the primary mission and the general intent of the statute is not at odds with the mission. Another circumstance that can foster creative implementation, despite vague statutes, is when there is no interest group that is heavily opposed to the administration of the program. Finally, when the effectiveness of lawmakers is in question, precise legislation is less appealing (Thompson, 2001).

Another variable is the public's acceptance. Policy implementation is susceptible to the responses of individuals that vary depending upon the extent that their self-interests are served or affected by the policy. Individuals who repudiate implementation may do so because it causes them to change their patterns of behavior or because they are frustrated. Federal protection for the safety of nursing-home residents is one example. Regulations were in place that were a result of public horror and outrage over the deplorable conditions of patients in long-term care facilities. Antiregulatory zealots who were tired of government interference began to attack proven regulatory mechanisms. The zealots attempted to impose restrictive new requirements on the overall process of issuing federal regulations and, at the same time, impose parallel antiregulatory moves at the state level. One proposal involved weakening the health care workforce regulation. Such proposals, however, outraged the opposition. Efforts to eliminate federal nursing home standards were met by a sustained and broad-based public outcry. The efforts to roll back existing federal regulation ultimately failed (Keepnews, 1997).

There is the possibility that the policy design was defective. Policy decisions may not be good for a variety of reasons. One example of a questionable policy decision was the Healthy People 2000 initiative, the only health initiative so far to come out of the second Bush presidency. The Bush administration's summary of goals for the future detailed the targets and goals set in Healthy People 1990 by the Carter administration. Unfortunately, very few targets had been met during the 1990 initiative. Interestingly, according to Garrett, 2000, the Healthy People 2000 initiative made no reference to the crisis in health care identified in the 1988 IOM report. The crisis identified access to health care issues, the rising number of underinsured and uninsured, and the future of Medicare and Medicaid. During the 1990 American Public Health Association Annual meeting, the organization's executive director stated, "The potential of Healthy People 2000 is sold short by the administration's timidity to address the tough issues involved with implementation. As it stands, Healthy People 2000 may be filled with good stuff, but the cup is half empty" (Garrett, 2000, p. 427). The executive director went on to say that the action plan is lacking in its ability to achieve the goals and objectives set and that the document "draws us a picture of the 'Emerald City', but never shows us a 'yellow brick road'" (Garrett, 2000, p. 427). The Healthy People 2000 report was abundant with health goals for American but stingy on financial resources to achieve the goals. The expectation was that goal achievement would happen through health promotion, not through expenditure on government services or regulation. Interestingly, the report indicated that unless uninsured Americans gained access to primary health care, the goals could not be reached. The report was correct. Little improvement was noted in basic health indicators at the time the draft of Healthy People 2010 was written (Garrett, 2000).

Citizens and policy makers alike assume that once Congress passes a bill and appropriates sufficient money and staff power, the effects of the policy will be what was originally intended. Policy makers, however, may not anticipate the circumstances under which the policy would have to operate. In addition, the costs in time and money may be underestimated deliberately by the decision makers in order to secure the approval for the policy (Quade, 1989).

Problems with Implementation

Problems of policy implementation are widespread in the United States. Certain types of programs present more of a problem than others. Policies that differ little from past policy are likely to meet less resistance. A common view of policy making is called *incrementalism*, which means the policy proceeds through long chains of political and analytical steps with no clear-cut beginning and end. Incrementalism assumes that the costs of delaying action are greater than the costs of error. Programs that are of a nonincremental nature are more difficult to implement but can be successful. One example is the State Children's Health Insurance Program (SCHIP), one of many programs that resulted from the Balanced Budget Act of 1997. SCHIP was appropriated generous funding, had strong presidential backing, and the historic rhetoric of insuring five million children (Smith, 2002). The organization responsible for implementing SCHIP was the Health Care Finance Administration (HCFA), renamed in 2001 as the Center for Medicaid and Medicare Services (CMS). HCFA wanted SCHIP to be a balance between an entitlement program (Medicaid) and a block grant (federal aid to states) and initially expected the implementation of SCHIP to be one of incremental amendments, largely to existing agencies. When the unexpectedly large authorization for funding was given, the implementing agency decided on the creation of whole new structures. A steering committee, comprising over a 100 members representing over 40 organizations within the Department of Health and Human Services, was formed. Smith (2002) believes that the role of the steering committee and the strategy guiding its organization contributed significantly to the ability of SCHIP to enroll two million children in the first 2 years of the program.

"When policies are implemented, tensions, strains, and conflicts are experienced by those who are implementing the policy and by those affected by the policy" (Quade, 1989, p. 343). Designing a public policy that looks good in print is not easy. One difficulty is the translation of the policy into words and slogans that political leaders like. Even more difficult is the implementation of the policy in a way that pleases others (Bardach, 1977). Thus, policy implementation may not achieve what was intended by the policy makers when any or a combination of these factors occur.

The majority of problems that interfere with policy implementation are people problems. Policy analysts refer to these types of problems as political problems. Many of the difficulties in the implementation process involve actors maneuvering with and against each other both for end results and strategic advantages. Bardach (1977) calls these maneuvers *games.*

Implementation Games

Games are classified according to the nature of their stakes, with control at the heart of the implementation process. Control is exercised through bargaining, persuasion, and maneuvering under conditions of uncertainty. The result is that control manifests itself as strategies and tactics. Thus, the implementation process involves assembling the elements required to produce a particular policy outcome while playing games that either withhold or deliver the elements to the policy process (Bardach, 1977).

Categories of maneuvers include the diversion of resources, deflection of goals, dilemmas of administration, and the dissipation of energies. The diversion of resources, especially money, manifests itself in several ways. Organizations and individuals who receive government money tend to provide less in the way of exchange services for that money (Bardach, 1977).

Playing the budget game is another diversion. Persons responsible for the budget do what they can to win favor in the eyes of elected and appointed officials who have power over their funding. Therefore, the incentives shaped for implementers by those who control their budgets influence what the implementers do with respect to executing policy mandates. Often, however, the less well the bureau performs, the larger the task left to perform; hence, more money is needed (Bardach, 1977).

Enormous pressure is placed on legislators to spread resources, usually money, around so as many constituents as possible can receive the benefits and the legislators gain political patronage. This game is called *pork barrel*. When resources need to be concentrated in order to reach some threshold level of effectiveness, this attempt to divert resources is counterproductive (Quade, 1989).

Deflection of goals is another game. In an important way, implementation is the continuation of policy-adoption politics by alternative means. During the implementation phase, goals often undergo some change. Some may feel the original goals were too ambiguous, that they were based on a weak consensus, or the goals were decided too hastily and, perhaps, insincerely. Interest groups that remained quiet during earlier points in the policy process may now come forward because they were counting on seizing the opportunities to achieve their own purposes.

Regulatory agencies are constantly being accused of being captured by the professions they are supposed to regulate. The Professional Services Review Organizations (PSROs) were established in local communities according to the design of legislative and administrative policy makers at the national level. The purpose of the PSROs was to introduce cost and quality controls in the delivery of federally supported medical care. According to Bardach (1977), the PSROs were likely to be captured by county medical societies. This capture could mean that the regulators, in this case the local medical society, would be too soft on the PSROs or that the PSRO could get the medical society to do its bidding. Although the process by which the capture occurs will differ somewhat in each locality, Bardach (1977) contends that the history of government efforts at regulation strongly suggest that, one way or another, capture will occur.

The dilemmas of administration also present problems for the implementation process. According to Bardach (1977), tokenism and massive resistance are the principal games that bring grief to administrators and administrations. Tokenism involves an attempt to appear to be contributing but, in reality, the contribution is a mere symbol or a small degree. An example is the 1990 Clean Air Act and the Emergency Planning and Community Right to Know statute. Congress reauthorizes all environmental laws every 5 years. When the Clear Air Act was reauthorized in 1990, Congress required industrial sites that use extremely hazardous substances to disclose worse-case accident scenarios as part of their risk-management plans. The intent of Congress was to post information about hazardous chemical threats on the Web so the public could be informed and protected. The chemical industry was opposed to the requirement and was seen as undermining the public's right to know. Unfortunately, the required risk-management plans used by the chemical industry deal with emergency planning, not accident prevention. According to Afzal (2003), the information has never been posted on the Web, and intentional barriers were created to prevent easy access to the information. A written procedure for how to locate and make an appointment to view the worse-case scenarios is available at the federal reading room. Part of the process requires calling either the EPA or the Department of Justice and providing them with information. An appointment for a reading room by the Department of Justice requires a 7-day advanced notice but, according to Afzal, "as limited as the current access is, the chemical industry would like to do away with the reading rooms altogether" (p. 26).

Massive resistance obstructs program implementation by withholding essential policy components. By overwhelming the agency with the need to enforce sanctions for noncompliance, massive resistance can cause the evasion of the responsibility mandated in the policy. An example of large-scale noncompliance included efforts to enforce the civil rights movement. Both tokenism and massive resistance can be detrimental to the process of implementation.

The last category of games is dissipation of energies. This mix of games has a common theme: The entities involved in the implementation process all waste a great deal of energy avoiding responsibility, defending themselves against others, and setting themselves up for advantageous situations. Bardach (1977) named these games Tenacity, Odd Man Out, Reputation, and Not Our Problem.

Tenacity is a game that can be played by anyone involved in implementation. This game takes the power to slow or stall the progress of a program until one's own terms are met. Tenacity can lead to delay, withdrawal of financial and political support, or the total collapse of a program. *Odd Man Out* is an implementation game normally played by actors in addition to whatever other games are being played. The actors attempt to maneuver other players into forfeiting their options while keeping the actors' own options to withdraw in check.

The *Reputation* game has various outcomes depending on the player's intent. Players seek reputation as a means of achieving other ends, such as getting elected, being promoted, or having a reputation for being good at Tenacity. Bureaucrats play the game *Not Our Problem* under several circumstances. One circumstance occurs when bureaucracies realize that the program will impose a heavy workload. Two other instances occur when the program takes the bureau into realms of controversy or the required tasks are too difficult for the bureau to perform. The agency will try to shift certain unattractive elements to different agencies. If nobody wants the responsibility, citizens get the runaround and each agency involved can claim it is not the problem.

Successful Implementation

So far, the discussion has centered on the variables of policy implementation and their effects. Mazmanian and Sabatier (1983) identified several elements that contribute to successful implementation:

- The program is based on sound theory relating changes in target group behavior to achievement of the desired end-state (objectives).

- The statute or basic policy decision contains unambiguous policy directives and structures the implementation process so as to maximize the likelihood that target groups will perform as desired.

- The leaders of the implementing agencies possess sufficient managerial skills and political skill and are committed to statutory goals.

- Throughout the implementation process, organized constituency groups and elected or appointed officials maintain active support.

- The ranking of statutory objectives remains stable over time so as to minimize conflicts in the environment that could undermine the statute.

The task of ensuring that the conditions are met is difficult. The implementation process is so complicated that it challenges all who attempt an analysis. Bardach (1977) believes the best approach is *scenario writing*. This involves inventing several plausible stories attempting to answer the question of "what will happen if. . . ." Through trial and error and successive redesign, a best-case scenario emerges (Bardach, 1977).

One important conclusion that appears from the study of implementation is that implementation is inherently unpredictable. During the process of implementation, forces may be in play to try and change the policy. These forces include interest groups, opposition parties, affected individuals and organizations, and the bureaucracy that has the responsibility for implementation. Individuals who study implementation have made the following observations. After all these years, implementation continues to be an afterthought in the study of the policy process. Interested individuals should look closely at the implementation issues raised by managed care and possible Medicare and Medicaid reform. States will continue to be a focal point for the study of implementation as more responsibility is given to them. The high levels of cynicism, mistrust, and partisan polarization in government perceived by the public may be a cause of concern for well-performing government institutions that thrive in an environment of civic trust and cooperation. What remains constant is that implementation issues continue to be the subject of great concern because they make a difference in our daily lives.

Effects of Implementation on APNs: A Case Study on Direct Reimbursement, Prescriptive Authority, and Physician Supervision

In the mid-to-late 1980s, the availability and accessibility of rural health services was gaining national attention. More health professionals were needed in rural areas, and there were no comprehensive government policies that attempted to recruit and retain a mixture of health professionals most appropriate in a rural health care delivery system. Each state can use considerable power to permit and facilitate the development of rural health care programs, regardless of the funding source.

A host of regulatory and political activities conjoined at the state level, including licensure of APNs, reimbursement levels for APNs from Medicare and third-party payers, health planning responsibilities, and medical society lobbying. The decisions made by state boards that regulate APNs are thought to have an effect on the availability and utilization of APNs in rural areas. What was not known at the time of the research by Wilken (1993) was whether certain characteristics of board structure affect policy decisions and whether policy decisions affect utilization of APNs.

The intent of the research was to determine whether the structure of the state boards affected the restrictiveness of three regulatory barriers for APNs:

1. direct third-party reimbursement
2. authority to prescribe
3. physician supervision

The researcher hoped to discover what effect such regulatory barriers had on the utilization of nurse practitioners (NPs) and certified nurse midwives (CNMs) in rural areas.

The research design was both descriptive and quantitative. The descriptive data were provided by a mailed questionnaire to all state boards of nursing and boards of medicine. The response rate was 87 percent. The quantitative component utilized selected variables chosen for their theoretical fit and potential power to explain. Logistic and multiple regression were used to produce statistical models, some of which are discussed here (Wilken, 1993).

Board Structure and Function

Typically, regulation of the health professions is carried out by state boards. *State boards* are agencies created by state legislatures to protect the public. A state board's governing administrative law comes from state statutes that are written in general, rather than specific, language. Such general language allows each state board to implement regulations at its own discretion. One result is that state boards will vary in the levels of restrictiveness applied to regulations, even though state statutes may read alike. Statutes that use a "laundry list" format run the risk of becoming immediately restrictive. The profession plays a role in regulation by setting and ensuring standards for the provision of safe, quality health services.

Four models of organization for state occupational licensing boards have been developed and become apparent when examining regulatory board structure. The models lie on a spectrum ranging from autonomous boards to central agencies. Autonomous boards, the first model, perform all administrative, budgetary, and disciplinary activities, and no central agency exists. The second model relies on a central agency to perform certain administrative duties but the board remains autonomous in other areas. In the third model, the central agency may have authority for such functions as budget, staff, and investigations. The fourth model is dependent upon the central agency for review and, in some cases, the board exists only in an advisory capacity but may be given certain housekeeping duties. More than 80 percent of the boards of nursing that responded to the mailed questionnaire indicated the level of the board's autonomy was either autonomous or a mix of autonomy and central control (Wilken, 1993).

APNs can see that the power a board exerts will affect policy implementation. Most boards have involvement with a central agency, such as the state department of health. Central agencies provide an additional accountability factor, which is the mechanism for multidisciplinary decision making. Such a mechanism can assist in resolving scope of practice boundary disputes (Wilken, 1993).

Historically, legislators have expressed confidence in the ability of the professions to regulate themselves in the public interest. Autonomous regulatory agencies have developed a uniqueness that many ordinary citizens do not fully understand. These agencies are empowered to promulgate rules that have the force of law, to implement laws, and to exercise sanctioning power over individuals within the agency's jurisdiction.

Political power is usually gained from the use of administrative law versus clientele or possession of knowledge. Administrative law is a form of rule making in which the regulatory agency has the power to fill in the details of the law. Administrative discretion about what is subject to public policy is apparent in such areas as the states' Medicaid reimbursement process. Wide variation among states regarding reimbursement exists for APNs (Wilken, 1993).

Another factor affecting policy implementation is the size of the regulatory agency. Small agencies are more likely to be controlled by the occupation's own self-interest, while larger agencies claim that no one occupation can control the agency. The employees of these agencies play roles in policy implementation. Larger agencies are thought to attract higher-quality employees who have a greater interest in regulation and create a more consumer-oriented regulatory agency. Other researchers have indicated that the larger the agency, the greater the number of decisions and, perhaps, the greater the chance for deviation from the policy intent.

Composition and organization of regulatory boards affect implementation. The individuals who serve on these boards are important actors in the development of professional licensing and regulation policy. State legislatures require consumer representation on occupational licensing boards to help discourage a monopoly of professional members on the board. The hope is that consumer members would serve as lobbyists for the people. Wilken (1993) noted that the presence of consumers on regulatory boards had a positive impact for both NPs and CNMs. For every unit increase in the percentage of consumers, an increase in direct third-party reimbursement for both NPs and CNMs was noted. These findings indicate that consumers can affect policy outcomes.

Another aspect of board composition is the presence of committees. Because no states have boards of nurse practitioners or nurse midwives, some state boards of nursing have committees for the regulation of NPs and CNMs. The presence of such committees indicates that a vehicle is present in the board structure that allows input from APNs to board members. This variable was considered to have a causal effect on restrictiveness of regulations. Wilken (1993) found that the presence of an NP or CNM committee affects the authority to prescribe for both groups. For every unit increase in the measure of NP and CNM committees, there is an increase in the authority to prescribe. The presence of a committee can be a powerful force affecting implementation. Committees often contain members with expertise and experience that can influence board members. This finding makes a strong case for all nurses in advanced practice to work toward the establishment of committees on boards of nursing.

Regulation and Utilization of APNs

There is no doubt about it: Lack of uniform regulation among states and strict guidelines for reimbursement, prescriptive authority, and physician supervision can be harmful both to the public that demands access to cost-effective primary health care and to the practitioners who wish to provide care (Wilken, 1993).

Access to health care is a major item on the U.S. political agenda. For rural Americans, the relative scarcity of health services is viewed as an issue of social justice. APNs are credited with providing health care services to rural Americans, but the presence of regulatory barriers has limited their availability and utilization. Advanced practice nursing has focused for some years on barriers to practice inherent in many state licensure and scope of practice laws and regulations. Scope of practice legislation has been attacked as unduly restrictive for many professions and an obstacle to accessing care. APNs have been battling restrictions in three areas: (1) direct third-party reimbursement, (2) prescriptive authority, and (3) physician supervision.

Americans want access to quality health care at low cost. One action that would directly improve access and quality at the same time and lower cost, especially for poor and rural people, would be to remove the barriers to practice faced by NPs and CNMs. These two groups of APNs have demonstrated their ability to provide 80 percent of American's primary health care needs at a cost lower than that of physicians and without sacrificing quality (Wilken, 1993; Office of Technology Assessment, 1986). Research has credited nurses in advanced practice for improving access to health care for rural Americans because of APN's willingness to practice in rural areas. Unfortunately, this willingness to locate in rural areas is declining, and APNs cite regulatory barriers as one reason for the decline (Wilken, 1993).

Direct Third-Party Reimbursement

The ability of APNs to practice independently or work on a collegial footing with physicians is dependent upon reimbursement. One of the major reasons expressed by CNMs for not engaging in nurse-midwifery practice was lack of direct third-party reimbursement. When the state of Washington implemented a policy to pay all providers the same rate for the same services, the policy had a significant effect on recruiting NPs and CNMs. The improved competitive fees were instrumental in bringing 33 percent more nurse practitioners into the state to staff clinics (Wilken, 1993).

The decision to reimburse APNS involves three elements: (1) what services, (2) at what level, and (3) whether third-party payments are made directly to the provider or through a physician. Because states regulate the insurance industry, reimbursement depends in large part on state statutes. Direct third-party reimbursement has an impact on availability of NPs. Wilken (1993) found that increases in direct third-party reimbursement for NPs led to increased availability of qualified health care providers. This finding indicates that equal pay for equal work may be a strong issue for NPs. In 1993, 26 states had passed mandatory benefit laws requiring private insurers to reimburse NPs directly. The range of reimbursement rates for Medicare, Medicaid, and private insurance is 75 to 100 percent of physician rates, depending upon the type of APN (Pearson, 1997).

Sometimes legislation leads to more legislation in order in ensure implementation. Not only are there differences among the states regarding direct third-party reimbursement, but there are differences within states regarding reimbursement. Some reimbursement rates for the same service differ for APNs versus physicians. The federal Health Care Financing Administration (HCFA) set the NP fee at 85 percent of the physician fee, except in federally designated rural health clinics where NPs are paid 100 percent. Physician assistants have been reimbursed at 100 percent by Medicaid for many years. Legislation was introduced in 1997 in the U.S. House of Representatives to provide the same type of direct reimbursement to APNs for Medicaid as is proposed under Medicare (Helminger and Whittaker, 1997). The American College of Nurse Practitioners (ACNP) hired a lobbyist to help persuade Congress to provide direct Medicare reimbursement for all nurse practitioners, regardless of geographic or practice setting, and payment levels closer to that of physicians. ANA also worked consistently on this issue. The reimbursement rates are 15 percent and 25 percent less than the rates for physicians, depending on the setting (Ventura, 1977). President Clinton's 1997 budget proposal included a provision to provide direct Medicare reimbursement to all clinical nurse specialists and nurse practitioners (Helminger and Whittaker, 1997). In January 1998, all nurse practitioners and clinical nurse specialists were able to bill for Medicare Part B directly.

APNs won a victory for reimbursement in New York. Columbia Presbyterian Medical Center signed agreements with two major health care plans to confer primary-care status to the hospital's APNs and to list APNs as primary-care providers in the directory. The plan reimburses APNs at physician rates (Canavan, 1997).

Authority to Prescribe

Regulatory boards make policy decisions about the power to prescribe. These policy decisions include determining which providers will be authorized to prescribe drugs and devices, what will be the extent of the authority conferred, and which agency will regulate. Many states severely limit prescriptive authority by imposing such restrictions as requiring written protocols and physician supervision or direction; restricting the types of drugs, usually by adopting a formulary; limiting the number of dosage units or refills that can be prescribed; and restricting prescriptive authority to certain geographical locations or institutions. Sometimes the agreements and protocols must be reviewed by the state board that authorizes the APN to prescribe (Wilken, 1993).

Historically, nurses prescribe if prescribing is defined as giving directions, either orally or in writing, for the administration of medication. The ability of APNs to provide drugs to patients, particularly in rural areas without pharmacy services, is essential for the delivery of effective health care. Clients are subject to delays in treatment and needless gaps in the continuity of their care if APNs cannot prescribe. Methods to deal with this problem include making a request to the physician for each prescription needed, utilizing presigned blank prescription forms, or telephoning prescriptions into the pharmacy using a supervising physician's name. Each of these methods has practical, and sometimes legal, problems. Having to consult a physician is time-consuming and annoying for the nurse, the physician, and the patient. Presigned prescription blanks are illegal in most states and could pose a further problem if they are stolen. The legality of telephoning prescriptions is unclear (Wilken, 1993). For CNMs, the often vague and conflicting state medical and nurse practice acts allow for growth in some instances by allowing physicians to delegate large portions of their legally sanctioned activities to nurses without violating the practice acts of either profession. However, this places the CNM in a precarious legal position of increased responsibility and liability without the corresponding increase in authority, serving as a block to autonomous nurse-midwifery practice (Wilken, 1993).

As of January 2003, all 50 states and the District of Columbia have some degree of prescriptive authority for APNs. In 12 states and the District of Columbia, APNs can prescribe, including schedule II narcotics, without physician involvement. In the other 38 states, the NP can prescribe with some physician delegation. "APNs in all states and the District of Columbia have authority to receive and/or dispense drug samples according to the authorized scope of practice, statute, or rules and regulations" (Pearson, 2003, p. 31).

According to Wilken (1993), authority to prescribe was a predictive variable. The data indicate that the availability of NPs decreased as the authority to prescribe increased. Possibly, the absence of authority to prescribe does not affect NP availability to the extent that direct third-party reimbursement does. NPs, on the whole, may be satisfied with their current authority to prescribe and may see the issue as unimportant (Wilken, 1993).

Physician Supervision

The requirement of physician supervision has a negative impact on the distribution of NPs in rural areas. The legal relationship of supervision between physicians and APNs varies from state to state. Requirements may include formalized practice relationships with physicians; written practice agreements, protocols, and collaboration guidelines; and physician direction and/or supervision. In addition, requirements may be placed on some sites and facilities or geographic areas. For example, federal standards for reimbursement to rural health clinics require the presence of a medical doctor once every 2 weeks in clinics staffed by APNs, but some statutes have more specific requirements for on-site physician supervision. Some states require mutually agreed-upon APN/MD written protocols that are reviewed annually and submitted to the board of nursing and/or board of medicine committees for approval and recording.

Certain exceptions may be made for "medically underserved areas" where physicians will not or do not practice but where APNs have stepped in to the fill the void. These exemptions make the statutes hypocritical and fundamentally indefensible, because exempting supervision in certain areas sends the message that the competence of APNs is determined by where they practice (Wilken, 1993).

States that were less restrictive in physician supervision requirements had greater numbers of nonphysician providers. As mention earlier, groups influence policy decisions and consequent implementation. Research indicates that state medical associations and the American Medical Association (AMA) provide powerful lobbying to resist the power of APNs to take control of their profession. A great part of the power of the medical community comes from the money they contribute to political action committees (PACs) and the professional organization, as well as the prestige in which society holds physicians (Wilken, 1993).

State Nurses Associations

State nurses associations, anxious to ensure that patients receive safe, quality nursing care, have moved forward with innovative adaptations of the ANA's Patient Safety Act (PSA), reintroduced in Congress in the spring of 1997. The PSA requires institutions to make available to the public the nursing staff levels, nursing staff mix, and patient outcomes. As a result of the PSA, state nurse's associations responded in varying ways to the interpretations and consequent implementation of this bill.

The Massachusetts Nurses Association developed legislation that requires reasonable standards for nurse staffing based on the patient's acuity and functional status and on the standards of nursing practice to which the nurse is accountable. Through the organized efforts of nurses in Massachusetts, a bill was passed requiring all health care workers to wear easy-to-read identification of their licensure status so that consumers know who is providing their care. The MNA is now recognized as a power player within the state on issues related to health care (Schildmeier, 1997).

The Tennessee and Kentucky nurses' associations worked within their states to draft relevant variations of the PSA. In 1996, the Florida Nurses Association influenced passage of legislation that required a task force to conduct a study on nurse staffing and outcomes data. The Pennsylvania Nurses Association, along with the ANA, succeeded in procuring the U.S. House of Representatives Committee on Health and Welfare to recommend that the state collect more data on rates of patient infections in hospitals, patient injuries, and incidence of pressure ulcers in relation to nurse staff levels (Helminger and Whittaker, 1997). Here we see a target group, the special interest group, seizing the opportunity to change the policy during implementation. Various state legislative committees have been influenced to recommend that more data be collected on hospital infections, pressure ulcers, and patient injuries, all which relate to patient safety.

Another aspect of the PSA implementation is that New Jersey, Oregon, Washington, Kentucky, and Massachusetts worked on legislation that required public disclosure of staffing levels, staff mix, and patient outcomes. The legislation also would provide for identification of unsafe patient conditions, lapses in hospital quality, and the health and safety effects of health care mergers and acquisitions (Keepnews, 1997).

Hospital mergers also were addressed as a result of the PSA. Massachusetts and Washington pursued legislation that required public hearings before the merger of health care facilities. The Massachusetts legislation also required notification to employees 60 days before jobs are changed or eliminated (Helminger and Whittaker, 1997).

Nurses throughout the country have won impressive victories in their efforts to eliminate or reduce restrictions on their practice and to ensure safe, cost-effective health care. They have achieved successes not through fundamental structural or systemic changes in health care workforce regulation, but by pressing for change through their state legislative and political processes—making their cases before policy makers, mounting grassroots political campaigns, and electing friends of nursing to state legislatures.

The Cost Factor

ANA's response to the Pew Health Professions Commission Report on Health Care Workforce Regulation addressed the issue of implementation. ANA repeatedly commented that the Pew task force report lacked discussion about how the recommendations and options were to be implemented. For example, the Pew task force recommended that states use standardized and understandable language for health-professions regulation, and its functions clearly describe rules for consumers, provider organizations, businesses, and the profession.

The ANA responded that the premise for this recommendation was logical and the goal was laudable, but the goal would be difficult to achieve. Such a standardization process would be costly. The regulation of APNs varies among the states. The reasons for the differences are due to the political climate within the state in which the regulation was developed. Different groups within jurisdictions are resistant to change, fearing loss of position and opportunity. The number of professions and special interest groups makes the enormity of the proposal obvious (NCSBN, 1996).

Policy Language

In 1995, legislation passed related to nonfamily caregivers. The original legislation was introduced to ensure cost-effective and efficient selection by patients of a caregiver who would be trained by the chosen home-care agency and who would work with the patient. This policy, however, was flawed. Language in the original bill required the board of nursing to approve individually, on a case-by-case basis, every patient designation of a nonfamily caregiver. This caused a dilemma for the board of nursing due to the lack of funding and staff to perform this function. In 1997, the state legislature revised the language in H. B. 2779 that would allow the board of nursing by board rule, rather than a lengthy and costly approval process, to execute the medical orders as provided by a physician or dentist. The changes made possible the original goal of cost-efficient selection by patients of qualified caregivers. This is an example of the power and influence that APNs can exert in the implementation of public policy (A. Jackson, executive director, Oregon Hospice Association, personal communication, November 4, 1997).

Personal Interpretation

Each state has written laws that serve as the basis for the states to govern in matters covering a broad spectrum of activities. One area covered in state law is the reporting of deaths. This topic is of interest, in part, because of the increasing number of deaths in the home as a result of the hospice movement. This increase in the number of deaths in the home has called into question the legal responsibility on the part of hospice organizations for dealing with such deaths.

A Personal Hospice Experience   Oregon hospice organizations look to the law for guidance as to the responsibility of nurses who deal with hospice deaths in the home. According to the state attorney general, the interpretation of the law is left up to each county's district attorney (DA). The statute under discussion is ORS 146.090 (Oregon Revised Statute), that deals with deaths requiring investigation. The statute reads: "The medical examiner shall investigate and certify the cause and manner of all human deaths: . . . (f) while not under the care of a physician during the period immediately previous to death." As one reads further, ORS 146.100 (5) exempts the former statute by stating that "The district medical examiner shall immediately notify the district attorney for the county where death occurs of all deaths requiring investigation EXCEPT for those specified by ORS 146.090 (1)(d) to (g)" (ORS 14-204,205).

District attorneys in 35 of the 36 counties in Oregon determined that the medical examiner does not need to investigate hospice deaths (hospice patients were under the care of a physician). Hospice nurses determine the patient's death and report the death to the appropriate officials. According to the state board of nursing in Oregon, a registered nurse is competent to make a nursing assessment that a patient is dead, record the assessment in the patient's chart, and notify the appropriate health care providers of such death.

One district attorney, however, interpreted this statute to mean that all hospice deaths must be treated as investigations, thus requiring that law enforcement be notified at the time of the patient's death. This meant that law enforcement must come to the deceased person's home and inspect the body to determine whether this death constitutes a crime scene. Hospice nurses in this county found that the presence of law enforcement in the home created unnecessary hardship on the family and, in some instances, emotional trauma to family members. The presence of law enforcement sends a message that the patient's death is suspect, especially since the body is inspected from head to toe for signs of trauma such as bruising, strangulation, or gunshot wounds. As if this were not bad enough, the family members are asked questions about the patient's condition at the time of death, as well as other seemingly irrelevant questions, such as the birth dates of family members, and, in one case, even the birth date of the hospice nurse. Waiting for law enforcement to come to the deceased person's home took up to 3 hours. This demonstrated needless waste of resources, time, and suffering as a result of one district attorney's interpretation of how the law should be implemented (Wilken, 1997).

The variable of public interest played a major role. First, a workshop was convened by the county board of health to discuss the issue with the county commissioners, the district attorney, law enforcement, and the hospice agencies. The public was invited to attend. After the news release about the workshop in the local papers, interested persons starting calling hospice to see how they could help. Over a period of 3 to 4 weeks, many letters to the editor appeared in the local newspapers opposing the presence of law enforcement in hospice deaths. The letters were written by nurses, concerned citizens, and officials such as the executive director of the Oregon Hospice Association. The district attorney received telephone calls by concerned nurses, hospice family members, and angry citizens. After several weeks, the district attorney reversed his decision, stating that it was no longer necessary for law enforcement to be involved in routine hospice deaths (Wilken, 1997).

In this case, the variables of public interest and interest groups played a significant role in the implementation process. Because hospice affects so many lives and deaths, many citizens could relate to the adverse implications of such a policy. Within a relatively short time, the implementation of this policy changed quite dramatically. The district attorney notified the local hospices that hospice deaths would not be investigated by law enforcement officers and the DA would interpret the statute as intended.

Conclusion

Policy implementation is a dynamic process, involving directed change that results in the accomplishment of policy goals. Implementation usually goes through a number of stages, which can be thought of as variables. Identifying the numerous variables involved and the interaction among them is complicated and complex. The basic forces affecting the process encompass legal, bureaucratic, and consensual aspects.

The courts can affect implementation in a variety of ways. The public can initiate a request to the courts through the initiative process. Legislators can draft legislation that refers issues back to the public for a vote in a form called a *referendum*. The courts listen to appeals and can issue temporary restraining orders and permanent injunctions that alter the implementation process.

Much bureaucratic behavior, with emphasis on workability, consistency, and organizational maintenance, may be explained by the legal structure, or lack of structure, imposed by the relevant statutes. The program for implementation should be simple and place as little reliance on bureaucratic processes as possible, because the greater the diversity of proscribed behavior by the policy statute, the greater the discretion of the persons involved in the implementation.

Implementation addresses who is to do what, when, and how. Organizations may be designed to carry out policy implementation if structures do not exist. Institutions can determine their own standards and programs while working within the policy. The effect of implementation on the organization and its staff must be considered. The response of the staff to implementation can vary considerably. Sometimes incentive schemes that promote cooperation can be designed, but the commitment and leadership skill of implementing officials are critical to implementation.

Environmental factors also affect policy implementation. Policies that are linked directly with technology are subject to changes over time as the state of the art advances. Continuous or periodic infusions of political and public support are needed. There is sufficient evidence to indicate that elected officials are influenced by public opinion and that agencies use opinion polls to help support policy positions.

Control is at the heart of the implementation process. Manifestations of control include maneuvers that are categorized as diversion of resources, deflection of goals, dilemmas of administration, and the dissipation of energies. Within each of the categories are strategies and tactics that are often referred to as implementation games.

Research specific to APNs identifies many of the variables involved in implementation. The structure and composition of boards of nursing have an effect on direct third-party reimbursement and prescriptive authority for APNs. Groups of APNs have influenced policy implementation in areas of patient safety, staff mix, and patient outcomes. In addition, consumers have been influential in the implementation process.

One certainty of implementation is that it is unpredictable. During the process, forces at work try to change policy and implementation does not proceed according to plan. These forces involve individuals, groups, organizations, and sometimes the bureaucracy that is responsible for the implementation. Even the best policy will not ensure successful implementation.

In 1997, the Delegate Assembly of the National Council of State Boards of Nursing took a monumental step toward future nurse licensure by proposing a "mutual recognition" concept. The concept means boards of nursing will agree to work toward an interstate compact that would allow a nurse with a license from one state to work in any state, provided she or he follows the respective state's scope of practice (Sharp, 1997). By the middle of the first decade of the 21st century, this movement gained momentum, and many states passed laws that would facilitate nurses working in more than one state with a single license. According to the NCSBN, there are currently 20 states that have enacted the nurse licensure compact (NCSBN, 2003).

The entire nursing community—individual nurses, the state and national nursing organizations, the academic world of nursing, the nurse lobbyists, and grassroots team members—can affect implementation. APNs are in a key position to be valuable players in the advancement of nursing practice.

Discussion Points

1. Describe how the factors of target groups and behavior changes affect the tractability of implementing a standard nurse practice act for APNs.
2. Identify attitudes and resources available from constituency groups that support APNs.
3. Discuss how APNs can affect revisions of basic statutes related to their practice.
4. How did policy decisions of various implementing agencies differ in regard to APN reimbursement?
5. Identify several ways to minimize variation in basic statute interpretations that affect APNs.
6. Discuss the politics of defensiveness used by players in the implementation of prescriptive authority and physician supervision for APNs.
7. Describe the impact (intended and unintended) of direct third-party reimbursement for APNs.
8. What bioethical models in nursing and health care can be extrapolated from the individual ethical problem to a societal ethical problem? In what ways does changing the focus from the individual to society change the model?

References

Afzal, B. (2003). Protecting the health of American communities: Access to information. *Policy, Politics & Nursing Practice* 4(1), 22–28.

American Nurses Association (ANA). (1995). American Nurses Association's response to the Pew task force on health care workforce regulation. *Nursing Trends & Issues* 2(1), 1–9.

American Nurse. (2003, March–April). Barriers to advanced practice outlined to FTC, p. 9 (no author). Testimony is available at http://www.ftc.gov/ogc/healthcarehearings/index.htm.

Bardach, E. (1977). *The Implementation Game: What Happens after a Bill Becomes a Law.* Cambridge, MA: MIT Press.

Blakeney, B. (2003, March–April). Life-altering experiences keep nurses growing. *The American Nurse* (4 pg).

Buchanan, L. and Powers, R. (1997). Establishing an NP-staffed minor emergency area. *The Nurse Practitioner* 22(4), 175–187.

Canavan, K. (1997). Columbia Presbyterian recognized APRNs as primary care providers. *The American Nurse* 29(2), 1.

Charters, K. (2003, Feb.). HIPPA's latest privacy rule. *Policy, Politics & Nursing Practice* *4*(1), 75–78.

Garrett, L. (2000). *Betrayal of Trust.* New York: Hyperion.

Gross, M. (2003). The second wave will drown us. *American Journal of Public Health* *93*(6), 872–881.

Harrington C. and Estes, C. (2001) *Health Policy: Crisis and Reform in the U.S. Health Care Delivery System 3rd ed.* Sudbury, MA: Jones & Bartlett.

Harrison, T. (2002, Nov.). Has the Americans with Disabilities Act made a difference? A policy analysis of quality of life in the post-Americans with Disabilities Act era. *Policy, Politics & Nursing Practice 3*(4), 333–347.

Helminger, C. and Whittaker, S. (1997). Washington watch. *American Journal of Nursing* *97*(2), 16.

Irvine, D., Sidani, H., O'Brien-Pallas, L., Simpson, B., McGillis, L., and Grayon (2000). Organizational factors influencing nurse practitioners' role implementation in acute care settings. *Canadian Journal of Nursing Leadership 13*(3). Retrieved June 6, 2003, from http://www.acen.cjonl.org/NL133/Nl133Dirvine.html.

Keepnews, D. (1997). Is health care regulation really dead? *American Journal of Nursing* *97*(2), 66–67.

Litman, T. and Robins, L. (1997). *Health Politics and Policy* (3rd ed.). Boston, MA: Delmar Publishers.

Locher, A. and Didion, J. (2003). Epidemic to endemic: The impact of HIV on health care policy and nursing practice. *Policy, Politics & Nursing Practice 4*(1), 62–69.

Mazmanian, D. and Sabatier, P. (1983). *Implementation and Public Policy.* Dallas, TX: Scott, Foresman and Co.

Nathan, R. (1993). *Turning Promises into Performance.* New York: Twentieth Century Fund.

National Council of State Boards of Nursing (NCSBN). (1996). National Council of State Boards of Nursing's response to the Pew task force on health care workforce regulation. *National Council of State Boards of Nursing,* pp. 1–6.

National Council of State Boards of Nursing (NCSBN). (2003). Retrieved July 2003 from http://www.ncsbn.org/public/nurselicensurecompact/nurselicensurecompact_index.htm.

Office of Technology Assessment. (1986). Nurse practitioners, physician assistants, and certified nurse-midwives: A policy analysis (Health Technology Case Study 37). OTA- HCS-37. Washington, DC: U.S. Government Printing Office.

Pearson, L. (1997). Annual update of how each state stands on legislative issues affecting advanced nursing practice. *The Nurse Practitioner 22*(1), 18–86.

Pearson, L. (2001). Annual legislative update: How each state stands on legislative issues affecting advanced nursing practice. *The Nurse Practitioner 26*(1), 7–57.

Pearson, L. (2002). The Fourteenth Annual Legislative Update. *The Nurse Practitioner* *27*(1), 10–22.

Pearson, L. (2003). Fifteenth annual legislative update. *The Nurse Practitioner 28*(1), 26–58.

Peterson, C. and Keepnews, D. (1997). Quality and staffing issues dominate the ANA agenda. *American Journal of Nursing 97*(2), 53–54.

Pew Health Professions Commission. (1995, Nov.). Critical challenges: Revitalizing the health professions for the twenty-first century (3rd report.). San Francisco, CA: UCSF Center for the Health Professions.

Quade, E. (1989). *Analysis for Public Decision* (2nd ed.). New York: Elsevier Science.

Reed, S. and Vanderbilt, M. (1997). Reimbursement, patient protection addressed. *American Journal of Nursing 97*(5), p. 20.

Rustia, J. and Bartek, J. (1997). Managed care credentialing of advanced practice nurses. *The Nurse Practitioner, 22*(9), 90–103.

Schildmeir, D. (1997). Using public opinion to protect nursing practice. *American Journal of Nursing, 97*(3), 56–58.

Sharp, N. (1997). Political news and views: Fall 1997. *The Nurse Practitioner 22*(10), 105–112.

Smith, D. (2002). *Entitlement Politics.* New York: Adeline de Gruyter.

Theoduolou, S. and Cahn, M. (1995). *Public Policy: The Essential Readings.* Englewood Cliffs, NJ: Prentice Hall.

Thompson, Frank J. (2001). *Federalism and Health Care Policy Towards Redefinition? In the New Politics of State Health Policy,* ed. R. Hackay and David Rochefort. Lawrence: Univ. Press Kansas.

Trossman, S. (2003). The return of smallpox vaccination. *The American Nurse* March/April, 2003, pp. 1–2, 12.

Trossman, S. (2003). Nurses' Rx for medication errors. *The American Nurse,* May/June, 2003, pp. 1, 2, 12.

Vedung, E. (1997). *Public Policy and Program Evaluation.* New Brunswick, NJ: Transaction Publishers.

Weissert, C. and Weissert, W. (2002). *Governing Health: The Politics of Health Policy* (2nd ed.). Baltimore, MD: The Johns Hopkins University Press.

Wilken, M. (1993). State regulatory boards, regulations, and midlevel practitioners in rural America. (doctoral dissertation). University of Nebraska–Lincoln. *Dissertation Abstracts International* 55-01, p. 14.

Program Evaluation

7

Ardith L. Sudduth, PhD, RN, FNP

Key Terms

Ethical evaluation   Assessment that follows the principals of good conduct and moral behavior.

Evaluation report   Compilation of the findings of the program evaluation study. Reports are presented in a variety of formats depending upon the needs of those requesting the evaluation. Common formats include written reports, electronic transfer, verbal presentations with multimedia enhancements, films, and video tapes.

Outcome evaluation   Assesses the extent to which a program achieves its outcome-oriented objectives. It focuses on outputs and outcomes to judge program effectiveness but may also assess program process to understand how outcomes are produced.

Policy   The purposeful, general plan of action developed to respond to a problem that includes authoritative guidelines. The plan directs human behavior toward specific goals.

Program evaluation   Analyzes social programs to gain an understanding of how well the interventions designed to solve a problem are meeting the objectives and goals set forth in the program's design.

Program evaluation design   The method selected to collect unbiased data for analysis to determine the extent that a social program is meeting its designated goals, objectives, and outcomes and to assess the social program's merit and worth.

Public policy   Provides a definitive course of action, or nonaction, developed by a governmental body that is goal directed.

Qualitative evaluation designs   Evaluation methods that assist the evaluator to determine the subjective meaning of the program and its interventions to the individual participants.

Quantitative evaluation design   Methods characterized as the "scientific model" of collecting measurable, objective data with an emphasis on explanation based upon well-defined expectations and observable events.

Social programs   Solutions developed to help solve an identified problem of human beings.

Theory   Used to design a program and its interventions and to explain and predict broad phenomena observed after data analysis.

Introduction

A dvanced practice nurses (APNs), such as nurse practitioners, school nurses, advanced practice critical care nurses, and others, are rapidly becoming key figures in the provision of health care or health care management of persons enrolled in governmentally funded programs. APNs that are providing care in rural clinics or inner-city clinics usually are there as a part of a program sponsored by the local, state, or federal government. When working with Medicare and Medicaid participants, APNs are participating in governmental programs. Programs funded by governments, nonprofit organizations, and most private foundations require that these programs be evaluated regularly to meet a variety of purposes, including ensuring that the program is being conducted as developed, that there is fiscal responsibility, that goals and objectives are being met and, increasingly, that the outcomes are examined. To assist the APN to meet the often-mandated requirements for program evaluation, this chapter will present some of the components of policy and program evaluation including conditions of evaluation, ethical considerations, potential design choices, and a few suggestions for reporting the results and recommendations of the evaluation.

APNs are not strangers to evaluation. They have long used evaluation in many clinical settings, including the evaluation of a patient's response to a nursing intervention, when using outcome-based clinical evaluations, the evaluation of a management strategy, or a self-evaluation for promotion. APNs are familiar with the use of evaluation in a practice setting. The transition to using these skills to evaluate a program is a natural evolution of nursing practice. The understanding of the process of policy and program evaluation will assist the APN to contribute to the evaluation of social programs by bringing the unique perspective of nursing practice to it. For a long time, the federal government has had a health care policy that has included the funding of hospitals and health care for the elderly. Policies also have funded programs to prepare advanced practice nursing. Health care policies are constantly being modified and in some cases expanded. An example of expansion occurred in the Balanced Budget Act of 1997 that expanded reimbursement to now allow nurse practitioners to bill Medicare directly for services provided. As evidence of additional areas an APN might function in evaluation, this writer examined how small rural hospitals in the Midwest adapted to changing health care policies of the 1980s and the sudden change to reimbursement formulas based on diagnostic-related groupings (Sudduth, 1992).

To meet the health-care needs of a population or to help solve a social problem in the community, the APN may decide to seek funding from a governmental agency, foundation, or other resource to develop a new or unique service. Funding resources, including governments and nonprofit companies, demand that the evaluation process be built into the proposal for funding (Fredricks et al., 2002). Often, it is the APN who studies the needs for a social program intervention, writes the proposal in collaboration with other interested parties, and works to develop the evaluation process. For example, APNs have written proposals for grant money to assist in health education of clients and in well-baby clinics. This author, shortly after joining the staff of a rural clinic, became a member of an evaluation team composed of another nurse practitioner, the sponsoring hospital financial officer, and hospital administrator to write a proposal for a grant to assist in providing an outreach rural clinic in an underserved county in Mississippi. Networks were established, consultation was sought from Mississippi's legislators regarding the need in rural Mississippi, the problem was defined, and a grant application was submitted.

Policy, Public Policy, and Social Programs

To start the discussion of the role of the APN in evaluation of a social program, it is helpful to start at the beginning and define *policy*. One definition of a policy is that it is a purposeful, overall plan of action or inaction developed to deal with a problem or a matter of concern in either the public or private sector. A policy includes the authoritative guidelines that direct human behavior toward a set of specific goals and provides the structure to guide action. Policy provides guidelines to levy sanctions that affect the conduct of affairs (Hanley, 1993). Policies can be determined by the private or public sector and together can have a significant and long-lasting impact on communities and individuals (Center for Health Improvement, 2001). It is also important to remember that public policies are a result of the politics and values of those determining the policy (Mason et al., 2002). One example that most nurses are familiar with is the policy manual found in most hospitals and clinics, which has been approved by authoritative figures such as a board of directors.

Public Policy

Public policy is developed by governments and the courts. A *public policy* becomes a definitive course of action, or sometimes a nonaction, developed by a governmental body that addresses public concerns or public problems (Hanley, 2002). It is goal directed toward some end and does not occur by chance. Public policy is determined by legislative bodies as they make laws, by executive bodies as they administer the laws, and by judicial bodies as they interpret these laws (ANA, 1997). Governments make public policy by making decisions regarding a health issue, such as requiring all children to be immunized before entering school. It may also be a policy for the government to act negatively by adopting a laissez-faire, or hands-off, policy and do nothing about an issue. The decision to do nothing may be as important as the decision to do something. In either case, some groups will be affected. Public policy gives direction to assist decision makers. Consider the thousands of decisions made by the Food and Drug Administration regarding the safety and effectiveness of consumer goods sold in the United States that includes the safety of drugs, vaccines, and the safety, purity, and nutritive value of foods (Anderson, 1975; ANA, 1997).

Public policies may be considered to be either positive or negative. Most programs that focus on the welfare of children; provision of safe water, food, and drugs; and public relief in times of disaster are considered quite favorably by the general public. However, public policies can have a flip side, because they also can create problems. Depending on one's point of view and individual circumstance, Medicare and home-health reform is cause for joy or sorrow. An example quite familiar to many APNs has been the changing policies regarding eligibility for home-health visits. These changes have been a concern of patients, families, home-health nurses, nurse practitioners, and other APNs as all affected parties have had to struggle to ensure essential care is provided. Although the idea of cost containment has been welcomed by some, the stresses and difficulties that are being met by patients, families, and nurses have made some question the wisdom of these changes. It is important that the results of policy changes be carefully evaluated for the multiple outcomes that can be a result of what may appear to be a positive change.

Even though public policy is developed by governmental bodies and officials, it is often influenced by multiple nongovernment persons and environmental factors. For example, in the 1960s, there was increasing concern about the access of affordable hospital care by the elderly. Families, labor unions, physicians, and many others were instrumental in creating the Medicare amendments to the Social Security Act. With the passage of these amendments, the federal government developed a policy of government assistance to provide hospital care to the nation's elderly. Over the years, there have been numerous changes to the initial amendments, many lobbied for by the ANA, but the overall goal of the federal policy of ensuring access to hospital and health care by the elderly, and now other group of citizens, has continued.

Another important dimension of public policy is that it is not limited to a specific law or legislative proposal. Public policy is a dynamic, evolving phenomenon with an ability to adapt as the needs and desires of its citizens change. One cannot go to a book in the federal government and find a listing of *the* American health care policy. Health care policy changes over time. An example is the changing emphasis that occurred in the last half of the

20th century. In the 1940s and 1950s, the focus was on access to hospital care, and Hill-Burton legislation provided funds for many rural hospitals. Medicare amendments were a further extension of access to health care. However, with the rising costs of the Medicare provisions, there has been a major push for cost containment since the 1970s with no end in sight (Jennings, 2001). Health care policy of the new millennium focuses not only on access, but on quality care provided at the lowest possible costs and determined by outcome evaluations. Outcome evaluations are those that focus on the benefits a program produces for the people who use the program (Young, 2000). Trends in health policy will continue to be driven by major trends in the health care delivery system which "is becoming more managed and consolidated, more cost and quality accountable, more consumer focused, and more communication and information technology driven" (Jennings, 2001, p. 224). Nurses can play an important role in the development of policies, including health care policy. In fact, the last revision of the ANA *Code of Ethics for Nurses* added a provision that states that nurses are "responsible for . . . shaping social policy" (Daly, 2002, p. 98).

Health care policy is complex and often influenced by multiple factors such as ethnic diversity, population demographics, finance, agriculture, education, transportation, energy, and housing (Jennings, 2001; Reutter and Duncan, 2002). It has been suggested that an important factor in improving the health of the nation is the development of a healthy public policy that is different from health care policy. A healthy public policy is one that arises apart from health care and recognizes social and environmental influences on health (Reutter and Duncan, 2002). The World Health Organization (WHO) in 1988 defined a healthy public policy as one in which "any course of action adopted and pursued (by a government, business, or other organization) can be anticipated to improve (or has improved) health and reduce inequities in health (Reutter and Duncan, 2002). Reutter and Duncan (2002) define *healthy public policy* as that which "includes but also goes beyond policies that support healthy personal behaviors (e.g. nonsmoking, exercise, nutrition) to policies that address socio-environmental risk conditions such as poverty and working conditions" (p. 295).

Social Programs

Social programs are public policy made visible. Once a problem has come to the attention of the appropriate governmental body, suggestions are made on how to solve the problem. After much deliberation, a solution or program is developed. If the matter is of sufficient concern to the legislative body and if the program has support, legislation is passed to authorize the development of the program and to fund it. Social policies and their effects on the health of individuals, families, and communities have been identified by the ANA Social Policy Statement as a part of nursing care and nursing research (Reutter and Duncan, 2002).

Usually at the legislative level, the goals and objectives of a program are only general in nature. Specifics are frequently left to the developers of the program that provides some flexibility. When Sudduth and her colleagues wrote an application for a rural health outreach grant, general criteria were published in the *Federal Register*. At a meeting of grantees, the diversity of programs that were funded by this agency was amazing. Some of the diverse grants that were awarded included mobile clinics, diabetes education clinics for Native Americans, and teen health in a school system. All the grants for programs identified specific goals, objectives, and projected outcomes that met the generalized goals of rural health outreach. To meet grant requirements, each program designed special methods of evaluation to ensure that the program and the enabling funds are used as outlined in the grant and approved by the Office of Rural Health Policy.

During the decade of the 1980s and 1990s, federal legislators began to return control of some policies to state and local governments in a process of "devolution," which has allowed the federal government to provide funds to the states for social purposes (Jansson, 1999). This allows states to determine how to use the resources with only minimal guidelines from the federal government. This devolution of authority has increased the complexity of social programs, and hence their evaluation, because the policies are interpreted by multiple stakeholders such as state legislators, county boards of supervisors, municipal governments, and sometimes nonprofit, community organizations.

Program Evaluation

A *social program* then is the set of resources and activities that have been directed toward one or more common goals. The resources and activities vary from program to program and can be as small as a few activities, a small budget, minimal other resources, and managed by a staff of one or two. Some programs can be very large with extensive resource allocation, complex activities, and implemented at several sites or two or more levels of government.

Nurses, by the nature of their profession, develop evaluation skills as they work in the health care delivery system in a wide range of roles. Although nurses are familiar with the concept of evaluation, which is the judging of the value, merit, or worth of something (Clarke, 1999), many APNs have not had the opportunity to participate in a formal, planned evaluation process of a policy or program. A formal evaluation has been described as a form of "disciplined inquiry" (Lincoln and Guba, 1985, p. 550) that applies scientific procedures to the collection and analysis of information about the content, structure, and outcomes of programs, projects and planned interventions (Clarke, 1999). Due to the practical nature of evaluation and the fact that it examines social programs established by political entities, program evaluation is influenced by political process and, in turn, influences the political outcomes.

Public policy has generated large numbers of programs intended to improve the lives of citizens in a broad range of life, including health, education, environment, and social services, that would have been unthinkable prior to the 1960s (Light, 2001). The growth of governmental programs at all levels of government has resulted in the need for program evaluation. The importance of program evaluation has also been underscored by federal legislation that mandates it as well as supplying the funding needed to meet the evaluation requirements. The National Performance Review and the Government Performance and Results Act (GPRA, 107 Stat.285, PL 103-62, 1993) was created to focus the evaluation process on accountability, performance measurement, and results. One section of the GPRA mandates performance measures for specified budgeted federal programs for fiscal year 1999 (Fredericks et al., 2002). Because many programs are funded by both federal and state money, states have also become very powerful in requiring evaluation of programs (Guzman and Feria, 2002).

Program evaluation has become a specialized field of inquiry and research over the past 40 years to meet the increasing needs for evaluation. Evaluation provides information to assist others in making judgments about a program, service, policy, organization, or whatever is being evaluated. Evaluation is used to examine the programs to gain an understanding of how the human services policies and programs are solving the social problems that they were designed to alleviate. Program evaluation may be conducted for a wide variety of reasons, many of which are particularly adaptable to the APN's practice. Some of the practical reasons that program evaluation may be conducted include the following (Posavac and Carey, 1992):

- Determine the extent and severity of a problem
- Choose among possible programs
- Monitor program operations
- Determine whether the program has resulted in desired change (outcomes)
- Document outcomes for program sustainability
- Account for funds
- Revise program interventions
- Answer requests for information
- Learn about unintended effects of program
- Meet accreditation requirements
- Determine the extent and severity of a problem

Evaluation designs are used to determine whether a problem is severe enough to require that a program be established to help solve it. In today's world of scarce resources—including time, money, trained personnel, and other valuable commodities—it is imperative that a well-documented program exists. Programs vie for resources, and the one that can show the best justification is the one most likely selected for implementation. Additional information must be supplied to show how the suggested program will solve the problem, what resources will need to be used to bring resolution to the problem, and how outcomes of the program will be evaluated. Resources that must be identified and justified include dollars, time, skilled personnel, equipment, and space to house the program and provide the intervention.

At a local level of examining a community problem and a solution, the author was part of a grant application team that decided to determine whether an underserved, rural county would benefit from a health clinic. Before submitting the application, a careful study of the county and its needs was conducted using published data from the state, emergency room utilization records from the closest hospital, and personal interviews. Based upon the needs study, the projected response to the establishment of a clinic was determined and a grant application was successfully written.

Emergency-room nurses in California were concerned about the potential for violence in emergency departments. A survey was conducted in 1990 by the California Emergency Nurses Association (ENA) Government Affairs Committee of emergency departments in California to determine the severity of violence against emergency-room nurses and what practices were being used to deal with the problem (Peek-Asa et al., 2002). This study was integral to the passage of the California Hospital Security Act (AB508) being implemented in 1993.

Choosing among Possible Programs

Evaluation data may be used to help make difficult administrative decisions. Over the years, there has been an exponential growth in social programs. For example, in just the area of programs for children, it is reported that there are more than 17,500 organizations providing youth programs (Lerner and Thompson, 2002.) All of these programs must compete with multiple other social programs in a community.

Often several excellent social programs have been established and are functioning in a community. When a request comes to add another program, difficult decisions must be made in these days of limited resources. A city may be sponsoring a homeless health care clinic, an after-hours sports program for inner city youth, and a lunch program for the elderly. When it becomes apparent that a program to deal with school violence may need to be added, it may be that it will be added only if another program is eliminated. Program evaluation that provides systematic, reliable, and valid information will certainly assist the administrative staff in making difficult decisions. Unless good program evaluation data exist, decisions are more likely to be made based upon perception, anecdotal evidence, or political pressure (Posavac and Carey, 1992).

Monitoring Program Operations

Monitoring a program has as its primary purpose the tracking and reporting of program outcomes that can provide feedback to the program sponsors and treatment team (Affholter, 1994). In general, new social programs are supported by authorizing legislation or private foundations. Rarely does the legislation or foundation specify in detail what the program is to be or how it is to be implemented. The sponsors or funding sources identify only a set of general goals and some broad guidelines concerning the kind of intervention program that is authorized. The details of program design and implementation are left to the agency or organization that has the authority to administer the program. Demonstration projects are one example of programs that are frequently established to meet general goals and objectives. They focus on a new approach to solving a problem, and if the demonstration project is successful, additional programs may be funded in other locations. Learning how the demonstration project is working to achieve its goals makes replication of the demonstration project easier.

Program monitoring is much easier when the program has been developed with clear, consistent, operational objectives that allow for direct and reliable measurement. The results of monitoring the program can help program managers pay particular attention to a specific performance problem or recognize outstanding achievements of the program. Data resources frequently used for program monitoring include direct observation by the evaluator, program records, surveys of program participants (and nonparticipants), and community surveys (Rossi et al., 1999). Some program sponsors have timely reports that must be submitted for evaluation. Other program sponsors will allow the recipient of a grant to alter the parts of the program sponsored by the grant as long as the intent is not changed. If a school APN develops a program to teach teenage fathers parenting skills and few boys enroll in the program, then the sponsoring agency might allow the program to be expanded to include teen mothers.

Another example of a reason to monitor a social program is the need to know the day-to-day operational difficulties as they occur. For example, during the start-up of a program, there are frequently unavoidable delays in portions of a program, for example, tables and chairs may not arrive at a clinic but the examining tables arrive on time. By keeping a close eye on the operations of the program, glitches can be caught quickly and alternative plans made. New ways to solve problems that were not anticipated, such as when the city closes the street in front of the clinic to widen the street, can be developed promptly.

Determining Whether the Program Has Resulted in Desired Change

Legislative bodies, most nonprofit organizations, and philanthropic organizations request feedback about the program to determine whether the program has achieved the stated goals. Organization officials want to know whether the desired change has occurred, or in other words, what are the outcomes of the program? This has become known as *outcome-based evaluation* and has received increasing attention as a result of the GPRA of 1993. According to the U.S. Accounting Office (GAO) (1998) outcome evaluation "assesses the extent to which a program achieves its outcome-oriented objectives. It focuses on outputs and outcomes . . . to judge program effectiveness, but may also assess program process to understand how outcomes are produced" (p. 5). Outcomes are those benefits the participant receives from participating in the program. The United Way of America provides guidelines readily available on the Web for conducting outcome-based evaluation (McNamara, 1998). See these guidelines at http://www.unitedway.org/outcomes/.

Outcome-based evaluation uses the term *program* to mean a series of services or activities that leads toward observable, intended changes for participants (Moen et al., 2002). A sponsoring agency may require data to show that a program designed to teach diabetic Native Americans better diet control has reached the targeted population and resulted in a reduction in blood-sugar measurements. It is not unusual for sponsoring agencies to require evaluation procedures to determine whether the outcomes observed were the results of the program or whether they would have occurred without the intervention or with an alternative program (Chelimsky, 1987). Systematic data collection for evaluation of goal attainment and fund management is much easier when the program design has included a detailed evaluation design.

Determining outcomes of a program may utilize a variety of techniques, including quantitative and qualitative data collection that is discussed later in the chapter. Impact analysis is one method of outcome evaluation that might be selected because it often uses statistics such as regression techniques to control for initial sample differences, provide unbiased estimates of intervention effects, control statistically for the influence of other explanatory variables, and to assess the impact of variables on the outcome. Statistical studies attempt to sort out the reasons for the observed change. In an impact analysis, the goals and objectives of the program, including the planned interventions, are examined (Schalock, 1995).

Documenting Outcomes for Program Sustainability

Periodic evaluation of the social program, including management, program outcomes, and financial solvency, becomes essential when a program has been designed to be maintained over a long period of time. Careful and precise documentation must be developed to show that the program should be continued because it is achieving the targeted outcomes. Many programs sponsored by governments and other resources provide start-up money, but expect that the program will be designed in such a way that the community, other interested parties, or the program itself will generate the financial, personnel, and other resources to keep it running long after the initial grant money has been used. To ensure additional funding from the same source, or to enable a program to seek additional funding from different government or private agencies, the viability of the program must be established. In today's extremely competitive environment, sustaining a social program requires careful documentation to demonstrate that the program is achieving its goals and objectives and creating positive outcomes. It is also wise for the staff to cultivate good political and public support for the program. Keeping interested persons fully informed of the achievements of the program requires additional work by the program staff, but it may be important in retaining the funding and other support needed to sustain the program. The program staff, including the APN, cannot assume that political or public support will be there just because the program is doing a good job.

Some programs use a cost-benefit or a cost-effectiveness analysis, or both, to relate a program's costs to its results (Levin, 2001). Costs are measured using market values or another technique that simulates market values (Levin, 1987). Cost-benefit analyses are expressed in monetary terms and work well for programs where the evaluator can determine the costs of providing a program balanced against the monetary gains that can be achieved. For example, a cost-benefit analysis of a program to mandate that all children wear bicycle helmets would focus on the difference between dollars spent on equipment and monitoring the use of bicycle helmets and the monetary savings from the medical and rehabilitative costs of trauma. Cost-benefit analysis allows the evaluator to determine whether costs exceed benefits; if they do, then there is reason to look at alternatives. Cost-benefit analysis allows policy makers to compare many programs and determine which programs should be continued or which should be eliminated.

Cost-effectiveness analysis, on the other hand, attempts to determine the benefits of outcomes that are difficult to convert to dollars (Kee, 1994). Cost-effectiveness evaluations are often used to measure outcomes in terms of alternatives that can reach a common goal. Levin (2001) cautions that cost-effectiveness analysis should be used to guide decisions but not to determine them. Feasibility of implementation is also a variable that must be considered.

Accountability in Program Evaluation

Funding Agencies

Grant applications submitted to governmental resources and private foundations require that the program develop methods to ensure that the money being spent on the program is used as directed in the grant. Careful accounting principals must be followed. Most government grants require at least an annual audit report be submitted regarding the use of funds. Some sponsoring governmental groups will make site visits to review financial records and to ensure that everything documented can be verified. However, some grant rules allow for the recipients of the grant to alter the use of funds with special permission of the granting agency. Some grants allow the principal program administrator to discuss the needs verbally, followed by written documentation of the request according to the agency policies and procedures.

The need to request a change in fund allocation can occur even with detailed and careful planning of the program. Circumstances and situations that were not known at the time of the grant application may occur, which require a change in the distribution of the grant moneys. For instance, inflation may raise the costs of an essential piece of equipment, such as the mobile van needed to provide outreach health care. Some grants allow requests to shift funds from one category to another, or within categories, based upon a specific formula. Likewise, if the cost of equipment is less than projected, provision may be made for using the additional funds for a different purpose. However, it is important to always check the rules of the granting agency to be sure financial compliance is maintained.

Revising Program Interventions

Program evaluation provides valuable feedback to provide the essential information needed to make necessary revisions. Programs are usually written by a group of individuals who have the best of intentions as they develop a program based upon the most recent and best data available at the time of writing. Often several months to even years can elapse between the development of an idea for a program and the receipt of funding or other resources allocated to the program. As time elapses, situations change; personnel are recruited with differing backgrounds, personalities, strengths and weaknesses; or the program is administered differently from the original design. It is important to evaluate periodically to ensure that the program is progressing as designed and that if change is needed, revisions are made appropriately.

An excellent example of needing to change the interventions occurred when a cost-effectiveness evaluation was conducted on the program for preventing perinatal human immunodeficiency virus (HIV) transmission (Stoto, 2001). Based on clinical trials published in 1994 that indicated that proper treatment of HIV in the mother could reduce perinatal transmission, specialists in preventive medicine and public health recommended counseling all women at risk of AIDS on the benefits of testing and voluntary testing. This intervention was successful, but in 1996 Congress instructed the Institute of Medicine (IOM) to evaluate how successful states had been in reducing perinatal HIV transmission. Data revealed that only about 60 to 94 percent of women were offered HIV testing during pregnancy. After careful cost-benefit analysis, the IOM concluded that universal testing was cost effective and that universal testing was the best intervention for preventing HIV transmission in the perinatal period. In 1999, the American College of Obstetricians and Gynecologists and the American Academy of Pediatrics issued a joint statement that adopted the universal testing approach of the IOM. The Center for Disease Control (CDC) recommends universal HIV testing for all pregnant women; testing remains a voluntary decision by the pregnant woman (CDC, 2001). This example demonstrates how evaluation can alter interventions and make a difference in a health policy.

Answering Requests for Information

Program evaluation and careful maintenance of records enable the project director to complete the large number of documents required by governmental agencies funding a social program. Periodic evaluation along with meticulous record keeping can provide a ready source for the data required. Otherwise, the person completing the surveys may find that she or he will be required to spend untold hours doing a manual search through the program files.

Learning about Unintended Effects of the Program

Program evaluations can also help discover any unintended effects of an intervention. As APNs know, medications can have good effects as well as negative side effects. Program evaluations are particularly valuable when they have built into them systems to detect unanticipated and unwanted outcomes of the treatment intervention (Posavac and Carey, 1992).

Accreditation Requirements

Many health care facilities are required to evaluate their facilities to meet accreditation standards, which usually have been authorized by legislation. Although meeting these standards may not predict the effectiveness of the programs offered, it does imply that the program meets the standards set by an official accrediting body that serves to increase public trust. APNs in their more advanced roles as nurse practitioners, clinical specialists, and such often are asked to assume a key role in preparing the accreditation self-report and to ensure that the agency and its programs meet the standards.

Theory: A Valuable Tool in Evaluation

The use of theory in program evaluation provides a map to guide the evaluation process. APNs have been using theory to guide their practice for many years, so the use of theory to guide evaluation of social programs is a normal extension of nursing knowledge and practice. *Theory* is defined in research and scientific inquiry as a set of interrelated concepts that explain and predict broad phenomena. A *concept* is an abstract idea about a part of the phenomena. The concepts may include definitions, empirical facts, or propositions that are related to help explain and predict the phenomena observed. Theories do not have the simplicity of laws, nor do they have the same level of certainty (Mason and Bramble, 1997). For example, a theory of illness held by ancients was that illness was the result of offending the gods; the belief that a special illness was the result of angering a particular god is a concept (Trussell et al., 1981). An ideal evaluation theory would describe and justify why certain evaluation practices lead to specific results across the many situations that program evaluators must confront (Shadish et al., 1995).

The use of theory in developing a program and its evaluation is beneficial for evaluators and program administrators. A clear statement of theory gives direction (McEwen, 2002). When a social program is designed, those persons responsible for its development and implementation have some basic ideas of what they plan to achieve (outcome) and have some ideas on how they believe such a program will function to achieve the desired results (Clarke, 1999). Theory-based evaluations provide substantive theory about the problem and help define the conceptual relationship between program implementation and expected outcomes. Theory may also allow the evaluator to have a broader role in the evaluation process than the detached observer (Caracelli, 2000).

A literature search can provide validation for identifying and using a particular theory in a program intervention or evaluation. Sometimes the literature search produces an alternative theory on which to base the program or its evaluation. The use of theory provides guidance in the selection of interventions and evaluation designs. It is helpful to remember that evaluation theory is not an exact science, but is often "made up of a combination of hunches, beliefs, intuitive assumptions, and knowledge founded on practical experience" (Clarke, 1999, p. 31). For example, the school APN who is developing a program to improve the health habits of overweight teenage girls must decide upon a focus of the program. If the APN uses a microeconomics theory that emphasizes the influence of monetary incentives, the program and its evaluation will be designed quite differently than if the APN chooses to use a group support concept of behavioral change (Scheirer, 1994).

Consider one example about the use of a theoretical framework to guide evaluation that comes from the work to meet the requirements of an advanced degree (Sudduth, 1992). The focus of the evaluation project was to examine the impact of the multiple changes in health care occurring in the 1980s on the survivability of small rural hospitals. It quickly became apparent in starting this task that there had to be a way to collect and examine the data to make some sort of sense out of it. After much searching, the evaluation study was organized using a theory of strategic adaptation and a theory of organizational structure used by organizations undergoing change. These theories gave focus to the types of data that would be collected and provided a framework on which to interpret the information learned. Theories help limit the scope of an evaluation project and give it direction, assist in the organization of large amounts of data, and help identify significant factors that need to be considered such as time, money, clarity, and conciseness.

Since the 1960s when evaluation research saw its sudden rise to prominence, the evolution of evaluation research has resulted in increasing diversification as evaluation research has matured. The first evaluation researchers were concerned about methodology and process because the methodological problems were so pressing. Later evaluators would recognize the impact of politics on program implementation. The field's first theoretical integration involved the evaluation of demonstration projects to test new ideas that could be incorporated into existing or new programs (Shadish et al., 1995).

Over time, evaluation theories changed and diversified to reflect accumulating practical experience. Evaluation research began to shift focus from process research to a concern with evaluating the quality of program implementation. By the late 1970s, the strict reliance on quantitative methodology began to include qualitative methods (Lincoln and Guba, 1985). The context of evaluation practice and fitting evaluation results into highly politicized and decentralized systems were part of evaluation research in the 1980s. Today's evaluation research theories recognize more complexities of evaluation practice and integrate more diverse concepts, methods, and practices.

Ethics and Evaluation

Program evaluation, by its very nature, evokes a sense of anxiety in most persons. Questions are asked such as: How does the program measure up? Are we doing a good job? What happens if the evaluator finds a problem with the program? Will the clients lose the service? Will I lose my job? How much information should I share with the evaluator? Will the evaluator be fair? From these questions, it can be seen that the role of the evaluator can create stress and the potential for ethical dilemmas for all involved in the evaluation process. Good program evaluation will plan for the potential for ethical conflict and develop strategies to avoid it or confront the conflicts as they arise during the evaluation process.

Potential Areas of Ethical Conflict

Ethical issues must be considered whenever an evaluation design is planned or an evaluation is conducted by an evaluator. Posavac and Carey (1992) identified several major areas of ethical concern that include the protection of the people treated, the danger of role conflicts by providers, threats to the quality of the evaluation, and the discovery of any negative effects resulting from the evaluation. Put into a slightly different context by Sieber (1980), ethical dilemmas occur in three major areas: (1) conflict between the roles of researcher, administrator, and advocate; (2) conflict between the right to know and the right of privacy; and (3) conflict between the demands of the evaluator, political officials, and/or other significant stakeholders. *Stakeholders* are either individuals or organizations that are either directly or indirectly affected by a social program's implementation or results and who believe they can make a difference the outcomes (Rossi et al., 1999; Sikma and Young, 2003). Nurses in the mid-20th century identified the need for ethical nursing care when the House of Delegates of the American Nurses Association adopted a code of ethics that has been continually updated to reflect changes in society and health care. The latest version now explicitly states the nurse's primary commitment "is to the patient, whether an individual, family, group, or community" (Daly, 2002, p. 98). The newest code reflects on the importance of the nurse's responsibility to participate as an equal in ethical debates (Daly, 2002). Although it can be difficult to confront other individuals involved in the evaluation process who may have higher rank or status than the APN, the *Code of Ethics for Nurses* provides guidance for ethical decision making that takes into account the protection of participants in the program and the role of the nurse.

Protection from Harm: An Ethical Priority

A central ethical concern is that the evaluation should not harm the participant or anyone else involved in the program. One of the first areas of evaluation will be to determine whether the program does any harm to someone receiving the program's intervention or whether the program harms the program staff in any way. Neither the participants nor the members of the program staff should be harmed.

In the process of evaluation, much information is collected to meet the requirements of either the program design or the persons that have commissioned the evaluation. An evaluator must use utmost care so that the program participants and staff do not have their privacy, anonymity, or confidentiality violated. This is particularly true since the passage of the Health Insurance Portability and Accountability Act (HIPPA) of 1996 that went into effect in 2003. HIPPA rules also recognize the privacy and security issues associated with electronic patient information that might be a data resource in a program evaluation (Cheung et al., 2002). A program evaluation researcher must maintain a high level of vigilance to ensure that privacy and security issues are not compromised in the process of data collection, data utilization, or data reporting.

The phenomenal growth of electronic record keeping that allows for the storage of data collected by all levels of government and private organizations has resulted in the ability to link various data sets. For example, data on individuals participating in a government-funded alcohol treatment program may be matched to outcome data in state employment records or law enforcement records. There are many benefits to this technological advance, but also many ethical challenges in terms of privacy and confidentiality (Caracelli, 2000).

Real dilemmas can arise if courts subpoena an evaluator's records and these records contain information that might identify the program participant who has been guaranteed confidentiality. If such a problem arises, the evaluator would need to consult legal counsel. According to Hatry and colleagues (1994), evaluators should continue cautiously and refrain from turning over subpoenaed information until the legality of such a request has been determined. One suggestion to reduce the possibility of identifying specific individuals and undermining confidentiality might include using a code known only to the individual, such as father's birthdate. If such a code were used, the project director would need to keep a master list of the individuals identified by the code in case the evaluator should ever need to access those individuals' records for a specific reason. Often group data are collected so individuals are not identifiable.

Informed consent is a recognized component of all care provided by the APN and is a method frequently used to protect people from harm (Norwood, 2000). Just as patients in clinics are informed about all aspects of a treatment and give permission to do the procedure or treatment, participants in the evaluation process should be informed of the evaluation, what it means, and given a choice to participate or not participate. As part of the informing process, each participant must be made fully aware of his or her role in the program and in the evaluation process. If the evaluation includes treatment and control groups, participants must be fully aware of what this may mean to them, both as a group and as an individual. The APN, whether participating as the evaluator or as a member of the program staff, should be certain that confidentiality and privacy of participants and program staff have been secured in the design and implementation of the evaluation and its report.

Role Conflict: Potential for an Ethical Dilemma

Potential for conflict exists at several levels in program development and implementation. The complexity of the institutional and political networks that have had to evolve among social service providers in order to attain and maintain funding resources in a constantly changing environment, is ripe for conflict as multiple groups form alliances to secure limited resources. (Fredericks et al., 2002). Interested persons in the social program being evaluated may comprise many diverse groups of persons, including the politicians who sponsored the funding legislation, the designers of the program, the recipients, and supporting members of the community. These supporters are often called *stakeholders* because they have a vested interest in the program. Stakeholders may view the program personally, as their "child," and try to protect the program and the participants from outside scrutiny during the evaluation process and the sharing of evaluation results.

Most social programs are designed to implement a larger public policy. As a result, there are many stakeholders who may become involved in the program evaluation process, including the political persons who first created the legislation to create the program, the administrators and other workers in the program, the recipients of the program, and the taxpayers funding the program. It is quickly apparent that many people have a stake in the success or failure of a program and, as a result, there is much opportunity for conflict. Ethical questions arise when some might wish a bad or even a mediocre program to continue when their jobs depend upon the program. Conversely, sometimes taxpayers want good programs ended to save tax dollars. Therefore, it behooves all evaluators to carefully determine the identity of the stakeholders, their concerns, and the real pressures they could bring to bear upon the evaluator and the completed evaluation report. After identifying potential conflicts, a plan can be developed that will avoid them or at least keep them to a minimum.

Dilemmas can occur when programs are developed to deal with socially and politically charged issues. For example, a social problem with moral, religious, political, and social overtones is that of teen pregnancy. Communities have a difficult time coming to a firm conclusion on the best approach to address this teen behavior, and no matter how the program has been developed, there will be stakeholders with conflicting views. This creates an important issue for evaluators to consider as they develop an evaluation plan that provides as clear a description as possible of the program objectives, goals, and outcomes (Guzman and Feria, 2002).

When the evaluator is also the administrator of the program, there is much potential for ethical conflict. It is difficult to wear two hats at one time. If the evaluator is the administrator of the program, it is possible to have role conflict between the role of administrator and evaluator. As the administrator, the role is to ensure that the program runs smoothly with the least amount of interruption. The role of evaluator requires that data collected to evaluate the program may require record examination, interviewing recipients of the program, and discussing the evaluation with staff.

The author had an opportunity to function as an APN nurse practitioner and worked simultaneously with the medical staff and administrator to evaluate the services provided in a rural health clinic. The evaluation team, who were all members of the clinic staff, worked to collect the data, performed the analysis, and wrote a report that included strengths, weaknesses, and suggestions for making the clinic better. The potential for conflict was great because the members of the evaluation team were also key players in the program. Some members of the group also carried more status and influence than others. This group worked hard to be objective in order to provide quality health care to the patients and because there was a high ethical standard among the group to be honest and sincere in the evaluation process. Group members recognized that change can only occur if an objective evaluation was performed.

Objective Program Evaluation: An Ethical Responsibility

Evaluators must conduct sound evaluation studies to answer the questions that have been included in the evaluation design. If the evaluator does not provide a trustworthy evaluation and report it in a timely manner, this may be considered by some as unethical (Posavac and Carey, 1992). Objective evaluation needs to include providing a fair and accurate description of how the program succeeded or how it failed from the perspective of all who were affected by the program (Morris, 1999).

Program evaluators must try to provide the best study possible by selecting the methods and evaluation tools that are most appropriate. It is critical that evaluators select tools for evaluation that are as accurate as possible. Making a mistake in identifying accurately the outcomes of a program, for example, might either allow the program to continue when it should be eliminated or, conversely, the program may be canceled when it should be continued. In both situations, the ethical dilemma is readily apparent.

Another area of ethical concern is to ensure that the evaluation design fits the needs of those who have requested the information (Posavac and Carey, 1992). If the evaluator cannot provide the answers needed by the persons requesting the information, then the evaluator must do the ethical thing and either decline to conduct the program evaluation or request that the evaluation tool be changed so that the evaluator can continue. For example, a program has been designed to help diabetics alter their lifestyles to prolong their lives. At the end of 1 year, the APN is asked to evaluate the program to determine whether the program has made a difference in life expectancy. This would be an impossible task. Good program evaluation could not be done to answer this question because a 1-year period of time is not long enough to determine life expectancy. To agree to do an evaluation to answer this question would create an ethical dilemma. A better question, albeit an extremely limited one, might be to request that the evaluation tool be revised to determine improved disease control as measured by hemoglobin A1C, lipid profiles, incidence of delayed healing, and other such parameters over the 1-year period as a measure of improved self-care.

An evaluator must also consider an ethical responsibility to provide a report promptly so that the results can be used while the program is being implemented. The design of the evaluation needs to be written with enough detail that the procedures used and the process of data analysis could be understood by the persons requesting the evaluation. The report must contain enough detail that someone else later could duplicate the evaluation or read the report and come to the same conclusions.

Reporting Negative Effects: An Ethical Requirement

An ethical dilemma occurs when the evaluator discovers that while many of the objectives of the program are being met, some aspects of the program may be having negative effects. The question becomes how to report these findings so that the data can be used by the program administrators to alter the program. If the negative effect is judged to be serious enough that the harm outweighs the benefits, the program should be ended or revised. An example of a negative result might be a program to establish transportation for the mentally handicapped. If the program's bus had big, bold letters on it that announced it was for the mentally handicapped, some might believe that this was demeaning. The program could be eliminated or altered so that the bus was not labeled and the program could continue.

Suggestions to Reduce Ethical Dilemmas in Program Evaluation

By the nature of social program evaluation, the possibility exists for ethical dilemmas to occur. One of the first things the APN can do to avoid ethical conflict in evaluation is to plan so that ethical dilemmas are avoided. The APN should consent to provide program evaluation only after carefully studying the request and establishing clear guidelines for the study. The APN does not need to determine the "right and wrong" of observed phenomena, but instead must create a working environment that does not compromise or create ethical dilemmas (Morris, 1999).

Good communication is essential throughout the evaluation process but is invaluable when avoiding conflict, especially ethical conflicts. One suggestion that may be helpful would be to establish written agreements between the evaluator, the program requesting evaluation, and any other significant stakeholders who have been identified in the evaluation design. In some cases, it may be helpful to include written agreements regarding the evaluation plan, its implementation, and methods of sharing the result. A clause that provides a mechanism for either party to withdraw from the relationship should be included if issues that cannot be resolved develop as the evaluation is conducted (Sieber, 1980).

It is also important for the evaluator to carefully assess his or her own strengths and weaknesses as well as strong beliefs. An evaluator must be extremely confident in his or her own beliefs and ethical standards and conduct. An evaluator who firmly believes that all homeless people are lazy probably should not be the person participating in the evaluation of a homeless shelter. When the program director and other members of the program staff select an evaluator, it is important that this person be selected carefully so that biases are discovered and another evaluator selected to provide an objective evaluation study.

Ethical-evaluation practice can be challenging in the real-world settings of program implementation. APNs who become involved with a social program or its evaluation must continue to function with clear ethical principals just as in clinical practice. It is imperative that the APN recognize the potential for ethical conflict and develop plans to confront these issues to bring resolution to them. Any comments or questions that cast a shadow on the program can sometimes be taken quite personally by the stakeholders.

The potential for role conflict is quite apparent when a person intimately involved in the program tries to do an objective evaluation of the program. For this reason, outside evaluators are often hired. However, even this group can find they are in a conflict, because to get information from the significant persons in the organization and program recipients, the evaluator must establish good rapport with them. The potential exists that in the process of not offending the persons with the information, the evaluator becomes one of the group and the objectivity is lost.

Suggestions to Avoid Conflict

Program evaluation is complex and involves multiple stakeholders, ranging from powerful political and social leaders to the program implementers and their support staff to the recipients of the program. All of the persons involved are interested in the program at various levels of interest. Five suggestions for program evaluators to assist in avoiding conflict were made by Smith et al. (as cited in Clarke, 1999, p. 17).

1. Recognize the potential conflicts between multiple stakeholders and deal with them in a diplomatic, efficient manner. Attempt to identify the primary and secondary stakeholders. Failure to examine potential and actual conflicts can easily lead to problems throughout the evaluation process.

2. Involve the multiple interest groups in the design of the evaluation study. If each group "owns" a portion of the design and is engaged as an active participant in the process, less chance exists for the varying groups of stakeholders to splinter off or create additional tensions in the evaluation process. Likewise, this approach recognizes the importance of each group and allows for compromises as needed.

3. Keep the multiple stakeholders and members of the evaluation team informed about the progress of the evaluation. It is easier to maintain cooperation among divergent groups if the groups are kept current with the project and given opportunity to provide feedback from their perspective.

4. Ensure that all stakeholders understand the goals and objectives of the program as they have been developed. This helps the stakeholders better understand exactly what the program was established to accomplish and identify the objectives that have been met and those that have not been met.

5. Identify the political and organizational environmental conditions in which the evaluation is being conducted. These situational factors are important to understand throughout the evaluation process in order to develop the design, implement the evaluation project, and disseminate the results.

Program Evaluation Design Options

As discussed earlier, the environment in which program evaluation takes place is often complex with a large number of stakeholders who have been involved in some manner in the development and implementation of a social program. This is especially true as governments have attempted to reduce their size and contain their expenditures. Frequently, government-sponsored programs are involved in a mosaic of community service organizations that have become the implementers or evaluators of the social programs (Guzman and Feria, 2002). It is the multilayered requirements of program evaluation that require careful development of evaluation plans that are acceptable to the many parties involved in the program and the process. Sometimes this requires multiple attempts to find a compromise plan that all stakeholders can accept. Due to the changes in elected governmental officials and often their political appointments to boards and other governing bodies, evaluation plans may need to be renegotiated during the evaluation process.

It is important to determine who holds the power to make decisions regarding evaluations, especially when there are multiple levels of stakeholders involved in the program. School-based programs are key examples of organizations with multiple stakeholders, all of whom interact with each other at varying levels. Federal, state, and local resources may be involved in significant ways with their multiple layers of decision makers. When an APN is asked to participate in the evaluation of a school-based health program, it would be essential that the APN consider the heads of the agencies sponsoring the program's priorities both politically and personally. Next, the school board and superintendent would be recognized as powerful decision makers. School principals, counselors, and teachers provide another layer of decision making. Parents have indirect authority as they can choose to allow their student to participate or not (Guzman and Feria, 2002). Students also influence the outcomes of the evaluation because they control the information that they share with the evaluator. Knowing the chain of command is essential when developing evaluation designs to make certain that decisions can be made to ensure the success of the evaluation process.

The earliest evaluation designs were based on the scientific approach that is founded on the principle of causation. This approach is sometimes characterized as collecting measurable, objective data with an emphasis on explanations based upon well-defined expectations and observable events. The goal of quantitative evaluation is to collect sufficient data to rule out rival hypotheses by such means as control or comparison groups or by statistical adjustments (Datta, 1994). Quantitative evaluation methods seek to be precise and to identify all the relevant variables prior to the data collection. The method also seeks to minimize the role of the evaluator or data collector in the collection of the evaluation data.

The quantitative data design continues to have merit. However, as the complexity of social programs was revealed, additional evaluation designs were needed to determine additional information about how a program was affecting the individual recipients of the program interventions. Evaluation designs began to incorporate the qualitative approach. The qualitative approach has as its basis the belief that it is the quality or the subjective reality that has true meaning in the events, lives, and behaviors of individuals (Datta, 1994; Fine et al., 2000). Qualitative data are used in much of life. It is qualitative reasoning that allows a reader to solve a mystery. The reader can conclude that the butler did it based upon data collected from a variety of sources and combining the information in a qualitative manner (Posavac and Carey, 1992).

Evaluators, using a qualitative approach, attempt to seek an understanding of the meaning of public policy, its attendant programs, and interventions from the perspective of the recipients of the program, the staff, community, and other significant persons (House, 1994). If an inner-city emergency room APN observed that many homeless persons used the waiting room as a shelter, he or she might approach the city to establish a shelter for the homeless. To establish a successful program, the design, implementation, and outcomes of the program would have to include not only the city's point of view but also the needs and views of the homeless themselves. Qualitative issues, such as desire for autonomy by the homeless, can make or break the best intentions of a social program.

The following short discussion of evaluation designs is intended to provide a brief overview of some of the choices that can be made using either a quantitative or qualitative design strategy. These summaries will illustrate the range of available designs that an APN might select when considering program evaluation. To be successful in achieving an evaluation that is useful to the persons who have requested it and to be beneficial to the social program and its recipients, the design of the evaluation must receive careful planning. A good design is like a good road map when planning a car trip from San Francisco to New York. It helps to decide where you are going, how to get there, how long it will take, and how many side trips can be made on a limited budget.

Quantitative Design Strategies

The design of a program evaluation must balance the need to take into account the demand for rigor to assure that relatively decisive conclusions can be reached with the practical considerations of time, money, cooperation, and the protection of the rights of human subjects. A guideline for selecting a design is the "good enough" rule proposed by Rossi and Freeman: "The good enough rule is that the evaluator should choose the best possible design from a methodological standpoint, having taken into account the potential importance of the program, the practicality and feasibility of each design, and the probability that the design chosen will produce useful and credible results" (1993, p. 220).

Experimental Design   The randomized experimental model has been the classic design used in evaluation research to determine the relative effectiveness of two or more interventions or to control conditions. The hallmarks of this design are the utilization of a randomly selected experimental group that experiences a treatment and compares their outcomes with those of a randomly selected control group that does not receive the treatment. Measurements of relevant criteria variable(s) are taken before the program starts and after it ends. Differences are computed and the program is deemed a success if the experimental group has improved more than the control group (Weiss, 1972). A variation of this design, sometimes used with recipients of social programs, is to give the control group the standard, or usual, treatment so that treatment is not denied.

Although the experimental design has often been considered the optimal design for research, this design has a number of limitations that must be carefully considered when used for program evaluation. As stated earlier, the major focus of program evaluation is for practical information on which to base conclusions. The experimental design can be quite expensive in terms of time, dollars, equipment, and personnel, and randomization of subjects difficult. Ethical considerations are also of concern in the selection of participants and the control groups.

Quasi-Experimental Designs   Practically speaking, the true experimental design for program evaluation is not often the design selected by an APN who is probably engaged in an evaluation of a program in which he or she is involved in some way. *Quasi-experimental designs* are studies that seek to establish a cause-and-effect relationship between a dependent and an independent variable with some of the true experimental characteristics missing. Usually the missing element is the random assignment to treatment and nontreatment groups. For example, it is not possible to obtain a control group if evaluating a program that affects an entire population, such as California emergency room nurses who all work under the California Hospital Security Act (AB508) passed in 1993 (Peek-Asa et al., 2002). Sometimes there are ethical constraints that do not permit random assignment to treatment and nontreatment groups such as might occur with new cancer treatment programs. At other times, there might be political opposition to a true experimental model. Quasi-experimental studies can be designed rigorously but with the limitations of the design recognized. A few of the most common quasi-experimental designs are discussed briefly here. For a complete discussion, it is suggested that readers consult one of the many excellent research texts available.

Time Series.   Time-series designs provide a way to measure outcomes and the effectiveness of a program. Cholesterol reduction programs in many clinics are managed by APNs. One design the APN might select to determine if the intense program of education and medication are able to reduce the cholesterol and lipids is a time-series design that allows the evaluator to take a series of measurements at periodic intervals before a program begins and after the program ends. If cholesterol and lipid studies improve, it can be inferred that it was the program that made a difference. In this case, each client would serve as his or her own control.

Comparison Groups.   APNs are often employed by social programs that are not able to use a random assignment to the program or a control group. To determine whether the interventions are successful, the APN may chose to use a comparison group as a control. The control group is "matched" to the intervention group prior to the beginning of the intervention program (Norwood, 2000). Control groups may be selected on an individual basis or in the aggregate. For example, the APN may be working on a program of assisting teenage parents to learn parenting skills. The young people participating in the program might be matched to young people in another school or town on as many similar traits as possible. If individual matching is not feasible, a similar group of teen parents might be matched as a group.

When comparison groups are extremely difficult to obtain, an alternate source of comparable individuals may be found in a timely data base such as statistical records, a survey done for Medicare, or other sources of recorded data (Cheung et al., 2002). This data base may provide a sufficiently large number of nonparticipants to function as a control group. One source of data sets is the collection held at the Inter-University Consortium of Political and Social Research at the University of Michigan (Rossi et al., 1999).

Ex Post Facto Studies.   Sometimes the APN becomes involved in the evaluation of a program after it has been established and functioning for some time. The evaluation design selected in this case may be an ex post facto, or "after the fact," design. This design seeks to determine cause-and-effect relationships between things that have happened already (Mason and Bramble, 1997). Ex post facto designs may be chosen when the selection of a comparison group before beginning the program was not feasible or was overlooked in the process of program development and implementation. A classic example was the evaluation of Head Start programs for disadvantaged children several years after they had been established in many communities (Posavac and Carey, 1992).

Pretest-Posttest.   A frequently used design in ex post facto evaluation is the pretest-posttest design. There are occasions when programs may be initiated and it is not feasible to develop a true experimental research design or to develop a random control group through matching or statistical means. For example, this occurs when nearly all of a significant population is affected by an intervention such as Medicare health insurance. Most senior citizens are eligible for Medicare coverage, so it becomes difficult to compare the health of covered versus noncovered elderly persons. A pretest-posttest design has as its basis of comparison the group itself; that is, two sets of data are collected from the same group. One set is collected and analyzed before the intervention and one set is collected and analyzed after the group members receive an intervention (Brockopp and Hastings-Tolsma, 2003). This design was selected by the writers of an outreach rural clinic grant as a method to evaluate the success or failure of the patient education component of services offered to patients and members of the community.

Pre- and posttest designs do have weaknesses. One weakness is that the results may be caused by something other than the program. Three common problems include changes occurring over time, the changes in secular trends between the two measurement periods, and interfering events that may occur between the two measurement periods (Rossi et al., 1999).

Expert Judgment as Shadow Controls. The use of experts, such as program administrators, respected authorities, or even participants themselves who have been consulted about the program, are known as *shadow controls* (Rossi et al., 1999). Experts (shadow controls) frequently use site visits on which to base their evaluation assessments. Data used include administrative records, observations of the project in operation, and interviews with participants and significant stakeholders and informants. Well-known to APNs are the program experts used by states to visit nursing educational programs to guarantee these programs meet the standards established by state law. APNs may find that they are considered the experts and be asked to participate in a program evaluation.

Even though the use of shadow controls may provide useful information about a program, limitations must be kept in mind and used with caution. Validity and reliability may be checked horizontally, that is, asking other people in the agency or program with technical knowledge of the program to review the evaluation report written by the experts. Checks can also be done vertically by having superiors at different levels in the evaluation office hierarchy review the evaluation report of the experts for such things as technical merit and organizational and political acceptability. At other times, when expert members of the program have conducted the evaluation, the evaluation report may be sent to outside peer reviewers (Averch, 1994).

Statistical Evaluation: Use in Program Evaluation

Statistical analysis is one method of organizing and interpreting a large amount of data into meaningful and understandable information, and it provides a means to summarize, reduce, evaluate, and communicate information (Norwood, 2000). As social programs have become more complex, statistical methods of evaluation have been developed. One approach has been the development of multivariate evaluation designs with intact groups, rather than strict experimental or control comparisons (Schalock, 1995). Often, program evaluators add a statistical consultant to the evaluation team to provide expertise and assistance with the statistical design, interpretation, and communication of this part of the evaluation process.

Qualitative Design Strategies

Qualitative program evaluation, by its very nature, is a flexible methodology. The evaluator using a qualitative approach is not always able to examine the program as a whole. At times, the evaluator must become involved in examining variables, goals, and parts of a program as separate entities (Silverman, 2000). The capacity of qualitative design to afford the evaluator the freedom to discover the unexpected, to change directions, or redesign the evaluation study is considered by some to be one of the major advantages of qualitative evaluation (Bryman, 1988).

Evaluator as Data Collecting Instrument   The success of qualitative evaluation design is quite dependent upon the skills of the evaluator from its inception to its completion. An evaluator uses multiple skills, including an open mind that allows field studies to be conducted without bias. The evaluator-observer, when possible, conducts the observations and interviews personally. When evaluation must be conducted by designated data collectors, they must be carefully trained so that these selected surrogates are as skilled as the evaluator (Caudle, 1994). The ability to remain open to all possibilities is important to the evaluator from inception of the evaluation project, through the conduction of the field study, to the interpretation of the results. It is the keen observations that allow the evaluator to alter the design as needed to ensure good program evaluation.

Interviewing in Qualitative Evaluation   Interviewing skills are an area in which most APNs have already been trained and have achieved a level of excellence based upon education and clinical practice. *Phenomenology*—a qualitative, inductive research method—uses systematic, in-depth interviews to gain insight into a participants personal interpretation of events he or she have experienced (Kerschner and Cohen, 2002). Qualitative evaluation believes the informant's perspective is valuable, meaningful, knowable, and able to be drawn out. Because this qualitative design is extremely flexible, the evaluator-observer must be able to think quickly, to phrase the next question to respond to the informant or to redirect the respondent (Lincoln and Guba, 1985).

Nonparticipant Observation   Sometimes, an evaluator will use nonparticipant observation to collect data to gain a broader and clearer understanding of the program, procedure, or policy being studied. The role of the nonparticipant observer is to be present in the situation without changing the social system. The nonparticipant observer-overt performs no function in the administration or delivery of the program, but identifies him- or herself as conducting research and describes the data that will be collected. The nonparticipant observer does not participate in the group, but watches passively (Nieswiadomy, 2002).

A nonparticipant observer-covert does not inform the subjects that they are being observed. This is considered unethical in most situations

(Nieswiadomy, 2002). Generally, it is best if the persons being observed have given informed consent. Special populations such as children, for example, would need parental consent to be observed. The use of one-way mirrors, hidden cameras, or other such devices may be used as long as the participants have given permission and are aware of their use. An example is a therapy group that may be observed from an adjacent room.

Participant Observation   Sometimes a program design requires a participant observer to collect data. The participant observer is open and candid regarding the observations to be made and the data to be collected. A participant observer has a legitimate role in the field setting, such as a teacher's helper in the classroom or a receptionist in a mental health clinic. As with all evaluation methodologies, issues of privacy and informed consent must be addressed.

Secondary Data Sources in Qualitative Design   Although qualitative evaluation uses direct observation as much as possible, evaluators may also wish to use secondary sources for additional data. Posavac and Carey (1992) use the term *program traces* to describe secondary sources such as physical remains and outcomes of the program or policy being evaluated. Secondary sources can be valuable, nonreactive, and fairly inexpensive. If a community health APN had been working to reduce raw garbage and rat infestations with a neighborhood clean-up program, examples of indirect resources could include the amount of graffiti on walls, evidence of garbage left on the street, planting of flower beds, or the condition of back yards. Examination of program traces can be conducted unobtrusively and without anyone associated with the program being involved. Photographs would be one way to document this type of data collection. This physical evidence plus other data sources such as interviews of residents provide additional depth to the evaluation of a clean-up program.

Selecting the Method for Program Evaluation

Each evaluation team will need to decide how it will evaluate a program. The major issues that determine design selection are needs of the stakeholders requiring the evaluation, skills of the staff to conduct the evaluation, budget (money available), and time limitations (National Science Foundation, 1997).

Selecting the method that best meets the needs of the decision makers or program sponsors is vital to the success of the evaluation process. The use of a combination of evaluation methods usually is needed to complete the evaluation process, especially with today's complex social programs sponsored and implemented by multiple stakeholders, serving an ever-diverse population. It is important for the evaluator to recognize when assistance is needed (McNamera, 2002). There are multiple resources available to assist with any portion of the process that include resources found on the Web; the use of boards and their committees; consultants, including university resources; and knowledgeable members of the community and program staff.

It is hoped that this brief overview of the wide scope of evaluation tools available to the APN will give some brief insights into choices that can be made to conduct program evaluation. It must be repeated that program evaluation designs must be able to provide effective, useful, reliable, and valid information as well as be conducted within the many constraints of real life, such as limitations of resources including time, money, personnel, and expertise.

Some down-to-earth suggestions by McNamara (1998, p. 11) seem particularly useful to the novice APN evaluator. His suggestions include:

1. Don't fear evaluation. Remember the 80/20 rule: The first 20 percent of the work will produce the first 80 percent of the plan. This is a an excellent start.

2. Remember that there is no "perfect" evaluation plan. Getting something done is better than waiting until every last detail has been identified.

3. Include a few interviews in evaluation methods. The stories provide powerful descriptions of the outcomes of the program.

4. Don't review just successes. Failures also give valuable insights into the function and outcomes of the program.

5. Keep the evaluation data after the report has been written. This data may be useful as the program continues and changes overtime.

Evaluation Reports: Sharing the Findings

After the social program has been evaluated, the results of the evaluation study need to be shared with those who have requested the evaluation: significant stakeholders, the staff of the program, the community, and/or sometimes the recipients of the program's interventions. Evaluation, as often mentioned, is time consuming and expensive. It is important that the results of such an important task be used so that the program may be continued, made better, or discontinued.

Six Principles of Reporting

Hendricks (1994) offers six principles of reporting that provide the best information to those who have requested the evaluation and enhance utilization of the report.

1. *The mode of writing and content of the evaluation report is the responsibility of the evaluator.* It is the responsibility of the evaluator to present the results of the evaluation in the form of a report in a timely and appropriate manner. The evaluator must select a format to report the evaluation data, its interpretation, and final recommendations that will be useful to those who have commissioned the evaluation. The evaluation report must be developed to meet the needs of the program, its staff, and the sponsors of the program. The task of presenting a meaningful evaluation report is up to the evaluator(s).

The results are reported factually and unbiased so that anyone can read the data and be able to come to a useful conclusion on their own. A separate section of the report will include the interpretation of the data by the author of the report. Last, the recommendations are presented. When evaluation reports are completed before a program had been targeted for closing, evaluation reports that are given to the staff and program sponsors can provide useful insights into how well the program is meeting its goals and objectives and give guidance for ways to improve the program. Effective communication is essential if the evaluation report is to be accepted and used. Part of the evaluation plan should include plans for communication with members of the program and other interested persons (Posavac and Carey, 1992). When possible, communication meetings should be planned and scheduled at mutually acceptable times and intervals. Evaluators must recognize that sometimes people associated with the program are fearful of the results of an evaluation. To allay some of this fear and potential for poor utilization of the evaluation report, one technique used by evaluators is to first present the report as a draft report. The early presentations provide key persons in the program an idea of the results of the data, some of the interpretations of the findings, and potential recommendations. The early meetings about a draft offer opportunities for valuable comments and discussion between evaluator and program staff and sponsors. After all inputs from the significant readers of the report are taken into account, a final report can be written.

2. *Provide multiple opportunities for presenting the evaluation reports.* Some evaluation reports will be more useful if they are presented to multiple audiences. If the APN has been selected to be the evaluator of a homeless shelter, the more audiences who can learn of the successes and areas of needed improvement, the more likely the APN is to build support for the program. The APN may seek to report to community groups, health care providers, city council members, and the like to reach a larger audience regarding the results of the evaluation. Frequently, community projects need to keep many diverse interested groups informed so that they will remain supportive of a good social program that is meeting its goals and objectives.

3. *Reports should be succinct, with the major points presented clearly.* Writing long, in-depth reports may result in these impressive documents being left on shelves to gather dust or languish in a computer file. Most persons associated with policy and social programs are busy with multiple demands on their time, so a report that addresses the major points quickly may receive more attention. Short, powerful sentences work best to grab the attention of decision makers (Jennings, 2003). The inclusion of an executive summary that gives a brief summary of the main findings and recommendations is appreciated (Clarke, 1999).

Reports are written for the sponsors and stakeholders and, as much as possible, technical terms need to be kept at a minimum. The language of the report is extremely important because "language either consciously or unconsciously shapes perceptions, defines 'reality,' and affects mutual understanding" (Patton, 2000, p. 15). Complex statistical interpretations may need to be simplified, depending upon the audience. Often, simple, descriptive statistics are more meaningful to a lay audience.

It is wise to avoid using jargon, whether evaluation or technical, in the discussion because the readers of the report may not be familiar with the terms and tend to skip over the report without really reading it. A glossary of terms may be helpful to the readers (Clarke, 1999). Many evaluators find that presenting findings in graph form is a useful method of communicating information in a condensed and visible form. Detailed, additional information that is important to the total evaluation process may be put in appendices for those interested in a more detailed and in-depth presentation.

4. *Write the report to catch the interests of the audience.* Whenever possible, the evaluator(s) will find that their evaluation report will have a wider audience if it can be written to address special interests and concerns of those persons who will be receiving the report. Tailoring the report to the audience is important. For example, consider a program developed to improve water quality due to chemical pollution of the groundwater. The APN has been involved in the program to assist families in learning to use only approved water for drinking and cooking. As a member of the evaluation team, the APN would recognize that the report would be written quite technically for the water pollution experts, but could be written more simply for presentation to the local residents of the community.

An evaluation report is also more likely to be used if it addresses some of the particular interests and concerns of key members of the program staff, sponsors, or program participants. If residents are worried about the red-iron color of the water, for example, then this concern should be addressed in the report.

5. *Give direction and provide guidelines for action in the form of recommendations.* The recipients of most evaluation reports want to learn what is good about the program and what areas need improvement. Recommendations for action often are best received if the program staff reports them in identifiable, practical, and achievable terms. General, nonspecific recommendations may be viewed as not helpful, so the report contents will not receive the attention that the report deserves. Unusual or unexpected outcomes must also be reported. If unusual outcomes are presented in a value-free approach with several suggestions for change, the need for improvements will be more readily acceptable.

The question can be asked: How specific should recommendations be? An absolute rule cannot be given to answer this question. In general, recommendations should always be presented as two or more options unless there is only one very obvious recommendation to be made. A specific topic with suggestions for the direction of change may be more effective because it gives those involved in the program direction and flexibility in choosing an approach or making a decision.

Whenever time, budget, and expertise allow, evaluation reports are able to target a larger audience if as many issues as possible are considered. Many recipients of the evaluation appreciate the evaluator giving some indication of the suggested recommendations, such as cost, acceptance, and/or the effects of the recommendations. This allows more of the persons involved in the program or its sponsorship to learn of specific recommendations and increases the likelihood that more of the recommendations will be considered or implemented.

6. *Use multiple communication techniques to disseminate results of the evaluation.* Whenever possible, the evaluator should consider using multiple communication techniques to disseminate the results of the evaluation research. Written reports may be delivered in printed or electronic format. Video tapes, personal briefings, and community meetings are just a few examples of other methods of sharing the results of a program evaluation. The technique(s) used should be appropriate to the audience or audiences.

Program evaluations may be utilized not only by those who have supported, developed, implemented, and/or used the program, but also by "policy entrepreneurs" who use the report as a resource to support new policy ideas (Cabatoff, 2000). A well-written report that defines the evaluation findings in clear, nonpartisan terms may be helpful to those engaged in seeking political support for changes in a broader, public policy (Cabatoff, 2000).

U.S. General Accounting Office (GAO) Requirements

The Hendricks general principles are useful in writing an evaluation report; however, specific guidelines have been developed by the GAO to meet the requirements of the Government Performance and Results Act of 1993 (GPRA) that was passed to hold executive agencies accountable for better management of programs. A detailed guide used by these agencies for their annual reports can be obtained at the GAO Web site (www.gao.gov/special.pubs/gg10120.pdf). Although these guidelines have been established particularly to meet GPRA requirements, they can provide guidance for an evaluator who is writing an evaluation report. These requirements (U.S. GAO, 1998) include the following: (1) identify annual performance goals and measures for each of an agency's programs, (2) discuss the strategies and resources needed to achieve annual performance goals, and (3) provide an explanation of the procedures the agency will use to verify and validate its performance data.

Conclusion

Advanced practice nurses have unlimited opportunities to participate or conduct public policy or program evaluation. Public policy is developed by governments and the courts. Public policy is determined by legislative bodies as they make laws, by executive bodies as they administer the laws, and by judicial bodies as they interpret these laws.

Public policy is determined by governments and put into practice by the development of social programs. Most governmental and other agencies that sponsor social programs require that these programs be evaluated. Evaluation may take many forms, including studying the extent and severity of a problem, determining whether the program is meeting its goals and objectives, conducting a financial audit, examining program outcomes, verifying program outcomes, and seeking information about needed changes in the program.

The tools for evaluation include the quantitative and qualitative methodologies used by social scientists, which are carried out with a rigor needed to meet the needs of the evaluation. Evaluation is expensive in time, money, skilled personnel, and other scarce resources, so it is imperative that the evaluation study be done skillfully and efficiently to meet the varying needs of multiple stakeholders.

After an evaluation has been conducted, the results of the study must be communicated. Some of the important principals of providing an evaluation report that is meaningful and useful include presenting the report to multiple audiences, providing multiple opportunities for others to learn about the evaluation report, writing the report succinctly with the interests of significant others included, giving guidelines for change, and using multiple presentation approaches when needed.

Evaluation of social programs is valuable and can provide very useful information to the APN who is providing care through a funded or sponsored social program. Evaluation can present exciting challenges for the APN who participates in program evaluation and the presentation of the results.

Discussion Points

1. When might an APN be called upon to do program evaluation?
2. Define how policy, public policy, and social programs may play a role in the APN's practice.
3. List the reasons an APN might be a participant or conduct a program evaluation.
4. Under what conditions might the APN use a quantitative evaluation design? Qualitative design? Combined quantitative and qualitative designs?
5. How can theory drive a program design and an evaluation design?
6. Identify the conditions in program evaluation that might lead to ethical conflict.
7. How might the APN avoid ethical conflict when participating or conducting a program evaluation?
8. Identify the components of a program evaluation report.
9. Suggest several ways that the APN might improve utilization of an evaluation report by the sponsors of the evaluation.

References

Affholter, D. P. (1994). Outcome monitoring. In J. S. Wholey, H. P. Hatry, and K. E. Newcomer (Eds.), *Handbook of Practical Program Evaluation* (pp. 96–118). San Francisco, CA: Jossey-Bass.

American Nurses Association (ANA). (1997). *Legislative and Regulatory Initiatives for the 105th Congress.* Washington, DC: American Nurses Publishing.

Anderson, J. E. (1975). *Public Policy-Making.* New York: Praeger.

Averch, H. A. (1994). The systematic use of expert judgment. In J. S. Wholey, H. P. Hatry, and K. E. Newcomer (Eds.), *Handbook of Practical Program Evaluation* (pp. 293–309). San Francisco, CA: Jossey-Bass.

Brockopp, D. Y. and Hastings-Tolsma, M. T. (2003). *Fundamentals of Nursing research,* 3rd ed. Boston, MA: Jones and Bartlett.

Bryman, A. (1988). *Quantity and Quality in Social Research.* London: Unwin Hyman.

Cabatoff, K. (2000). Translating evaluation findings into "policy language." In R. K. Hoopson (Ed.), How and why language matters in evaluation. *New Directions for Evaluation 86,* pp. 43–54.

Caracelli, V. J. (2000). Evaluation use at the threshold of the twenty-first century. In V. J. Caracelli and H. Preskill (Eds.), The expanding scope of evaluation use. *New Directions for Evaluation 88,* pp. 99–111.

Caudle, S. L. (1994). Using qualitative approaches. In J. S. Whole, H. P. Hatry, and K. E. Newcomer (Eds.), *Handbook of Practical Program Evaluation* (pp. 69–95). San Francisco, CA: Jossey-Bass.

Center for Disease Control (CDC). (2001, Nov. 9). Recommendations and reports: Revised recommendations for HIV screening of pregnant women. Retrieved June 20, 2003, from http://www.cdc.gov/mmwr/preview/mmwrhtml/rr5019a2.htm.

Center for Health Improvement. (2001). Sacramento, CA. Retrieved June 12, 2003, from http://www.healthpolicycoach.org/doc.asp?id=5213.

Chelimsky, E. (1987). The politics of program evaluation in evaluation. In D. S. Cordray, H. S. Bloom, and R. J. Light (Eds.), *Evaluation Practice in Review 34,* pp. 5–21. San Francisco, CA: Jossey-Bass.

Cheung, R. B., Moody L. E., and Cockram, C. (2002). Data mining strategies for shaping nursing and health policy agendas. *Policy, Politics, & Nursing Practice 3,* pp. 248–260.

Clarke, A. (with Dawson, R.). (1999). *Evaluation Research: An Introduction to Principles, Methods and Practice.* London: Sage Publications.

Daly, B. J. (2002). Moving forward: A new code of ethics. *Nursing Outlook 50,* pp. 97–99.

Datta, L. (1994, Spring). Paradigm wars: A basis for peaceful coexistence and beyond. In C. S. Reichardt and S. F. Rallis (Eds.), *The Qualitative-Quantitative Debate: New Perspectives 61,* pp. 53–70.

Fine, M., Weiss, L., Weseen, S., and Wong, L. (2000). For whom? Qualitative research, representations, and social responsibilities. In N. K. Denzin and Y. S. Lincoln (Eds.), *Handbook of Qualitative Research,* 2nd ed. Thousand Oaks, CA: Sage Publications, pp. 107–131.

Fredericks, K. A., Carman, J. G., and Birkland, T. A. (2002, Fall). Program evaluation in a challenging authorizing environment: Intergovernmental and interorganizational factors. In R. Mohan, D. Bernstien, and M. Whitsett (Eds.), *New Directions for Evaluation,* 95, pp. 5–21.

Greipp, M. E. (2002). Forces driving health care decisions. *Policy, Politics & Nursing Practice 3,* pp. 35–42.

Guzman, B. L. and Feria, A. (2002, Fall). Community-based organizations and state initiatives: The negotiation process of program evaluation. In R. Mohan, D. Bernstein, and M. Whitsett (Eds.), *New Directions for Evaluation,* 95, pp. 57–72.

Hanley, B. (1993). Policy development and analysis. In D. J. Mason et al. (Eds.), *Policy and Politics for Nurses* (pp. 3–17). Philadelphia, PA: W.B. Saunders.

Hanley, B. E. (2002). Policy development and analysis. In D. J. Mason, S. W. Talbott, and J. K. Leavitt (Eds.), *Policy & Politics in Nursing and Health Care*, 4th ed., pp. 55–69. St. Louis, MO: Saunders.

Hatry, H. P., Newcomer, K. E., and Wholey, K. E. (1994). Improving evaluation activities and results: An introduction. In J. S. Wholey, H. P. Hatry, and K. E. Newcomer (Eds.), *Handbook of Practical Program Evaluation*. San Francisco, CA: Jossey-Bass.

Hendricks, M. (1994). Making a splash: Reporting evaluation results effectively. In J. S. Wholey, H. P. Hatry, and K. E. Newcomer (Eds.), *Handbook of Practical Program Evaluation* pp. 549–575. San Francisco, CA: Jossey-Bass.

House, E. R. (1994, Spring). Integrating the quantitative and qualitative. In C. S. Reichardt and S. F. Rallis (Eds.), *The Qualitative-Quantitative Debate: New Perspectives 61*, pp. 13–22.

Jansson, B. S. (1999). *Becoming an Effective Policy Advocate*. 3rd ed. Pacific Grove, CA: Brooks/Cole.

Jennings, B. M. (2003). A half-dozen health policy hints. *Nursing Outlook 51*, pp. 92–93.

Jennings, C. P. (2001). The evolution of U.S. health policy and the impact of future trends. *Policy, Politics, & Nursing Practice 2*, pp. 218–227.

Kee, J. E. (1994). Benefit-cost analysis in program evaluation. In J. S. Wholey, H. P. Hatry, and K. E. Newcomer (Eds.), *Handbook of Practical Program Evaluation* (pp. 456–487). San Francisco, CA: Jossey-Bass.

Kerschner, S. W. and Cohen, J. A. (2002). Legislative decision making and health policy: A phenomenological study of state legislators and individual decision making. *Policy, Politics & Nursing Practice 3*, pp. 118–128.

Leavitt, J. K. and Mason, D. J. (Eds.) (1998). Policy and politics: A framework for action. *Policy and Politics in Nursing and Health Care*, 3rd ed., pp. 3–28. Philadelphia: W. B. Saunders.

Lerner, R. M. and Thompson, L. S. (2002). Promoting healthy adolescent behavior and development: Issues in the design and evaluation of effective youth programs. *Journal of Pediatric Nursing 17*, pp. 338–344.

Levin, H. M. (2001). Waiting for Godot: Cost-effectiveness analysis in education. In R. J. Light (Ed.), Evaluation findings that surprise. *New Directions for Evaluation 90*, pp. 55–68.

Levin, H. M. (1987, Summer). Cost-benefit and cost-effectiveness analyses. In D. S. Cordray, H. S. Bloom, and R. J. Light (Eds.), *Evaluation Practice in Review 34*, pp. 83–97. San Francisco, CA: Jossey-Bass.

Light, R. J. (2001). Editors Notes. Evaluation findings that surprise. *New Directions for Evaluation 90*, pp. 1–2.

Lincoln, Y. S. and Guba, E. (1985). *Naturalistic Inquiry*. Beverly Hills, CA: Sage Publications, p. 550.

Mason, D. J., Leavitt, J. K., and Chaffee, M. W. (2002). *Policy & Politics in Nursing and Health Care* (4th ed., pp. 1–18). St. Louis, MO: Saunders.

Mason, E. J. and Bramble, W. J. (1997). *Research in Education and the Behavioral Sciences*. Madison, WI: Brown & Benchmark.

McEwen, M. (2002). Overview of theory in nursing. In M. McEwen and E. M. Wills (Eds.), *Theoretical Basis for Nursing* (pp. 23–47). Philadelphia: Lippincott Williams & Wilkins.

McNamara, C. (1998). Basic guide to program evaluation. Retrieved May 25, 2003, from http://mapnp.org/libraryu/evaluatn/fnl_eval.htm.

McNamara, C. (2002). *Nuts and Bolts Guide to Nonprofit Program Design, Marketing and Evaluation*. Minneapolis, MN: Authenticity Consulting.

Moen, W., Simpson, C., Mason, F., and Wetherbee, L., (2002, December 10). A white paper on outcomes evaluation: Concepts, strategies, and practical applications. *The Texas Center for Digital Knowledge, University of North Texas*. Retrieved July 22, 2003, from Project web site, www.unt.edu/needz. www.unt.edu/needz/EvaluationPaper/EvaluationWhitePaperFinal10Dec2002.d

Morris, M. (1999). Research on evaluation ethics: What we have learned and why it is important. In J. L. Fitzpatrick and M. Morris (Eds.), Current and emerging ethical challenges in evaluation. *New Directions for Evaluation 82* (pp. 15–24). San Francisco, CA: Jossey-Bass.

National Science Foundation. (1997). National Science Foundation's Handbook, 1997. Retrieved June 20, 2003, from www.ehr.nsf.gov/EHR/REC/pubs/NSF97–153/CHAP_1.HTM.

Nieswiadomy, R. M. (2002). *Foundations of Nursing Research*, 4th ed. Upper Saddle River, NJ: Prentice Hall.

Norwood, S. L. (2000). *Research Strategies for Advanced Practice Nurses*. Upper Saddle River, NJ: Prentice Hall Health.

Patton, M. Q. (2000). Overview: Language matters. *New Directions for Evaluation 86*, pp. 5–16.

Peek-Asa, C., Cubbin, O., and Hubbell, K. (2002). Violent events and security programs in California emergency departments before and after the 1993 hospital security act. *Journal of Emergency Nursing 28*, pp. 420–426.

Posavac, E. J. and Carey, R. G. (1992). *Program Evaluation: Methods and Case Studies*, 4th ed. Englewood Cliffs, NJ: Prentice Hall.

Reutter, L. and Duncan, S. (2002). Preparing nurses to promote health enhancing public policies. *Policy, Politics, & Nursing Practice 3*, pp. 294–305.

Rossi, P. H. and Freeman, H. E. (1993). *Evaluation: A Systematic Approach*, 5th ed. Newbury Park, CA: Sage Publications.

Rossi, P. H., Freeman, H. E., and Lipsy, M. W. (1999) *Evaluation: A Systematic Approach* (6th ed.). Thousand Oaks, CA: Sage Publications.

Schalock, R. L. (1995). *Outcome-Based Evaluation*. New York: Plenum Press.

Scheirer, M. A. (1994). Designing and using process evaluation. In J. S. Wholey, H. P. Hatry, and K. E. Newcomer (Eds.), *Handbook of Practical Program Evaluation*. San Francisco, CA: Jossey-Bass.

Shadish, W. R., Jr., Cook, T. D., and Leviton, L. C. (1995). *Foundations of Program Evaluation: Theories of Practice*. Newbury Park, CA: Sage Publications.

Sieber, J. E. (1980). Being ethical: Professional and personal decisions in program evaluation. *New Directions for Program Evaluation 7*, pp. 51–61.

Sikma, S. K. and Young, H. M. (2003). Nurse delegation in Washington state: A case study of concurrent policy implementation and evaluation. *Policy, Politics & Nursing Practice 4*, pp. 53–61.

Silverman, D. (2000). *Doing Qualitative Research: A Practical Handbook.* Thousand Oaks, CA: Sage Publications.

Stoto, M. A. (2001). Preventing perinatal transmission of HIV: Target programs, not people. In R. J. Light (Ed.), *New Directions for Evaluation 90*, pp. 41–53.

Sudduth, A. L. (1992). Rural hospitals use of strategic adaptation in a changing health care environment (unpublished doctoral dissertation). University of Nebraska, Lincoln.

Trussell, P., Brandt, A., and Knopp, S. (1981). *Using Nursing Research: Discovery, Analysis, and Interpretation.* Wakefield, MA: Nursing Resources.

U.S. General Accounting Office (GAO). (1998, April). *The Results Act: An Evaluators Guide* to *Assessing Agency Annual Performance Plans.* Retrieved June 20, 2003, from www.gao.gov/special.pubs/gg10120.pdf.

Weiss, C. (1972). *Evaluation Research: Methods of Assessing Program Effectiveness.* Englewood Cliffs, NJ: Prentice Hall.

Young, D. (2000). Outcome-based planning and evaluation: What are they and why should I care? *Rehabilitation Review 11.* Retrieved June 20, 2003, from http://www.vrri.org/rhb0500.htm.

Online Resources

AcademyHealth. Provides links to 3,200 health services researchers in health policy http://www.academyhealth.org/.

Agency for Healthcare Research and Quality (AHRQ) home page. Provides links to multiple resources, http://ahcpr.gov/.

Authenticity Consulting. Free management library with over 675 online resources for program evaluation, personal, professional, and organization development. Many detailed guidelines, work sheets, etc., http://www.managementhelp.org/.

CDC Evaluation Working Group. Multiple links to program evaluation information, www.cdc.gov/eval/resources.htm.

Center for Health Care Policy and Evaluation. Helpful health services research and policy links, http://www.centerhcpe.com/links.html.

United Cerebral Palsy Association, Greater Utica, New York, area. Multiple links to outcome measurement and program evaluation, http://www.ucp-utica.org/uwlinks/outcomes/html.

United Way of America. Outcome measurement resource network with resources for methods in evaluation and social research. Free resources for methods in evaluation and social research, including how-to-do-evaluation research, http://gsociology.icaap.org/methods/.

University of Illinois at Chicago evaluation team. A guide to using evaluation reports, http://www.uic.edu/depts/psch/idhs/User's Manual.htm.

The Internet and Health Care Policy Information

8

Ramona Nelson, PhD, RN

Key Terms

Bookmark   A browser function that saves the URL for an Internet site on the user's computer. The user can then return to the site by clicking on the bookmark.

Browser   A software application that displays information found on the Internet. Examples include Netscape and Internet Explorer.

Home page   The starting point or first page for a Web site. This page usually provides an overview of what is available on the site.

Host   Any computer system connected to the Internet. A host is indicated by its domain name. With virtual hosting, it is possible for a single computer to host several different domains.

Hyper text markup language (HTML)   A coding language used to create Web pages on the Internet. It provides the links to other Web materials, as well as formatting instructions for how the screen should be displayed.

Internet site   An Internet location usually consisting of a collection of documents.

Link   A word, phrase, graphic, or address that, when clicked on, loads a related Web page.

Search engine   A computer program or group of programs that search a database relating the term or group of terms selected by the user to locate information in the database. The Internet is a database of Internet sites and can be searched with a search engine.

Signature file   A user-created file that will insert a message at the bottom of an e-mail message identifying the sender.

Uniform Resource Locator (URL)   Resource locators used by the World Wide Web as addresses for information. The URL will connect the user directly to a particular document or page.

User interface   Screens that are presented to the user when that user interacts with a computer program. If the set of screens presented to the user makes it easy for the user to interact with the software program, the program is referred to as *user friendly.*

Web page   A site on the Internet that uses HTML as its interface. Web pages are viewed with a browser. A page may include graphics, text, sounds, and video.

Introduction

With hands-on experience of the realities of health care, the advanced practice nurse (APN) is in a position to truly understand the need for new health care policies and the impact of current health care policies. However, it is impossible for the APN to effectively act as a health-policy advocate for the patient, the family, and the community if the APN does not understand the process for developing and implementing health policy. Knowledge of the policy process requires an understanding of the whole process, from agenda setting through policy and program evaluation. Understanding the process makes it possible for APNs to provide the needed leadership—individually and collectively—through professional and other interest groups. Leadership demands anticipatory performance in which the APN foresees health problems and solutions and initiates appropriate movement in the public sector. It is incumbent on the nurse in advanced practice to know how to access data, to present information, and to build a case to which public officials will listen. The APN must be information-literate and possess the skills needed to access, evaluate, and use information resources. Many of these resources can be tapped electronically through computers at home or at work. Electronic resources allow expert nurses to expand their comprehension of a problem, frame an argument, suggest one or more solutions, recommend policy tools in designing those solutions, and construct evaluation models for determining success or for making administrative decisions about continuation, change, or termination of a program.

This chapter introduces the APN to key health policy Internet sites and the process of using an Internet browser to search for health care policy data. These sites include government, universities, and organizations. The chapter explores how the Internet is changing the development of health care policy. The author does not assume the reader is an experienced Internet user; however, she assumes that the reader has access to an Internet browser and a basic understanding of how to use that browser. A *browser* is a software program that makes it possible to view documents on the World Wide Web (WWW). The browser "reads" the coded pages that reside at an Internet site and translates the code into a Web page as seen by the user.

Information Literacy and Health Policy

Information Literacy Defined

In 2000, the American Library Association approved information literacy standards for higher education. They defined *information literacy* as a set of abilities requiring individuals to "recognize when information is needed and have the ability to locate, evaluate, and use effectively the needed information" (Association of College and Research Libraries, 2000, p. 2). An information-literate person is able to:

- Determine the information needed
- Access the needed information
- Evaluate the accessed information
- Incorporate the information into what is already known
- Use the information in achieving a goal
- Access and use information ethically and legally

These standards apply to all graduates of a baccalaureate or higher degree education program. An APN should be able to apply these standards in accessing and using health-policy data in all steps of the health-policy development process from agenda setting through policy and program evaluation.

Using the Internet to Locate Information on the World Wide Web

As of January 2003, there were over 72 million hosts on the Internet (Internet Software Consortium, 2003). Historically, a *host* was defined as the main computer system to which users are connected. Each machine had its own domain name indicated by the URL. However, the definition of a host has changed in recent years. It is now possible for a single machine to provide a home for multiple hosts. Referred to as *virtual hosting*, a single machine acts like multiple systems and has multiple domain names and IP addresses. Each host can include numerous Web pages. For example, if a user is connected to Slippery Rock University, the Internet address or URL for the host is http://www.sru.edu. At this site, there are several Web pages related to the university.

A *Web page* is the screen that is seen when the Internet site is accessed. A *home page* is the first Web page of an Internet site, often thought of as a "front door" to the site. Traditionally, a home page contains an introduction to the site, an overview of the resources available at the site, and connecting links. A home page may have several links to Web pages that are part of the site or to Internet sites located elsewhere.

A *URL* is the Internet address for a site on the Internet. It functions as a traditional post office address. Each host on the Internet has a unique URL. If the user already knows the URL of a site, typing this information directly into the browser will immediately access that site. For example, Duke University maintains an excellent health-policy resource site. The URL is http://www.hpolicy.duke.edu. Typing this URL in the browser will provide immediate access to the Duke University health-policy home page. The home page links with several other Web pages on this site as well as other hosts and pages with health-policy information.

Using Search Engines   If the nurse knows the topic he or she is interested in, but does not know specific sites, a search engine and/or directory site is needed. The main function of a search engine site is to find Internet resources based on specific criteria, such as topic, date, or agency. These sites can offer both a search engine and/or a directory of related topics. The directories have information about sites and are organized by topics. The search engines provide the opportunity to look up references or sites based on key words. Search engine sites may offer both directories and online searching or only the online searching function.

Search engines and directories are designed and maintained on the Internet by various companies. Each company that provides a search engine has its own URL. Some examples include Google (http://www.google.com), Altavista (http://www.altavista.com), and Lycos (http://www.lycos.com). Several sites on the Internet maintain a list of search engines with links to the engines. One example can be located at http://www.sru.edu/pages/3128.asp.

Directories are usually more useful at the beginning of a search when background information about a topic is needed or when one is not sure where to start. Although directories are organized by topics in hierarchical structures, there are no standards to how these are structured. Sometimes it is useful to browse the directories or even search them with a search engine because health-policy data can be located in several areas. For example, the topic "health policy" can be located under medicine, government, or community.

Even though the overall functions offered by a search engine are similar, each company has taken a different approach to offering these functions. Each of the search engines and Web pages located on Internet requires time, effort, and money. Each company or institution that maintains a search engine expends this time, effort, and money for a reason. The search engine may be a commercial venture or it can be an attempt by a government agency to make citizen access more effective and efficient. The motivation behind the search engine has a major impact on how it is designed and functions. Each engine has a different user interface. This means that the screens will not be identical and the method of entering key words will vary. Search engines can also vary in the type of information they provide, how they locate information, and how they present the information they have located. These types of sites contain tutorials and help pages that explain how to use their sites.

Many people who prefer a specific search engine will bookmark the URL. When a site is bookmarked, the URL is saved in the browser and the user will not need to remember or type in the URL again. The bookmark function can be accessed through the main menu across the top of the browser. Click on the term *Bookmark* in Netscape or *Favorites* in Internet Explorer. Select ADD from the submenu. The URL will now be saved as part of the submenu and can be selected again in the future. To access the URL at a point in the future, return to BOOKMARK or FAVORITES and click on the saved URL.

With any Internet site, you may receive a message that "the server is down or not responding." This will happen if the site is busy or if the sponsor of the site is having technical problems or updating the site. The best approach in this situation is to try the site at a later time. Another problem is that Internet sites disappear or reorganize and previously located files can disappear. When this happens, you will get a message looking somewhat like this:

The page cannot be displayed.
The page you are looking for is currently unavailable. The Web site might be experiencing technical difficulties, or you may need to adjust your browser settings.

Sometimes it is possible to locate a document by searching the site if it still exists. Other times, the document is gone forever. That is why it is a good idea to print a copy of documents you are planning to cite or use in future research.

Locating Search Engines   Several different types of information exist on the Internet. These include Web pages, listservers, and people data. A general search engine may search for any and all of these or be limited to a specific type of information. A search engine also can be designed to search a specific site. For example, the URL for the U.S. Government Printing Office (GPO) is http://www.gpo.gov/. This site, referred to as GPO, disseminates official information from all three branches of the federal government using both a directory and site-specific search engine.

Another approach to locating and using general search engines is the use of megasearch sites. There are two types of megasearch sites. One provides a consistent interface to searching several different search engines. The ALLIN1 search page located at http://www.allin1.com/about/about.htm offers an example of this approach. A second approach is to search using a number of search engines at once. One example of this type of site is Dogpile, located at http://dogpile.com/info.dogpl/. Dogpile is a meta-search engine that searches other search engines such as About, Ask Jeeves, FAST, FindWhat, Google, LookSmart, Overture, and many more (InfoSpace, 2003). There are also sites that list sites of search engines. Exhibit 8–1 displays several of these types of sites. Many of these sites include information about using search engines. The last site provides a list of search engines that seeks government documents. A general or topic specific search engine will search for Web pages; there are also search engines that search for specific types of information such as listservers, people data, and health sites.

Listservers   A *listserver* is a virtual group of people with a common area of interest who communicate by means of a distribution electronic mail (e-mail) list. A virtual group exists on the Internet but not in the traditional spatial dimension. Individuals with an area of common interest join a list by subscribing to the listserver. Once they have joined the list, members read messages posted to the list or send messages to other subscribers. Those who reply to listserver messages should be aware that these messages are read by all subscribers; that

---

EXHIBIT 8–1 **List of Search Engines**

Home Page for the Site
http://www.searchengines.com/

http://searchenginewatch.com/

http://www.allsearchengines.com/
http://www.beaucoup.com/
http://lplcat.lacrosse.lib.wi.us/reference/

URL for the List of Lists
http://www.searchengines.com/
searchengine_listings.html
http://searchenginewatch.com/
links/article.php/2156221
http://www.allsearchengines.com/
http://www.beaucoup.com/
http://lplcat.lacrosse.lib.wi.us/
reference/govengines.htm

BOX 8–1 **Search Engines for Finding Listservers**

http://www.tss.qld.edu.au/resource/list98.htm

http://www.lsoft.com/catalist.html

http://tile.net/search.php

http://groups.yahoo.com/

---

is, replies should not be made unless the sender wants the whole listserver to read them. Subscribers also can send or post messages to individual members on the list by using the Internet e-mail address of the individual. In this way, a reader can respond specifically to another listserver member with some degree of confidentiality and without all members reading the response.

Box 8–1 lists four Internet sites that can be used to search for listservers focused on policy-related issues.

Many of these sites also explain how a listserver works and the process for subscribing. The APN may want to search different search engines using the key words "health policy." If health policy does not produce a successful result, try searching for a list with just the term "policy." With each of these search engines, the APN will find several different listserver groups. The search engines will return overlapping, but different, results. Some of the listserver groups focus on specific areas of health policy while others are more general. If a specific listserver looks interesting, it is usually possible to learn more about the list before subscribing. Exhibit 8–2 is a screen shot with an example of the kind of information that can be available.

People Data Several search engines on the Internet are specific to finding people. These are search engines that can be used when the APN has a name and needs to find the person's phone number, e-mail, or postal address. It is also possible to do a reverse lookup by entering the phone number and searching for the person's name. A list of these search engines for finding people is included in Box 8–2.

EXHIBIT 8-2

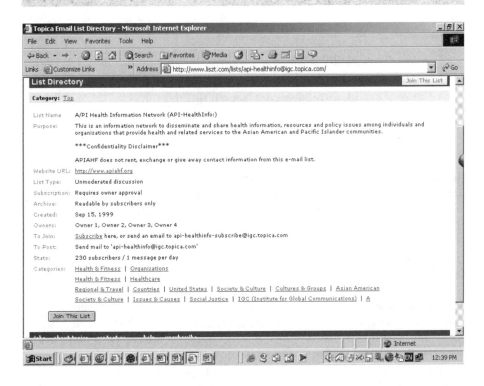

BOX 8-2   Search Engines for Finding People

http://people.yahoo.com/

http://www.whowhere.lycos.com/

http://www.anywho.com/

http://www.bigfoot.com/

http://www.peoplesearch.net/

These lists are sometimes referred to as the *white pages*. If the person the nurse is looking for is not located in the first search engine site, try searching at another site. Each search engine accesses a different database; therefore, the search results will vary. Most educational institutions and government sites maintain a directory of individuals who are employed at that institution. However, these types of directories are much less common at health care institutions and commercial sites.

Health Sites Search engine sites may also be topic specific. There are several that are specific to health. Like general search engine sites, topic-specific sites can include a directory and a search engine. Lists of health-specific search engine can be located at the following URLs:

- http://doradus.einet.net/galaxy/Medicine.html
- http://www-sci.lib.uci.edu/~martindale/Medical.html
- http://www.virtualfreesites.com/search.health.html
- http://www.medexplorer.com/

Key Words in a Search for Health Policy-Related Resources

Health care policy is an interdisciplinary field. It is of interest to health care providers, administrators and consumers, employers who provide health care benefits, companies that provide health care services and products, elected and appointed government officials, and academic and not-for-profit institutions that study or fund the study of health care policy issues. These interested parties can focus on a specific health problem or they can focus on the delivery of health care services. Depending on the specific issue, a wide range of terms can be used to search for health-policy data on the Internet. Regardless of the issues, there are some general terms that tend to locate health-policy data. These include administration, economics, law, management, policy, and statistics proceeded by the terms *health* or *medical.* How these words are combined can have a major impact on the results that are returned.

When doing a search, the most common problem is to have too many hits, many of which are not of interest. There are several approaches that can be used to narrow the search, thereby making the search results much more specific. In the majority of search engines, enclosing the terms in quotes (e.g., "health law" or "medical economics") identifies the term as a phrase resulting in a more specific search. If these are not in quotes, documents that include both or even either of these terms may be listed in the results.

Boolean operators are often used to construct queries or searches in data-based materials. These operators consist of a number of conjunctions (i.e., AND, OR, NOT, or ADJ). Their function is based on the work of George Boole who established the field of symbolic logic.

Using the Boolean operator AND between terms will also narrow the search. For example, health law AND children AND smoking will return documents that include all three of these terms or phases. A document with the terms *children* and *smoking* but missing the phase *health law* would not be in the former search results. Putting a plus sign (+) in front of a term has the same impact as using AND between terms. This approach would appear as health law + children + smoking. Some search engines will let the user select the option "all of the terms" when entering search terms. This also functions as an AND operator between the terms. However, the use of a term in a document does not always mean that the document contains information on that term. For example, a document that includes the notation, "This article focuses on health law and smoking as it applies to adults. Health law and smoking related to children is not discussed" would be included in the search results.

The more terms that are used with the AND operator and the more specific these terms are, the more likely the search will return the specific documents that are of interest. However, there are also times when the search results are too few. In this case, it is necessary to expand the search. Decreasing the number of terms and phases between the AND operator and using less specific terms will increase the search results. Using the Boolean operator OR can also expand the results. For example, the search for children OR kids OR pediatric will return documents that include any of these terms. In other words, if one document discussed pediatric patients and smoking, and a second document discussed children and smoking, both documents would be returned in a search if the operator OR had been used. Search engines often include the option "any of the terms" when entering a search. This option has the same effect as using the OR operator.

Evaluating Internet Resources

The Internet can provide almost unlimited access to information. However, access to information does not ensure the quality or credibility of the information. The Internet is open to all. Anyone with a limited knowledge of hypertext markup language (HTML) can design and post a Web page on the Internet. Anyone with access to e-mail can send a message to a listserver group or post to a newsgroup. On the Internet, the information of the highest quality is mixed with the worst of misinformation. It is the responsibility of the user to evaluate the information and separate quality information from misinformation. APNs know the existence of misinformation is not unique to the Internet. The evaluation of health-related information is not a new process for the APN who has years of education and experience in this process.

Much of the background has been gained by evaluating printed materials from a variety of sources as well as verbal data from colleagues and clients. These experiences have provided the APN with a set of informal criteria that are quickly used when presented with new information. For example, the advantages of a new treatment protocol are viewed differently when seen on a nightly news show than when presented at a professional conference. Health-related information is frequently presented in vanity publications and advertising materials. The APN will be more confident about the accuracy of information about the same topic if the information is presented in a professional journal article. However, on the Internet, many of the cues used by APNs are missing or altered. For example, a publication from a major research university could be considered a reliable source. However, a Web page located at the same university could be a very unreliable source. The Web page could be the personal home page of a student with no supervision, knowledge, or experience related to the topic. Therefore, the APN needs to apply criteria that are sensitive to Web-based issues. Two types of criteria can be identified: (1) criteria for evaluating information in general, and (2) criteria that are specific to health information. A great deal of work has been done in developing and applying criteria for health information on the Internet.

However, much of this work is directed at consumers of health care services, and the criteria do not apply well to health-policy information. The criteria for evaluating information in general is much more applicable.

Links versus Content   Many of the URLs presented in this chapter are "lists of lists." This means that most of the sites identified provide a list of pointers to other sites. These other sites contain primary source data as well as links to other related Web pages. Some of these links to other Web pages even point back to the URL that was included in this chapter. The Internet is organized by interlinking data. The URLs selected for this chapter were chosen because they are considered quality sites. However, this does not ensure the quality of the information at the linked site. A site can decide what links or pointers to include on its Web page. A site does not have control over the content or the links at the linked site. In other words, the APN may start at a reliable site and, by following links, end up at an inaccurate data source. Use the links to move around the Internet; however, when a primary data source is reached, it is at this point the APN should apply Internet evaluation criteria.

Internet Evaluation Criteria

Author. If the material being reviewed is a document, the first step is to determine the reliability of the author. Is the author of the information named? If the author is named, can the academic credentials, professional reputation, and affiliation be established? This information may be included on the Web page. There may even be a link to the curriculum vitae. The fact that author data are included does not ensure that the author data are accurate or current. Many universities, foundations, organizations, and government agencies include directories on the Net. Directories can be accessed to validate the author data. One can also use search engines for people data presented in this chapter. From these sources, the APN can obtain the phone number, e-mail, and/or postal address of the author. If the author of the document is not available, the Internet site may provide clues about the accuracy and reliability of the information.

Sometimes the source of the information is a Web page. Initial information about the site can be identified from the URL. The extensions or domains used to represent the type of organization include edu for education, com for company, gov for government, and org for organization. Directly in front of the domain extension is the institution's name, usually in abbreviated format. Information in front of the institution name indicates the specific location of the Web page at that institution. For example, the Slippery Rock University home page URL is http://www.sru.edu. Remember that the existence of a Web page at a site does not ensure that there is any overview process related to the individual Web page. For example, universities rarely supervise faculty or student home pages. What can be even more confusing is that sometimes a URL is sold to a new organization with a completely different mission. For example, the URL for the Computer-Based Patient Record

Institute was http://www.cpri.org. This URL now returns a blank page, but for a period of time, it returned a pornographic site.

Many times it is important to learn more about the specific organization sponsoring the Web page. On the home page, look for a link that uses the term *about* or a similar term. This link should provide information about the mission of the organization, the funding, structure, leadership, and history. If this information is not available, be careful. Always remember: Someone is paying for that Web site, and it is important to know the source of your data. For example, use of the search engines for a Internet search using the terms abortion AND health policy. Note the wide range of organizations that have posted information on this topic.

Timeliness. Even good information can become outdated misinformation. If you have located a site using a search engine, you may have noticed a date in the search engine results. The date indicates the last time there was a physical change made to the Web page. It does not indicate that the information on the page was updated. Many Web pages include the date of the last update as well as the author of that update. Sometimes there are dates included in the content on the Web page that provide a clue as to the currency of the information. If there is no update date and no dates referenced in the content, it is impossible to know how old the information may be.

Content. Important parts of health-policy information are opinions and viewpoints. Review the content to determine whether it is presenting facts or opinions. Evaluate whether the information presented is well-written and easy to understand. Determine whether the depth and breadth of the content are appropriate. If the information is accurate, it should be consistent with other sources. The APN should be able to validate Internet information with information from other sources. If the information that the APN has accessed on the Internet is timely content from a reliable source and consistent with information from other sources, then the information can be useful in the process of developing health policy.

Internet Evaluation Criteria Sites   The Internet provides an overwhelming amount of information mixed with misinformation. As the need increased for the user to determine what quality information is and what misinformation is, Internet sites related to this question evolved. Box 8–3 includes selected sites with evaluation criteria and tools for evaluating all types of information on the Internet.

BOX 8–3   **Criteria for Evaluating Information on the Internet**

http://www.ciolek.com/WWWVL-InfoQuality.html

http://www.library.jhu.edu/elp/useit/evaluate/

http://www.library.ubc.ca/home/evaluating/

http://school.discovery.com/schrockguide/eval.html

> **BOX 8–4** **Criteria for Evaluating Health Information on the Internet**
>
> http://www.uic.edu/depts/lib/lhsu/resources/guides/web-evaluation.shtml
>
> http://www.bettycjung.net/Quality.htm
>
> http://www.cancer.gov/clinical_trials/doc.aspx?viewid=C68637AF-2AEB-479D-AB60-228118D9674E
>
> http://www.aarp.org/health/Articles/a2003-03-17-wwwhealth.html
>
> http://www.healthfinder.gov/aboutus/selectionpolicy.htm

Box 8–4 includes Web sites for evaluating health care information on the Internet.

Key Health Policy-Related Sites on the Internet

Two questions guide the organization of key health-policy sites on the Internet. The first question asks who develops and who uses the sites. The answer to this question includes those interested in health care policy, including health care providers, administrators, and consumers; employers who provide health care benefits; companies that provide health care services and products; elected and appointed government officials; and academic and not-for-profit institutions that study or fund the study of health care policy issues. The second question asks what type of data and information are used in studying or developing health policy. These data and information can be grouped into four areas:

1. data related to the regulatory and legislative process
2. viewpoints and policy positions from interested groups, including businesses, health-related organizations, and universities
3. statistical and research results used in developing health policy, and
4. funding or granting agencies including foundations, insurance agencies, and government.

When selecting sites for inclusion in this section of the chapter, the author used three guidelines. First, Internet sites appear and disappear with great frequency. The sites noted in this chapter are reliable sources and can be expected to be maintained over a period of time. It is important that the APN realizes that at least one URL referred to in this chapter will be nonfunctional by the time the chapter is printed. That is why the first part of this chapter covering information literacy is important. As the Internet constantly changes, the reader must be able to find new and evolving sites. The second guideline was to select sites that included access to large databases or well-developed lists of links to key sites. This helps to preserve the credibility of the data and increases the probability that the nurse can access additional data from many points. The third guideline pertained to selecting sites of general value to health policy and not limiting them to a specific issue within the field of health policy. In this way, the APN can take the broadest approach to finding information and begin to narrow the list, rather than become stymied if a first, narrow search is nonproductive.

Four general sites—government-related, academic, health-policy organizations, and health-law resources—contain URLs to sites that can provide the APN with a wide range of information. Each is described briefly, and common URLs are provided.

Government-Related Sites

Government-related sites include sites from the executive, legislative, and judicial branches of the federal government, state government sources, local government sources, and international government sources.

GPO Access (http://www.access.gpo.gov). This is a service of the U.S. Government Printing Office that provides access to a wealth of important information and products distributed by the federal government. GPO Access is one of the leading online sources for free, official government information. The available resources cover all three branches of the federal government. Included are more than 2,800 separate databases through more than 80 applications including the *Congressional Record*, the U.S. Code, General Accounting Office (GAO) reports, congressional bills and reports, public laws, the *Federal Register*, and many more. In total, more than 145,000 titles are available on GPO servers, and more than 92,000 additional titles are linked from GPO Access (U.S. Government Printing Office, 2003). The home page for GPO Access organizes information into the following categories:

- Legislative resources (i.e., congressional bills, U.S. Code)
- Executive resources (i.e., code of federal regulations)
- Judicial resources (i.e., Supreme Court Web site)
- A comprehensive list of all federal resources available via GPO
- Local federal repository library location
- U.S. Government online bookstore
- *Ben's Guide to the U.S. Government* (an age-appropriate resource for understanding the structure and function of the U.S. government)
- GPO Access user support

In most cases the electronic documents appear on the day of publication, exactly as they appear in print. These electronic documents, like the print versions, are the official published versions.

National Technical Information Service (http://www.ntis.gov). The service is a branch of the U.S. Department of Commerce. It is the official resource for government-sponsored U.S. and worldwide scientific, technical, engineering, and business-related information. The National Technical Information Service is the largest central resource for government-funded scientific, technical, engineering, and business-related information available today. Each year it receives on average more than 1,000 new publications, technical reports, and other health care-related products (National Technical Information Service, 2003).

Duke Center for Health Policy, Law, and Management (http://www.hpolicy .duke.edu/cyberexchange/Whatleg.htm). This site provides extensive links to the legislative branch of the federal government as well as links to Senate standing committees, House committees, and joint committees. Included are links to:

- THOMAS—Federal Legislative Information (Library of Congress)
- U.S. House of Representatives Internet Law Library
- U.S. Legislative Branch (Library of Congress)
- Congressional directory
- U.S. House of Representative Web sites
- U.S. Senate Web sites
- U.S. Code (contains the text of all general and permanent laws of the United States enacted by Congress)
- VOTENET (with information for tracking local congresspersons' voting records and contacts)

World Health Organization (http://www.who.ch). This site is the home page for the organization. It provides electronic access to numerous reports on international health programs. WHO Library Information System (WHOLIS) is the World Health Organization's library database available on the Web. Included are indexes of all WHO publications from 1948 to date.

Note: *The World Health Report 2002, Reducing risks, Promoting Healthy Life* is one of the largest research projects ever undertaken by the World Health Organization. The report measures the amount of disease, disability, and death in the world today that can be attributed to some of the most important risks to human health. WHO then calculates how much of this present burden could be avoided in the next 20 years (WHO, 2003).

WHO Statistical Information System (WHOSI) is a guide to epidemiological and statistical information available from WHO.

The National Conference of State Legislators (http://www.ncsl.org/) and The Forum for State Health Policy Leadership (http://www.ncsl.org/ programs/health/forum/forum.htm). The first group was founded in 1975 as a resource for lawmakers and staffs of the 50 states. The forum was established in 1995 under the direction of the National Conference of State Legislators. In an effort to help state legislators and their staff stay current on health care policy issues, the Web site includes links to workshops, issues briefs, and newsletters.

The National Association of County and City Health Officials (NACCHO) (http://www.naccho.org/). NACCHO is a nonprofit membership organization serving and representing local public health agencies (including city, county, metro, district, and tribal agencies). NACCHO provides education, information, research, and technical assistance to local health departments and facilitates partnerships among local, state, and federal agencies in order to promote and strengthen public health. This site includes current information about health-policy issues as well as links and tools for understanding the process for influencing health policy. For example, a link to http://www.healthpolicycoach.org/ takes you to the Health Policy Coach. The Health Policy Coach is designed to equip you with the tools, strategies, and information necessary to create policy change in the community.

Academic Sites

A number of universities and research institutions have established health policy-related sites. These sites include links to a number of other government and non-government-related sites.

Duke Center for Health Policy, Law, and Management (http://www.hpolicy .duke.edu/cyberexchange). This site contains extensive links to a wide range of government and nongovernment health policy-related links. It includes links to U.S. health care system profiles and general health information sources.

Center for Health Law Studies at the Saint Louis University School of Law (http://law.slu.edu/healthlaw/research/links/topical.html). The center maintains an extensive list of links to Internet resources about health policy. Included are links to specific topics, such as aging and elder law, foundations, health financing, and public-health laws.

University of California, Los Angeles (UCLA) Center for Health Policy Research (http://www.healthpolicy.ucla.edu/). The center focuses on understanding and advancing public-health policies that can improve access to health care as well as promote good health among diverse populations in California and the nation. Key areas of interest include:

- Access to health care and insurance coverage
- Health promotion and disease prevention
- Management of chronic conditions
- Public programs and the finance and systems of health care

As part of its public service mission, the center maintains online access to its research data and results. These are made available at no cost to the public through reports, policy briefs, and fact sheets.

Ohio University (http://www.library.ohiou.edu/libinfo/depts/hsl/ htpoly.htm). The site is maintained by Cheryl Ewing at the university library in Athens, Ohio. It includes links to health policy-related associations, companies, directories, institutes, organizations, U.S. government sources, universities, articles, reports, and journals.

Universtiy of Pennsylvania Center for Bioethics & Department of Medical Ethics (http://www.bioethics.upenn.edu). This site is a key resource for evaluating the ethical issues within health policy. The center's stated mission is "to promote scholarly and public understanding of the ethical, legal, social and public policy implications of advances in the life sciences and medicine." This site includes an introductory course on bioethics with several resources for learning more about this topic as well as links to other Internet resources.

University of Wisconsin Center for the Study of Bioethics and Office of Research (http://www.mcw.edu/bioethics/). One of the primary resources is the Bioethics Abstract Service. This is the largest, free, searchable database of abstracts of key bioethics journal articles in the world. It is updated regularly and includes abstracts from bioethics journal articles, legislative actions, and court decisions that are not easily accessible elsewhere.

Edmund S. Muskie School of Public Service, Institute for Health Policy (http://muskie.usm.maine.edu/research/research_institutes_ihp.jsp). This site is a resource for APNs who are concerned with research and health policy. "The Muskie School's Institute for Health Policy conducts nationally recognized research and policy analysis to identify and promote solutions to complex health care challenges." Major areas of focus include children's health, health care finance and access, mental health, rural health, chronic illness, health care quality, and public health. The site contains a reference list of published papers and a list describing several funded research studies.

National Health Policy Forum (NHPF) (http://www.nhpf.org/). The forum is housed at Georgetown University. The site is designed to support informed decision making and informal off-the-record communication on issues surrounding health care policy. It serves mainly senior staff in Congress, the executive branch, and congressional support agencies. The site provides access to a wide range of issue briefs that are short, analytical reports on a wide range of health-policy issues, information on site visits around the United States, and an extensive list of links to other Internet resources.

Health Policy Organizations

AcademyHealth (http://www.academyhealth.org/index.htm). Previously the Academy for Health Services Research and Health Policy, AcademyHealth is a professional society consisting of 4,000 individuals and 125 affiliated organizations. AcademyHealth was established in June 2000 following a merger between the Alpha Center and the Association for Health Services Research (AHSR). The members are health-services researchers, policy analysts, and practitioners. The mission of the society is to be a leading, nonpartisan resource for the best in health research and policy: "AcademyHealth promotes interaction across the health research and policy arenas by bringing together a broad spectrum of players to share their perspectives, learn from each other, and strengthen their working relationships."

Moving Ideas Network (MIN) (http://www.movingideas.org/). Formally known as the Electronic Policy Network, MIN is interested in "explaining and popularizing complex policy ideas to a broader audience." The goal is to improve collaboration and dialogue between policy and grassroots organizations and to promote their work to journalists and legislators. Some examples of key sections of the Internet site include:

- "Weekly Round Up" features research, articles, and other resources from member organizations.
- "The Blitz" supplies facts from member organizations and others.
- Feature articles present original articles and op-eds from member organizations, other progressive organizations, and independent writers on current sociopolitical events.
- "In the Spotlight" includes quick news bites, statistical data, and timely articles from around the Web. This is updated 5 days a week.
- "Moving Ideas Network" is a project of *The American Prospect* magazine. Links from the home page explain this relationship, other resources offered by this organization, and the aim of the magazine.

Health Law Resources

Legal Information Institute at Cornell University (http://www.law.cornell .edu/). The institute offers one of the most extensive collections of legal information on the Web and links to a wide array of U.S. and international legal reference Web sites. It includes Internet-accessible sources of constitutions, statutes, judicial opinions, and regulations. For example, this site archive contains all opinions of the court issued since May 1990.

FindLaw (http://www.findlaw.com). This site is not limited to health-related information. It includes an extensive directory of links to legal information and sites as well as a law-focused search engine.

Impact of the Internet on the Process of Developing Health Policy

The Internet is changing the process of health-policy development in four primary ways:

1. improved access to health data and information
2. development of large electronic databases that can be data mined
3. better communication between all stakeholders
4. provides new opportunities for all citizens to participate in health-policy development

The following initiatives demonstrate the federal and state governments efforts to improve communication and policy development in all areas including health care.

FirstGov.gov (http://www.firstgov.gov/index.shtml). It is designed as an easy-to-use portal that provides access to all Internet-posted documents of the federal and state government. A portal approach to government documents provides a centralized place to find all information located on U.S. local, state, and federal government agency Web sites. To improve communication and search results, the developers are working with government agencies to encourage portals organized around customer groups and topics, instead of agency names. Examples of cross-agency portals include seniors and people with disabilities.

Regulations.gov (http://www.regulations.gov/). At this site, citizens can review and submit comments on federal regulations that are open for public comment and published in the *Federal Register.* The site makes it easy to determine what regulations are open for comment. Comments may be linked to the regulation or submitted to the appropriate agency. This site recorded 184,177 hits during June 2003 with an average of 6,139 hits per day (E-Gov Home, 2003).

E-Gov (http://www.whitehouse.gov/omb/egov/). This site provides an overview of the president's e-government initiatives. The goal of this project is to improve Internet-based technology, thereby making it easy for citizens and businesses to interact with the government, save taxpayer dollars, and streamline citizen-to-government communications (E-Gov Home, 2003).

U.S. Department of Health and Human Services (http://aspe.hhs.gov/sp/nhii/faq.html). The National Health Information Infrastructure (NHII) can be envisioned as a national electronic health care system. NHII infrastructure will enable enterprise-wide integration of information among all sectors of the health care industry. It will consist of three overlapping focused areas. These are:

1. personal health—includes a personal health record that is created and controlled by the individual or family
2. health care delivery—includes information such as provider notes, clinical orders, decision-support programs, digital prescribing programs, and practice guidelines
3. Public health—enables sharing of information, such as vital statistics, population-health risks, and disease registries, to improve the clinical management of populations of patients

Conclusion

This chapter has introduced the reader to a number of key health policy-related sites on the Internet. The first section prepared the reader for searching and locating new and interesting health-policy sites. Each of the sites selected for inclusion includes links to a number of other important health-policy sites. Because the Internet is a network and not a hierarchical structure, the links will interweave and overlap. In other words, the reader may reach any of the health-policy resources included here from several different starting points or through many juxtapositions. The Internet and the various links within the

Internet are constantly changing. The existence, location, and content of sites change frequently. The information-literate APN can use these sites to access enormous amounts of data and information as well as evaluate the quality of the data and the usefulness of the information. Through this information, the APN can use that data to effectively influence current public policy makers and thereby improve the health care of individuals, families, and communities.

Discussion Points

1. Using the terms health policy AND research AND nursing, conduct a search on the Google search engine located at http://www.google.com. Repeat the search using the same terms at the Lycos site located at http://www.lycos.com. Compare the results from these two searches. Which search engine found the greatest number of sites? Which search engine found the most useful list of sites? How does each site differ in presentation of information about the sites found? Both of these sites will let you do a more focused search. Look at the home page for both of these search engines to determine how to conduct a more focused search. Conduct the searches on both search engines and compare your results.

2. Use the listserver search engines to search for a listserver group that is of interest to you. Find the directions for signing on to the listserver. Once you have signed on, you will begin to receive e-mails that were posted to the group. Select a topic that is being discussed by the participants on the listserver and conduct a literature search on this topic. You may find MEDLINE, CINAHL, or Lexis-Nexis to be a useful resource for doing your literature search. Do the data that you found in your literature search support or contradict the point made by the participants on the listserver? Why do you think this would occur?

3. Use the Internet to identify your elected representatives to both houses of the U.S. Congress, and locate the e-mail addresses for these representatives. Send an e-mail to each of the representatives asking his or her position on third-party payment for advanced practice nurses. Compare the responses. Look at who responded to your e-mail. Was it the representative or one of his or her staff? Was the response individualized to your question or was it an e-mail version of a form letter? Did the representative or the staff person express an interest in your opinions about this issue?

4. Each state decided on prescriptive authority for advanced practice nurses. How can you use the Internet to locate individuals and organizations that support prescriptive authority in your state?

5. Both the U.S. House of Representative and the Senate maintain a home page on the Internet. Locate these home pages. Both houses use a committee and subcommittee structure for the purpose of considering legislation, conducting hearings and investigations, or carrying out other assignments. In both houses, health-policy issues are considered in a number of different committees and subcommittees. Use the located home pages to identify the names of all committees and subcommittees that would consider health-policy issues. You will also find the names of all committee members. Use these sites to identify what current health-policy issues are being considered in the various subcommittees and what representatives are important contacts. If you are accessing the Internet from a computer that has the capability, find the C-SPAN link and attend a hearing.

6. Select a health-policy topic that is of interest to you. For example, you might select smoking or access to health care for children. Locate the home page for the

Library of Congress. You may find the name Thomas Jefferson of help in your search. The Library of Congress has several different databases that you may search. Determine whether either the House of Representatives or the Senate is considering any current bills related to your topic. Search the catalogs of the library to determine whether there are related references in the collection. What other resources at this site provide you with information about your topic?

7. The U.S. House of Representatives Internet Law Library contains the text of current public laws enacted by Congress and is searchable. Locate this site. Be sure to read the introduction to this site so you know what codes are located there. Using your topic from Question 6, identify what current laws already exist. From this site, can you find any state laws that apply to your topic?

8. Almost all current Supreme Court opinions are on the Internet. One of the most complete collections is maintained by the Cornell law school. Find this site and determine which Supreme Court opinions relate to your topic.

9. Another key resource for understanding laws and regulations that relate to your topic are the executive orders from the executive branch of the federal government. These can be found in the White House Virtual Library. Locate this site, and then search the site for any executive orders related to your topic.

10. This chapter contained several sites focused on health-policy research. Locate these sites, and determine whether there are any current or published research studies related to your topic. Are there any researchers interested in your topic?

11. Use the FirstGov.gov site to determine whether there are other federal or state documents pertinent to your topic and not located on the sites you have already reviewed.

References

Association of College and Research Libraries. (2000). *Information Literacy Competency Standards for Higher Education.* Chicago: American Library Association.

E-Gov Home. (2003). Home page. Retrieved July 27, 2003, from http://www.whitehouse.gov/omb/egov/.

Internet Software Consortium. (2003). Internet domain survey FAQ. Retrieved July 6, 2003, from http://www.isc.org/ds/faq.html.

InfoSpace. (2003). About Dogpile. Retrieved July 8, 2003, from http://www.dogpile.com/_1_2T58UGNO3E81HEW__info.dogpl/about/corporate/about.htm.

National Technical Information Service. (2003). Subject coverage of the NTIS collection. Retrieved July 24, 2003, from http://www.ntis.gov/about/coverage.asp?loc=6–4–0.

U.S. Government Printing Office. (2003). Fact sheet. Retrieved July 19, 2003, from http://www.access.gpo.gov/public-affairs/gpofacts.html.

WHO. (2003). *World Health Report.* Retrieved July 20, 2003, from http://www.who.int/whr/en/.

Global Connections

9

Jeri A. Milstead, PhD, RN, FAAN

Key Terms

Grassroots response   Spontaneous reply to a social problem, often in contrast to a planned answer prepared by a formal organization.

Problem fading   A tendency for interest in a current problem to diminish. Declining attention can occur due to inaction, replacement by a more important issue, or lack of mobilization of resources.

Softening up   A political process in which ideas are discussed in an attempt to gain acceptance. Alternative solutions are considered in a variety of situations, opposition is identified, and counterarguments are developed.

Storefront program   A social program situated in a building.

Street program   A social program that is operated, literally, on the street. For example, workers in a needle-exchange program conduct the trading on the sidewalk rather than in a building.

Introduction

McLuhan and Fiore (1968) described the world as a global village in which each one affected all inhabitants. Although the majority of this book assumes a federal or state focus, Chapter 9 considers the global reality of health care today. The comparative approach to research is explained and a model is presented for the study of nursing and health policy at an international level. Comparative analysis of two needle-exchange programs in the United States and one in the Netherlands offers an example of how the model can be used.

Many nursing and health-policy issues are international issues. For example, bioterrorism, communicable disease and immunization, family planning, and acquired immune deficiency syndrome (AIDS) are health concerns that all countries must address. Nurses work with vulnerable populations of all types—abused, poor, and disenfranchised. Nurses are conducting research within international settings and developing models for cultural competence (Campinha-Bacote, 2002; Villarruel et al., 2003; Ross, 2000). One group of researchers has translated and validated a French version of a tool to permit cross-cultural research in perinatal health (Goulet et al., 2003). International health issues have economic, political, and sociocultural dimensions. The allocation of resources is at least a political decision. Today, advanced practice nurses (APNs) must have a deep knowledge of health, illness, and wellness plus an understanding of the broader social and political context within which these conditions exist. Issues of social justice, the relief of health disparities, and support for those with stigmatized disease or disability are integral to APNs' practices. Research is needed to help nurses and policy makers understand the extent of health problems, cultural and other variables that affect treatment, and political systems and players. There have been no comprehensive models for studying nursing and health policy from an international perspective. One approach to the study of systems from different countries is known as the *comparative analysis*.

Comparative Analysis

"Comparative analysis is a powerful and versatile tool. It enhances our ability to describe and understand political processes and political change in any country by offering concepts and reference points from a broader perspective" (Almond and Powell, 1992, p. 4). Because decisions about health care—who gets what, how, where, when, and at what cost—are essentially political, comparison of health care systems is framed within comparative politics.

Comparing issues and problems between countries can be an antidote to ethnocentrism, especially if the researcher is someone who is an outsider or who does not live in the situation. Commonly accepted values in one country are not necessarily universal, even though the country may be quite large or the values deeply ingrained. Comparative analysis searches for differences and diversity in addition to commonalities. Experimentation that is possible in a controlled laboratory is not possible in a human environment. "The comparative method was perceived by John Stuart Mill, Auguste Comte, and Emile Durkheim as the best substitute for the experimental method in the social sciences" (Dogan and Pelassy, 1984, p. 13).

The Relationship Between Nursing and Political Science

APNs can recognize the value of using concepts from political science in many ways. Whether through their interest in the allocation of resources for the public good or their concern with the maldistribution of health care, nurses and political scientists share a common regard and commitment to political activity. The quest for rigor and specification in research followed similar patterns in each discipline through the era of logical positivism and behavioralism. Quantification of data, sophisticated computer and statistical techniques, recognition and control of bias, and a search for theory certainly moved the knowledge base of both nursing and political science forward. In addition, the failures of logical positivism became a guide for further definition and refinement of each discipline. For example, the focus on civic culture in political science occurred at approximately the same time that Leininger (1991) founded the field of transcultural nursing. Both movements recaptured the meaning and context of what each discipline defined.

A third generation of political science researchers renewed the link of politics to policy and rekindled a responsibility for policy decisions and a desire for integration and collaboration with other social sciences (Cantori, 1974). APNs and political scientists have a natural and necessary interest in the process of public policy. Comparative public policy "illuminates the various ways in which politics works to produce choices of a collective or social nature" (Heidenheimer et al., 1983). Nurses in advanced practice understand the impact of health problems on society. APNs must integrate political concepts and theories into nursing practice in order to articulate nursing's positions to elected and appointed officials. APNs must have a working knowledge of the components of the policy process so that nurses can bring health problems to the attention of government, structure alternatives for governmental response, and evaluate the results. There is no better place for nurses to take leadership roles in health care than at the international level. Mechanic urges nurses to become effective spokespersons who "can articulate the issues for broader populations" (1990, p. 186). This articulation demands a thorough knowledge of policy processes, international issues and contexts, and cost-effective alternative solutions. However, APNs need a model to help them structure international health care research.

The Milstead Model

The Milstead model (Milstead, 1993) was developed to guide researchers in analysis of complex health issues within an international framework. Essential components of the model include selecting the international setting, specifying the problem or policy, analyzing the sociocultural system, clarifying the economic and political systems, and evaluating the specific health system. The Milstead model provides a comprehensive approach to the study of nursing and health-policy issues across countries and cultures and integrates the policy components of political science with the roles of the nurse in advanced practice.

International Setting   The choice of country for one's personal research can be guided by previous travel, a possible health crisis occurring in that country, a particular population, or something unique to the country that is worth studying. The researcher should ascertain for purposes of context whether the country is a developed democracy, second world or communist (or former communist) country, or third world or developing country. The investigator should describe the general governmental structure of the country. The choice of the national, provincial, regional, state, or local level may involve defining each of those terms to understand the scope of the study.

The Policy Process   A policy or program must be selected for study. Policy can be thought of as both directives and processes. There are four major components to the policy process.

1. *Agenda setting.* An *agenda* is a list of problems to which government pays attention. Agenda setting is a fluid, dynamic process in which problem, policy, and political streams couple and uncouple in an effort to link problems to solutions. The central tasks are to define a problem and consider alternatives. Five criteria ascertain the likelihood that a problem will reach or maintain agenda status: (1) technical feasibility, (2) tolerable cost of solutions, and the value of the problem and concomitant solutions as seen by (3) policy makers, (4) the public, and (5) elected decision makers (Kingdon, 1995).

2. *Government response.* This usually occurs as laws, regulations, or programs. Goals are proposed, program objectives are determined, a target group is specified, and potential cost is estimated. The use of policy tools is instrumental in designing laws, regulations, and programs.

3. *Program implementation.* Scholars focused on single case studies or models of top-down, bottom-up, and forward-backward "mapping" scenarios (Elmore, 1979–1980; Lipsky, 1980; Mazmanian and Sabatier, 1983; Pressman and Wildavsky, 1973; Van Meter and Van Horn, 1975), but few have placed research in a comprehensive analytical framework. Implementation games may be identified.

4. *Program evaluation.* Researchers analyze programs to determine success and failure. Measures include program conceptualization and design, monitoring implementation, and assessing impact and efficiency (Mohr, 1980; Quade, 1982; Rossi and Freeman, 1995).

Even though the components of the policy process do not follow a linear sequence and many times blend with each other, APNs can choose the component to focus their research and study concepts inherent in that component.

Sociocultural Systems   The researcher should examine elements of the social and cultural systems in order to place the policy or program within a realistic context (Pye and Verba, 1965). Policies that are studied without regard to the human systems within which they function have little relevance. One must start by identifying the values of those who affect and are affected by the policy. The researcher can identify music, dance, clothing, art, language, food, and work. It is important to discern the general attitudes of the population. Are the people healthy? How do they demonstrate feelings? Are they clean (according to what standards)? Is there a clear system of patriarchy or matriarchy? Does family hold special meaning? Is the family a nuclear unit or an extended family? What is the degree of spirituality of the population? What is the underlying philosophy about health, and how is it manifested in public policy? How do people access the system? How does one's level of health relate to other segments of life, such as work and relationships with others? Assuming the researcher is studying health policy, how is the policy or program influenced by other governmental policies such as education and transportation?

A competent scholar will identify ethnic groups and minorities within the general population. What is the history of the majority and minority groups? What strategies does the scholar use to account for cultural bias on the part of the target population and the scholar? What is the relevant history of the area? What is the geography of the immediate area? In what way have the history and geography contributed to the problem that is being studied?

Economic Political Systems   The researcher who is studying an issue regarding health care or nursing must place the issue within a framework that includes economic and political factors. Although no systems operate as pure systems, an understanding of the basic principles of economic theory will help the nurse ground the policy being studied within a framework in which analysis can be directed. Is there economic stability? Is an economic crisis occurring that has major impact on the issue? The nurse researcher can use measures of gross national product (GNP), gross domestic product (GDP), national debt, or a variety of health care cost figures to place the policy in a relevant economic perspective.

The nurse also must describe the political ideologies and their influence on the policy or program under study. Legal structures, interest groups, the role of the media, and the relationship between public and private enterprise are areas of investigation for the researcher.

The Health System   The nurse researcher should describe the health care system being studied. Is there a national health care delivery system? Is there national health insurance? Is there access to health care for all residents or citizens? What are the similarities between or among the systems being studied? If the health care systems are significantly diverse, what indicators will be used for comparison?

Often a researchable problem surfaces as an "irritation" or concern that has been encountered by the researcher. For example, in the United States, tobacco use is becoming regulated through government bans on smoking in public buildings or whole cities such as New York City in 2003. Violence in schools, homes, and on the street is becoming commonplace in many countries and can be studied as a health problem.

A focus on cure, disease prevention, or a holistic approach to health may be evident. Analysis of health care workers is a fertile field for the nurse policy analyst. Who provides health care can be an indicator of sociocultural, eco-nomic, and political interweavings. Nurses, physicians, feldshers, curanderas, Chinese barefoot doctors, and folk healers all reflect the philosophy and val-ues as translated into public policies related to health care. The education of health care providers is broad and inconsistent among countries and often within a single country.

Programs may be centered around formal structures such as community health, home health, hospice, long-term care, hospital acute care, maternity centers, clinics, information centers, and nurse- or physician-managed health centers. Programs also may be situated in informal or spontaneous circum-stances. The researcher must be attentive to the names that programs are given in different countries. Community-based programs are not necessarily the same as community programs. Clinics in other countries may provide ser-vices and carry connotations different from those in the United States.

The scholar should describe the extent to which technology is used in the unit of investigation. A discussion of the adequacy of infrastructure and techni-cal support, training, and maintenance can shed light on some health problems.

Implementation of Three Needle-Exchange Programs: Application of the Milstead Model

Implementation of three needle-exchange programs will be examined vis-à-vis the Milstead model in an effort to demonstrate the utility of the model for the nurse researcher. The model is not complete, but models are representations of reality that evolve as situations change. This study was conducted to discover how needle-exchange programs (NEPs) were implemented. *NEPs* are defined as organizational arrangements in which sterile (also known as clean) medical supply hypodermic needles and syringes are exchanged for those that have been used at least once and, thus, are considered contaminated or "dirty."

The policy process assumes a government response to a public problem (Milstead, 1993). The major health problem at the end of the 20th century was human immunodeficiency virus (HIV) and AIDS. In the early 1990s, drug users who shared needles and syringes (hereafter referred to as needles) to inject drugs intravenously had the highest proportion of HIV/AIDS of any group (Grund et al., 1991; Inciardi, 1990; "New York State AIDS," 1988). Intra-venous drug users not only transmit the virus among themselves through con-taminated needles but, once infected, transmit the disease through sexual contact to others who may not use drugs or, in the case of pregnant women, through the placenta to a fetus.

Needle-exchange programs are one response to reduce the spread of HIV/AIDS. Early research found that NEPs do no harm, reduce the spread of HIV, and are cost effective (Ginzburg, 1989; Joseph and Des Jarlais, 1989; "Needle Swap," 1991; "Tacoma Supports," 1989). In the mid-1990s, NEPs were illegal in the United States, although they were an accepted, legal component of drug programs in other countries (e.g., the Netherlands). The U.S. programs are implemented primarily by volunteers who operate outside the formal health care system. Most programs are financed by private donations and function with minimal resources. Most volunteers are not health care professionals.

In many states in the United States, laws restrict possession of a needle and syringe unless the carrier has a prescription written by a physician for medication that requires a syringe. For example, diabetics who use insulin may carry needles and syringes legally. If apprehended by the police, an individual who carries a needle and syringe without a prescription can be charged with a crime. Because NEPs were not considered legal programs in the United States, how did they develop? What was the motivation to disobey the law and to create controversial programs? Two sites in Tacoma, Washington, two sites in New York City (in the Bronx and Harlem), and several sites in Rotterdam, the Netherlands, were selected for investigation.

The research questions addressed included: What are the barriers and facilitators to implementing needle-exchange programs, and what program design is most effective? A qualitative cross-cultural approach was used to study the three NEPs. The researcher interviewed 41 policy makers and service providers using elite interview techniques (Dexter, 1970) and limited participant observation at NEP sites. Informants were protected through standard procedures for the protection of human subjects. The researcher did not speak Dutch, but most Dutch people speak English well and there was an interpreter available at each site.

International Setting   The United States and the Netherlands are developed democracies, although with different political structures. Three cities were selected, each a large, urban center. The study was comparative in that NEPs in the three cities were examined in relation to each other. Policy decisions in one country may affect or be affected by decisions in another. Lessons learned in one country might be applicable to another (Rose, 1991). The possibility of examining a health program in another country could explicate similar or different cultural and political values and highlight tools that may be transferable.

The Netherlands is a constitutional monarchy with a bicameral parliamentary system (Upper and Lower Chambers). Queen Beatrix is the head of state. The Constitution established the right of all residents to health care and, since 1919, equal rights for women. The queen and ministers constitute the Crown. The sovereign appoints ministers on the recommendation of the prime minister. Under the Constitution, the ministers are responsible to Parliament. All legislation is submitted to the council of state and is approved by Parliament to become law. Political coalitions form parties and divide up the number of ministerial positions based on the number of seats they control in Parliament.

The U.S. system is a democratic republic. Ideally, each state retains rights, and the federal government is empowered to attend to those problems that are beyond the states' jurisdictions or for which states have requested assistance. At the federal level, there is a bicameral legislature (House of Representatives and Senate) of elected officials. The president is chief executive of the administrative agencies. The Constitution established separation of the powers of the executive, judicial, and legislative branches. The Constitution did not establish health as a right.

The focus of this study was at the local level in three cities. However, state levels of government became involved. The three programs are described briefly.

Rotterdam. The Netherlands has a national health insurance plan that is funded by the central government and administered through private and government programs (Brasker, 1989; Buning and Verheijen, 1990; *Fact Sheet,* 1989). The Dutch NEP was supported legally from its beginning in 1986 as a response to a hepatitis-B epidemic. The Rotterdam NEPs exist in a variety of settings such as street, storefront, and community organizations. Contrary to popular belief, drug use is not legal in Holland.

Tacoma. The Tacoma, Washington, NEP was selected for the sample for several reasons. First, it is one of the first programs in the United States and was started in 1988 (King, 1988). In 1990, the program came under the direction of the joint city-county health department, which agreed to provide funding even though the legality of the program was questionable ("Tacoma Supports," 1989). In February 1991, the program was "approved" for operation through a court ruling (Shatzkin, 1990a), although the paraphernalia law remained unchanged. The process of creating a covert program and moving it to legal status was important to investigate.

Second, the program was developed by one person with his own money and objectives. This singular grassroots effort at policy making prompted investigation.

Third, this program is primarily a "street" program; that is, service workers park a van at a regular site on a city street, and clients exchange needles at the van. However, a "delivery service" also was available, in which requests for clean needles were made to the cellular phone in the van and needles delivered to an arranged site (Maples, 1991). A small exchange also was available at the health department pharmacy. The structure, variety, and innovation are important to investigate to determine what kinds of structures are effective.

Fourth, the target group is varied. In the early 1990s Tacoma-Pierce County was composed of 6.6 percent African Americans, 3.9 percent Asians, 3.8 percent Hispanics, 1.2 percent indigenous people (mostly Native American and some Aleuts from nearby Alaska), and 83.2 percent Caucasian (*Fact Sheet,* 1992). Members of all groups participated in the program. The number of IV drug users in Pierce County was estimated at 3,000, and approximately 35,000 needles were provided free to clients every month (Rosenwald, 1989).

New York City. The New York City program was included in the sample for several reasons. First, the scope of the drug problem in the city clearly was unique. According to interview data and media reports, drug availability and use was pervasive in New York City (Gonzalez, 1992). Streets and homes had become unsafe for residents due to the presence of drug dealers and users. Over and over, respondents talked about how New York City neighborhoods were embedded in the drug culture. In many families, all family members used drugs. In many neighborhoods, an individual was considered "abnormal" or "deviant" if he or she did not "do drugs" ("The World," 1992). Drug use was so pervasive that behavior could not be categorized as "normal," because there were no guidelines for defining it. To use IV drugs has status, not stigma, in this subculture. Interviewees stated that drugs were sold on the street, in school yards, in abandoned buildings, in cars, and in businesses. Age is not a factor in determining who uses drugs; children as young as 5 years old and the elderly are involved (Goldman, 1989).

Second, the number of IV drug users is greater than that in any other city in the United States. Of 260,000 injectors in the state of New York in 1992, 200,000 lived in New York City (Evans, 1988b). An additional 350,000 people used other drugs such as cocaine and crack (a cocaine derivative). Most IV drug users are multidrug users; that is, they do not have a single "drug of choice," as was the case in the 1960s, but use a variety of drugs.

Third, the phrase, "twin epidemics of drug abuse and HIV," is an apt description of the intertwining of the two problems in New York City (Goldman, 1989). It was estimated that 50 percent of the IV drug users in the city were HIV positive (Milstead, 1993). Approximately half of all African-American and Hispanic men and women with AIDS in New York City have been drug users. Needle sharing directly accounted for 36 percent of the reported cases of AIDS among men and 61 percent among women. Eighty percent of pediatric AIDS cases in New York City resulted from one or both parents' use of IV drugs. There are communities of orphans and grandparents in which most of the people between 20 and 40 years of age have died of AIDS.

Fourth, the program had been clandestine until June 1992. Like the state of Washington, New York had a drug paraphernalia law, making it a crime to buy, sell, or possess drug equipment without a prescription. Originally begun by AIDS activists as an underground transaction in 1988, the needle-exchange program became quasi-legal as a pilot program under the aegis of the New York State Health Department from November 1988 through February 1990. After this program closed, a clandestine program was operated by Rod Sorge and six to eight other activists until June 1, 1992, when a waiver was granted by the state commissioner of health for official approval of a second attempt at an authorized program. This study addressed the program as it evolved prior to that waiver.

Fifth, as in the Tacoma program, the New York City program was a street program in which service workers stand on the sidewalk and exchange dirty needles for clean ones. However, there was no volume delivery or pharmacy service, and the program was not administered through a health department.

The Policy Process The component of the policy process on which this study focused was implementation. The issue in implementation often is the extent to which the policy activities are consistent with the original legislative intent. Because the NEPs in the United States were outside the aegis of government, actually in opposition to current laws, this policy component might seem a moot point. However, these programs were examined from the perspective of those who actually initiated and implemented the programs.

New York City Pilot Program.   The program in Rotterdam was and is a top-down approach of typical bureaucratic style. Although there is no public health department in the Netherlands, the central government provides funds to regions for distribution to private health agencies. Large black boxes, the size of big U.S. refrigerators, house the needles. Drug users simply insert their dirty needles and get back clean ones, one for one. These machines are available throughout the city in rehabilitation centers, near train stations, and at other sites. Rehabilitation agency staff also distribute needles whenever intravenous drug users (IDUs) bring them in.

The New York program began as a grassroots response of the gay community to a growing belief that the government was not responding to this emergency as it has to other public health emergencies. The AIDS Coalition to Unleash Power (ACTUP) and the Association for Drug Abuse, Prevention, and Treatment (ADAPT) began meeting with the city health commissioner and provided data and ideas that were incorporated into proposals for exchange programs that were sent to the state for approval (Evans, 1988b).

Although the state, not the city, would fund the program, political support for the program from both state and city officials was crucial. Officials took sides in the issue. The governor and state assembly Republican minority, the New York City chief of police and his staff, all five New York City district attorneys, the Manhattan borough president, and the former special narcotics prosecutor were vigorous opponents of the program (Elovich and Sorge, 1991; "New York State Health Commissioner," 1988; "New York State Assembly's," 1988; Private Drug Abuse Agency, 1988). They feared an increase in drug traffic, drug use, crime, and violence.

National political figures became extremely vocal. The U.S. Surgeon General and the Secretary of Health and Human Services supported the concept ("Dr. Louis Sullivan," 1989; Evans, 1988a). The head of the Bush administration's antidrug program adamantly opposed federal plans to support needle exchange ("Aides," 1989), as did the U.S. representative from Harlem, Charles Rangel.

Planning for a pilot program went forward. Because of a demand from black leadership to be involved in planning programs that affected largely black and Hispanic populations and because of state-local political tensions that had been a part of New York's political history for decades, several groups were involved in negotiating the final program over the 2-year period of 1987 and 1988.

A legal loophole was found in the law that criminalizes needle sale or possession. The law allowed the state health commissioner to exempt organizations or individuals (Elovich and Sorge, 1991) and the commissioner issued a limited waiver to allow the pilot program. The original program, conceived as having a sample of 6,000 (large enough to obtain statistical significance), was whittled to 400. Kingdon (1995) noted that in light of huge budget problems, inexpensive programs have an easier time of being accepted. A small pilot program, especially one this controversial, had a greater probability for approval than one with a large budget. A budget of $240,000 was appropriated.

The press reported that the program would be based in a neighborhood, but several neighborhoods complained loudly to city hall that they did not want it there. The planners had rejected a street model (in which needles were handed out on street corners), fearing a lack of control, in favor of an attempt to legitimize and control the program through a public health organization. The health department was selected as the site. However, the New York City mayor surprised public health officials and declared that there would be no exchange within 1,000 feet (about two and a half city blocks) of a school due to recently uncovered legal restrictions. This posed a big problem, because health stations deliberately were built near schools during the rebuilding of slum areas of the city in the early part of the 20th century. Local health departments, therefore, could not be used as sites. The New York City Department of Health discovered an abandoned former x-ray clinic where the program could be housed. This site was in downtown Manhattan and was not convenient to the sample because it was distant from the site where most drug addicts live and most IDUs do not have money for transportation.

However, the building was next door to "the tombs," the municipal building that housed the city jail and the courtroom in which drug addicts were tried. Clients would be asked to come to an area in which police and prosecuting attorneys would be present in large numbers. Because the state code of laws made it illegal to possess or sell drugs or drug equipment, it was probable that clients would be in possession of illegal substances or supplies, which would put them at great risk for arrest. A plan to provide identification cards marking clients as participants in the pilot study did little to encourage attendance.

The program did not advertise, even in areas of high drug use. Policies were developed that limited eligibility to people who were on waiting lists for drug treatment programs, and the waiting lists were long. Treatment programs mailed invitations to IDUs, many of whom were homeless and had no address; response was sparse. Outreach programs conducted by other service and research groups such as ADAPT became the primary source of clients. This meant that an IDU had to be signed up in a local neighborhood on a waiting list for treatment, then driven by a volunteer to the program site in Manhattan where the IV drug user had to fill out many forms regarding informed consent and treatment options that took long, complicated explanations. The red tape did not portend easy access, and street-level bureaucrats (those who actually operated current programs) were not consulted for their input. The client also was subjected to various blood tests. After lengthy processing, the exchange was limited to only one needle and syringe per client per trip.

The pilot program was doomed to failure, according to all respondents who discussed it, by the twin concepts of influence and power. Lerner and Wanat (1983) explain that failure often is due to a mismatch between bureaucrats' and program administrators' definitions of benefits and needs. Pressure on politicians and public officials was substantial while the program was being considered. The newly elected governor reportedly supported the program, but opposition came from several channels ("Cuomo," 1988). In distinct contrast to Tacoma and Rotterdam, opposition was intense, polarized, and vocal. Within the political stream, there was much confusion among politicians, bureaucrats, and the public about AIDS and how HIV was spread. Myths were believed as truths; education was spotty and informal, if available at all. Political forces were outspoken and the mood was negative in many quarters.

The program was started November 7, 1988, the day after George H. W. Bush was elected to the presidency. An interviewee who was involved in the start-up said the time was selected in the hope that the story would get lost amid the big political news. The program ran for 14 months, and less than 300 people participated. In January 1990, newly elected Mayor Dinkins closed the exchange program shortly after he took office, following through on a political promise he had made during his campaign. Getting on bandwagons early or joining a cause late in order to tip the balance toward the importance of an item are common techniques in the political stream (Bowen, 1982). This researcher observed the latter strategy in New York City where some politicians "came late to the dance" after the initial flurry of opposition was extinguished.

The current program is a grassroots effort, developed by AIDS activists who put their grave concern about the epidemic into action, selected two sites in drug-active neighborhoods and showed up every Saturday morning, snow or shine, to distribute needles, brochures about AIDS, condoms, and material to clean IV "works": clean water, bleach, and cotton balls. Workers meet in a narrow cellar lit with a single bare bulb on Friday nights to fill two-ounce containers with bleach or water, place cotton balls in bags, and fill grocery sacks with their materials, which they took to the sites by car or on the subway.

Tacoma. Clearly a grassroots program, the Tacoma NEP also had the quiet knowledge of many city officials. The originator of the needle-exchange program in Tacoma, Dave Purchase, worked as a drug counselor for many years and had strong ties with many service workers and agency heads. By the mid-1980s, Purchase had become convinced that AIDS was going to be "the biggest health crisis known to humankind" (Milstead, 1993, p. 123). He read articles about HIV and its relationship to IV drug use. He also read a brief report about the Dutch needle-exchange program and decided that, regardless of the lack of compelling results at the time, the program made intuitive sense as a means to reduce the transmission of HIV. Although there were approximately 2,000 IDUs and 100 cases of AIDS in Tacoma in the early 1990s, Purchase decided to start an exchange program with his own money (Milstead, 1993). Kingdon (1995) speaks of needing visibility to propel a concern to problem status. Purchase determined that he would allow himself to become the visible catalyst to get attention for his cause.

Tractability of the Problem   Mazmanian and Sabatier (1983) noted that technical difficulties in the approach to solutions is one challenge to solving problems. They also identified three aspects of the target group that can make solutions more or less difficult: (1) diversity of the target group, (2) percentage of the total population, and (3) the extent of change required in the target population. The AIDS epidemic is the epitome of an intractable problem due to the characteristics of those who contract HIV/AIDS. Some IDUs and people who engage in both homosexual and heterosexual sex practices may not be identifiable groups who can be targeted with education and other incentives. The incidence of HIV/AIDS was rising rapidly. Homosexual IDUs may resist drug treatment and changes in sexual behavior.

Implementation Tools and Games   Bardach (1977) wrote of games played by public officials and interest groups during implementation. A twist to the "Reputation" game (in which players seek to enhance their chances of reelection, promotion, or deference) occurred in Tacoma with Purchase. He was described by himself and many others as "a ham," "a glib SOB," "spacey," "a lone bandit who is offensive and crude and gets away with it," and "a true hero who believes needle exchange is saving lives" (Milstead, 1993, p. 217). He had a flowing gray beard, dressed in jeans and t-shirts, used 1960s "hip" language, and carried a cellular phone. He acknowledged a shrewd political sense that he used "to get things done." He used his adeptness with colorful phrases to get his ideas into the media. Rather than promoting his own reputation for personal good, he risked his reputation to bring the issue of needle exchange to the political agenda.

Policy tools are mechanisms that are used to plan the structure and functions of a policy or program (Schneider and Ingram, 1990). Tools are classified according to five categories:

1. *Authority tools* have the force of government behind them. Incentives, either positive or negative, include inducements such as tax breaks, subsidies, grants and loans, fines, and sanctions (Milstead, 1997).

2. *Capacity tools* provide information and training to policy makers.

3. *Symbolic tools* rely on linking policy preferences to personal values.

4. *Learning tools* are used in uncertain situations.

5. *Innovative tools* in the use of language were developed to address the political reality that surrounded the threat of NEPs.

To educate the Tacoma board of health members, Purchase used street language, such as "cookers" and "works," to defuse discomfort upon hearing them. Metaphors were used to combat metaphors. For example, one member challenged that giving an addict a needle was like giving an alcoholic a drink. Staff responded that it was more like giving an alcoholic a clean glass. The term *bridge to treatment* was coined by one health department social worker. This concept legitimized needle exchange as a means for linking addicts to medical care, information, bleach, condoms, and drug treatment. The phrase has been adopted widely and today appears in language and print throughout the world.

Sensitivity to specific words was noted. All Tacoma informants talked about the needle exchange as being clandestine or covert; only one spoke of the program as illegal (Milstead, 1993). This was a deliberate conceptual strategy, not a semantic exercise. All but one informant believed that the current law was immoral and should not be obeyed. They also referred to drug users, not addicts. Again, this was a deliberate choice of words that conveys tolerance, if not acceptance, and lessens the pejorative tone.

Activists use symbolism to call attention to their cause. In the 1980s they adopted the pink triangle that homosexuals were forced to wear in Hitler's concentration camps, and added the words, "SILENCE=DEATH" (Zonana, 1989). They became experts in acts of civil disobedience, or "zaps" as they are now called. ACTUP members updated the 1960s civil disobedience tactics to include teaching demonstrators to talk in "sound bites" (focused, short comments). Activists were interviewed about their activities. However, the report often was only a 10-second clip on the evening news or a 2-inch column in the local newspaper. Advocates of NEPs became experts in the game of "Help the Media" by preparing material to use as quotes. They also were unafraid to clog the courts with arrests to make their point that paraphernalia laws are immoral and that exchanging needles is preferable to dying of AIDS.

Several incentive tools were designed to increase participation in the program. In addition to needles and referrals to treatment, providers told clients where they could get free meals, overnight shelter, and spiritual guidance. Blood testing for HIV was not done at the sites, but clients who sought testing were sent to appropriate places that offered counseling. Providers may have given clients tokens for bus service occasionally, but the rule was that providers did not give clients money. Workers provided voter registration at the Tacoma sites. In Tacoma, the health department used its connections with other public agencies to provide incentives and rewards for participation. Sunglasses, foot powder, and soap were distributed at the exchange site. Sometimes sanitary napkins and toothbrushes were available, although not on a regular basis.

New York City informants discussed personal incentives for implementing programs (Milstead, 1993). Some found work in which they excel. They developed skills in management, assertiveness and other communication techniques, media relations, and business. They learned how to maneuver through the legislative and court systems and the bureaucracy. One informant noted that when the New York City program becomes a legal program, an organization must be developed and administered in a much more formal manner than at present. The group of activists will have to document what they do, keep minutes of meetings, and hire a program director. The informant expressed concern that the "whole operation will change, and I'm not sure in what direction" (Milstead, 1993, p. 223). An articulate researcher who was one of the early street workers confided that a common fear is losing the individual contact with clients that occurs presently at the exchange sites. He expressed strong feelings about the "joy" (Milstead, 1993, p. 262) the workers feel during the one-to-one contact with the street people. Workers acknowledge that speaking to groups and performing other fund-raising activities are important, but they do not want to get sidetracked from their original focus. Several talked about their occasional discomfort with new people who want to work in the program. On the one hand, they need the assistance, but on the other hand, they question where these people were "three years ago when mucus was freezing on my lips and we didn't have car fare to get to the exchange site" (Milstead, 1993, p. 263).

Education is a tool that was used by the policy entrepreneur in Tacoma. Purchase taught himself about HIV/AIDS and convinced a small cadre of colleagues about the positive aspects of the program. These people became a core committed to teaching others, especially the board of directors of the health department. Formal study sessions were held prior to board meetings in which information was shared about AIDS, HIV transmission, current demographic and epidemiological data, and treatment and prevention efforts. Both board members and educators noted an intensity in the barrage of information. The workers discussed myths and their own fears about the disease in an open forum. Health department staff and other experts were available at the sessions to answer questions.

Other educative tools included public hearings and speeches to service organizations. Purchase initiated a North American Syringe Exchange Conference (Milstead, 1993) as he began to hear from people in other cities around the country about their efforts (most often clandestine) at needle exchange. In this way, he provided a "softening up" period in which "far out" ideas began to be seen as not so unusual or, at least, were being tried out by others. That people in other U.S. cities were implementing NEPs without discussions with each other seems to be a simultaneous response to dissemination of articles and research from Amsterdam and other places, rather than an example of the process of punctuated equilibria (sudden new forms springing up simultaneously and without connection) as Durant and Diehl (1989) suggest.

Kingdon described a "primeval policy soup" (1995, p. 122) as a process in which problems, alternatives, and solutions mix together as they are discussed among bureaucrats, elected officials, and interest groups. Solutions may be available before there are problems to which they may apply, and alternatives may connect and disconnect throughout the process as specific points are considered or new information is added or shifted. As solutions join with problems, details are worked out through draft proposals and bills. This researcher observed that a similar process occurred with the implementation phase of NEPs. As NEPs are designed and implemented through legal channels, elected officials need time to change their perspective of the program from its being an "illegal" program to being a program not only condoned but designed by government.

Implementation of old programs may be in full swing by the time legislators are involved in designing new programs. The "soup" of ideas and options needs time to simmer. Policy windows and opportunities for action in which problems and solutions join also are described in the agenda-setting literature.

This researcher observed windows also as entities in the implementation phase. Rather than wait for a window of opportunity, Purchase forced open a window in Tacoma. Rather than wait for a window of opportunity, Sorge and his colleagues forced open a window of opportunity in New York City. The window already was open in Rotterdam, because the NEP was being implemented, although for a different problem.

There was no softening-up period in Rotterdam; top administrators believed the program would work, so they implemented it without fanfare. The softening-up process in New York City served to increase fear and anxiety about the needle-exchange program. In this case, the softening-up period allowed time for the opponents to solidify their positions and gain a louder voice in dissent, a reverse of Kingdon's informants. New York City policy makers rejected the Amsterdam program as lacking compelling evidence that needle exchange would not lead to more drug use and would reduce HIV transmission. The incentive to be the first in the country to begin a program that was considered radical and controversial was not palatable to New York policy makers. In contrast, Tacomans thought the idea of being "first" with NEPs was progressive (Milstead, 1993).

Sociocultural Systems

Values   A strong value was expressed by all the of informants: the moral certainty in the "rightness" of what they were doing (Milstead, 1993, pp. 195, 204). All informants (except one in Tacoma) stated that U.S. laws restricting needle possession were wrong, illegal, or barbaric. Rationale for these types of laws centered on a fear that possession of needles created increased drug use and, conversely, restricting needle possession would decrease drug use. There was no evidence that these laws have been effective because drug use has increased significantly throughout the years. U.S. respondents felt an ethical and moral responsibility to oppose the law and to implement NEPs for the greater good of reducing the spread of HIV. The more opposition to their work that they encountered, the more firm their resolve was to continue. Their evangelistic fervor was consistent with the integrity of their beliefs; they wanted to talk about HIV/AIDS, IDUs, NEPs, and to convince others of the truth of their own convictions.

There are no laws in the Netherlands that criminalize possession or sale of drug paraphernalia. Drug use is illegal in the Netherlands as it is in the United States. However, some drugs, such as marijuana, are defined as *soft*, and small amounts for personal use are tolerated by the police and courts. Controlled drugs (those regulated by international standards) are not legal without prescription and enforcement is strict. Of the users in the Netherlands, 20 to 30 percent inject. Heroin is the primary substance, although some cocaine is injected.

Risk was a value that was expressed often by U.S. informants as a willingness to take significant personal chances. An NEP was considered outside the letter of the law. One respondent stated he took "a lot of risks for a bureaucrat" because he could have been fired for placing a public agency in direct confrontation with a state law (Milstead, 1993, p. 127). New York City activists were willing to risk criminal prosecution to force a change in the law. In addition, clients of NEPs risked being arrested for needle possession. Informants related incidents in which IDUs were arrested within one block of the NEP.

Lack of risk for carrying drug paraphernalia is illustrated by some Dutch coffee houses that sell small amounts of soft drugs and are identified by a marijuana leaf symbol on the front window. Police do not arrest individuals who purchase drugs in these places unless the person is making trouble, that is, fighting or disturbing others. One government official confided that about every 4 years (near election time), the issue of legalizing drugs surfaces but fades without action.

Courage, in the form of support for the program, was a value expressed by nearly all respondents. In Tacoma, informants stated that there is "danger in opportunity" (Milstead, 1993, p. 126) and that the program was a "make-or-break" issue. One health department worker felt his professional reputation and credibility rested on being able to convince enough people early on that the venture was "right" and appropriate. Several informants believed that the chairman of the board of health (who also was mayor) lost personal friends over his stand for the program. People who might not have had a great interest in the program but who knew about it through media attention questioned the ethics and moral code of the chairman. Some people believed that drug use was immoral and that a program that acceded to drug use was unethical. People feared that providing clean needles would condone drug use. One person countered, "How can being dead be a moral issue? AIDS is a health issue!" (Milstead, 1993, p. 127).

Values provided a major barrier to the services of the New York City NEP. All respondents talked about the twin epidemics of drug abuse and HIV/AIDS and the values that emerged about both. Opposition to needle exchange came from those who believe that drug use is a moral issue and that the only correct response is to "just say no" (the slogan of the U.S. drug policy in the 1990s). Needle exchange was perceived by these groups as encouraging or condoning drug use. In both New York City and Tacoma, the concept of needle exchange was taboo at first and was later viewed as possibly appropriate, but only if connected to drug treatment.

A concept emerged of imagery, emotional as well as metaphorical. Interviewees expressed in many ways that needle exchange is a different emotional issue for African Americans and Hispanics than for whites. Informants in New York City pointed out that African Americans and Hispanics live in neighborhoods where drugs are sold and used, and most residents have witnessed many deaths from substance abuse. When a family member dies of an overdose, it is hard for other family members to condone giving needles to anyone. Many families had been ripped off by family members who have stolen money or other items to sell in order to buy drugs (Milstead, 1993, p. 133). One respondent noted that these scenes are reality, and one cannot expect a person to go beyond that emotion and think rationally about the positive aspects of needle exchange. On the other hand, many families depend on drug money as their major or sole source of income. One New York respondent noted that it was not unusual for a 15-year-old drug runner to support a whole household or several families from his or her drug earnings. Drug traffic is big business in New York City, and many people who live in the neighborhoods are involved as a means of earning money and supporting a way of life.

Images are important in determining alternatives. A common value held in the United States, according to informants, was that a needle-exchange program would serve as a magnet that would draw other IDUs to the area, which, by extension, would enlarge and intensify drug use and attendant crime and violence. A pied-piper effect reflected concern that neighborhoods with relatively little drug traffic would become overrun with sellers and users, and those neighborhoods already trafficking heavily would spread. Few people wanted NEPs in their neighborhoods, and many opposed such programs (Evans, 1988a). In contrast, prevention teams were established in Rotterdam in which pairs of volunteers would patrol their own neighborhoods for discarded dirty needles. The teams were trained to handle the contaminated waste and could dispose of it properly. Neighborhoods became environmentally cleaner and safer. The strategy seemed to work, because people did not complain "so long as there were no dirty needles in my neighborhood." Elected policy makers saw the program as efficient in that it could be added to an existing drug treatment program and required little additional training of personnel and a moderate budget.

An interesting folk hero emerged from Tacoma. Purchase's brashness and ability to paint visionary pictures with words are part of his charisma. He used personal anecdotes to make points, which lent a certain benign storyteller aura to his persona. Most informants told how he began the needle exchange with a card table and lawn chair (Milstead, 1993). Even though not entirely accurate, the commonness of even the furniture added a certain storybook fantasy and a folksy aura to him.

Purchase deliberately provoked others by using challenging language such as "AIDS is a holocaust in slow motion," "This is a new world order with disposable humanity," and "The largest single policy problem with AIDS is a lack of leadership [at the national level] and it is willful, a crime of omission" (Milstead, 1993, p. 157). All are quotes that incite emotion, provide shock value, and force people to consider the problem at hand. The language pushed people to confront their own values. The emotional part of the issue was where Purchase believed the conflict arose. He was involved actively with people in the policy and business communities as he challenged them and hammered home his issue. His behavior emphasizes the importance of using the softening-up period as a forum for activity. Softening up may be a passive time for reflection about conflicting values, but it also is a time for action, an opportunity to convince others of the merits of an idea.

Discrimination in various forms was voiced in relation to drug use. Many respondents noted that in 1992 New York City had the largest number of IDUs and persons with HIV/AIDS of any city in the United States and that most of these were people of color (Milstead, 1993). Nearly all also noted that drugs are as much an economic problem as a racial one. One respondent noted that

African-American drug users were not treated well by other African Americans. She reported that black physicians and other health care professionals at a large hospital in a major black section of the city had invented a code word for a drug user who comes for emergency services. Providers called out, "Here comes another SCHPOS" (an acronym for subhuman piece of shit). This term, and the attitude with which it is spoken, dehumanized the person, was insulting because it was said within the patient's hearing, and indicated at least a measure of indifference, if not disgust, in the provision of treatment. Slow treatment was noted by one informant who recounted that often as many as eight women drug users (mostly women of color) were scheduled for gynecologic exams at the same hour and had to wait, sometimes six to eight hours, to be seen by clinic physicians.

Value acceptability of NEPs to elected policy makers became emotional and negative in New York City. National and state politicians of color began equating the program to the infamous Tuskegee (Alabama) study of the 1930s in which a control group of blacks was not given a new treatment (antibiotics) to cure syphilis (Thomas and Quinn, 1991). U.S. Representative Charles Rangel, Harlem, was especially outspoken and used the terms "genocide" and "guinea pigs" to accuse supporters of NEPs as demonstrating deliberate, conscious racism against people of color, especially African Americans (Nicholson, 1988). Black New York City Police Commissioner Benjamin Ward echoed this fear of genocide (Evans, 1988a). The Tuskegee 'experiment' holds tremendous emotional force, especially in the African-American community. The press, according to several informants, played into the issue irresponsibly and ridiculously by using tactics that continued to sensationalize the point. Rangel, chair of the U.S. House Select Committee on Narcotic Abuse and Control, questioned whether dispensing centers would be located only in poor neighborhoods and whether programs would be 'entitlement' programs with a means test required so that only poor drug addicts are eligible (Nicholson, 1988). He also asked whether there would be an age limit or whether needles would be available to minors. All of these questions conjured up negative emotional images intended to draw fire. Symbolism often provided visibility and emotional impact for issues.

Drug Treatment Philosophy　The value of acceptance of personal differences and personal responsibility for one's own behavior was evident in relation to two opposing philosophies about drug treatment. Dutch informants expressed amazement over American "ridigity" and "puritanical" approach to drugs. They either smiled or shook their heads when discussing the U.S. "war on drugs" policy. Several Dutch informants commented that the "war" seemed directed at the "victims" (users) rather than the drugs (dealers and importers). The Dutch espouse the philosophy of harm reduction that was formalized as a policy within the Dutch drug and alcohol rehabilitation community of policy specialists. The concept of personal responsibility was supported by both major Dutch political parties and served as the cornerstone of health services. This idea accepts that people may choose behaviors that others perceive as dangerous or damaging to one's health. The Dutch believe the role of the provider of health services is to support the personal choices of the individual and to help the person live in such as way as to reduce the harm that may be a consequence of the behavior. For example, even though drugs can be harmful, proponents of this philosophy believe that a person cannot be forced to give up drugs and will not be successful in treatment if the person does not have a commitment to the program. Harm reduction directs that injectors should be taught safe injection techniques, how to recognize and obtain treatment for abscesses, and how to clean IV works and not share them. An extension of this philosophy is seen in the free provision of condoms and literature on how to clean IV works, the dangers of sharing works with others, and how to avoid transmitting HIV.

In contrast, the official American policy for drug treatment is abstinence. Narcotics Anonymous and similar programs espouse this policy. Most American respondents agree with harm reduction, although many believe that abstinence should be tried first. In New York City, if a person is in a methadone treatment program and a random drug test shows positive for any drug (not just heroin), the person is terminated from the program. Abstinence from all drugs is required; the concept of harm reduction, in which drug use is tolerated, is not accepted by the political community. Informants bemoaned that there was no methadone-type treatment available for cocaine users. For heroin users, methadone can be substituted to reduce physical addiction and emotional dependence. Respondents also repeated that most drug users in 1992 were multidrug users; that is, they used a variety of drugs throughout the day.

Problem Fading   Kingdon (1995) speaks of the potential for problems to fade from the government agenda. This researcher found that related problems also may arise during implementation. For example, while funding for exchange programs in Rotterdam came from one ministry, another ministry became involved tangentially in exchange programs. Program administrators and service providers were aware of environmental hazards of dirty needles. They also had become aware that the sharps containers contain cadmium, a product that is hazardous to the environment. One foundation proposed research toward the development of an environmentally safe container, but the minister of health could not find funds to support the project. However, the foundation director pursued the idea with the minister of environmental safety, and funding was provided by this department. This project was unique to Rotterdam at the time. The director agreed that this was a creative method of moving between jurisdictions within the government. It is an example of second-order change or reframing (Watzlawick et al., 1974), a tool not often discussed in the policy literature. Again, the idea of "rightness" and merit and of new ideas surfaced. Kingdon states that policy makers often are intrigued with creative ideas that package old problems in new ways; Kingdon calls this a relief from the intellectual boredom of rational problem solving. Certainly policy makers, foundation directors, workers, and junkies in Rotterdam have not been bored.

At other times, problems may not fade but are redefined. Dutch health organization prevention teams of two people educate IDUs at exchange or clinic sites about health hazards and healthy practices. Teams also patrol exchange sites and neighborhoods where they pick up dirty needles and dispose of them in safe containers. Informants believe that this strategy increases local residents' support of the concept of needle exchange. Neighbors become partners with the NEPs in cleaning up neighborhoods. Individuals are encouraged to bring in needles if they find them in their vicinities or may call a prevention team to pick them up. The neighbors are provided with information about drug use and needle exchange, which often decreases opposition and has resulted in a cadre of supporters for the program.

Supporters of the New York City NEP wanted the publicity that surrounded the original needle-exchange program to fade. The negative emotions that were stirred worked against the efforts of activists who believed the concept was right and were committed to continuing the effort. In contrast, Purchase was concerned that the issue of needle exchange would fade from people's minds in Tacoma (Milstead, 1993). He feared that it would become "hip" to have an exchange program but that the program would not work in some places; that is, he feared the junkies would not participate if an exchange were not "user friendly" for them. He felt it was important that NEPs be located near the place where drugs are obtained and not be placed in buildings where those who live on the streets will not go because of their discomfort with confined spaces and regimented schedules. He noted that if this occurred, interest would wane and funding may be jeopardized.

Problems may fade because of lack of supporters. Traditionally, IDUs are not well organized. Informants noted that white-collar IDUs usually do not make known to others that they are users, because drug use is illegal. Informants also reported that the stereotype of a drug user is a dirty, poor, disheveled person with matted hair who stands around on the street. Politicians do not perceive IDUs as voters; thus, users are considered an invisible constituency. In New York City, the gay community came to the assistance of the large IDU population that was seen as disenfranchised. Gay activists have been the initial and continuing force behind needle-exchange programs in New York City.

In contrast, programs in Tacoma certainly would have been delayed if a single policy entrepreneur had not seized the moment. Informants reported that some funding from the state Omnibus AIDS bill had been appropriated for AIDS-related programs, but there was no organized program such as the needle exchange. The exchange program was considered a radical concept and carried some political cost in Tacoma, much political cost in New York City, and minimal political cost in Rotterdam.

Economic-Political Systems

Economic Systems   The Netherlands operates as a free market economic system within the European Union (Milstead, 1993). In 1992, sixty-seven percent of the labor force worked in the service sector, 28 percent in industry, and 5 percent in agriculture. The unit of currency is the euro. Thirty-three percent of

European Union goods that are transported by sea are loaded or unloaded in Dutch ports, mainly in Rotterdam (Buning and Verheijen, 1990), which is the largest port in the world. After having been bombed nearly to extinction during World War II, major portions of Rotterdam were rebuilt.

Data indicate that concern over budgets does not lessen during the implementation phase and may intensify after programs get started, because money must be appropriated for program continuation or expansion. The Rotterdam program was added to existing comprehensive drug rehabilitation programs in which support was offered and treatment was not required. Program officials reported that funding was a continuous problem. With the move of the central government toward a more decentralized or regionalized system, major municipalities faced the problem of prioritizing funding. Cities must negotiate their budgets with the ministry knowing that other municipalities also are doing the same thing. The municipal committee members discuss the current state of drug use in the region, plan programs, and negotiate a budget. The alderman has final budget authority for the completed regional budget. The cost of health care services is increasing in the Netherlands as well as in the United States. All Dutch informants said they like their system and do not regret the high tax rate that accompanies it, but they agree that costs must be contained and that there must be reform in the system.

Interviewees spoke often of the small cost of needle exchanges in relation to the cost of care and treatment of AIDS patients. Costs of the Rotterdam program were small when determined in light of the perceived seriousness of the potential AIDS problem and the limited number of IDUs in Rotterdam. Many informants commented on the general cost, three cents for each syringe and needle compared with 35,000 euros (approximately $40,000) for treatment of one patient with AIDS. A pragmatic philosophy was linked to the concept of prevention of HIV transmission as service providers and policy makers alike spoke of the cost effectiveness of NEPs.

The overwhelming failure of the New York City pilot program did little to encourage funding for current needle exchanges. In contrast, much money and effort were expended to oppose these programs, according to respondents. Control of illegal equipment and disposal of medically hazardous waste became issues related not only to dollars but to social and political costs. Some costs were defrayed in the current New York City program by agreeing to try out new types of syringes provided free by manufacturers of medical supplies. Although there was no controlled study, workers asked clients to try out the supplies and let workers know how the needles worked "next week when you bring them back." This subtle request encouraged clients both to continue the program and to return the needles. Comments from clients provided a rough survey of satisfaction from those who use needles every day. In turn, the workers relayed that information to the supply representatives.

In New York City, the extremely large number of IDUs placed great demands on resources for any program funded and operated by the state. With over 200,000 IDUs in New York City in 1992 (Milstead, 1993), there were only 50,000 drug treatment slots available. Waiting lists were of nearly 8 months' duration and were limited to methadone treatment, a traditional method of weaning addicts off heroin but one that does not address multiple drug use, which was the norm. In contrast to the IDUs in Rotterdam, those in New York City were perceived to be extremely disruptive to the general society because of the attendant crime and violence.

Cost was expressed through fear as interviewees related stories about future concerns that already had arrived. Communities of children orphaned by parents who have died of AIDS, predicted as early as the mid-1980s, were confirmed already in New York City, according to informants, who included a member of the New York State Assembly, a New York City bureaucrat, and a legislative aide to a New York state senator. Grandmothers were left to rear children who may be siblings, cousins, or other family members. A population of infants, known as "boarder babies," abandoned in the hospital by HIV/AIDS mothers who were too sick to care for them or did not have the resources, was identified in New York City as early as 1988. The state has become burdened with the costs of providing hospital care and housing for these babies, and adoption agencies were approached to seek volunteers to serve as foster parents. The cost of long-term medical and social care of boarder babies who are at risk for developing AIDS can only be guessed. However, this factor was not included in assessing the cost of NEPs.

The costs of the original Tacoma program were borne by one man who used his own money and enlisted contributions from friends. The entrepreneur did consider lost opportunity costs of those who would die early from AIDS if transmission rates were not reduced. Purchase considered the initial cost of the program ($25,000) versus the cost of treatment of an AIDS patient from diagnosis to death. Figures cited by several informants ranged from $50,000 to $102,000, although many reminded the interviewer that the cost of care will increase because the patients are being treated and live longer.

Problems often focus on budgetary matters. Although the city-county health department in Tacoma funded the program as part of its overall services, funds were sought from other sources. Purchase and others became fund-raisers. Some used the cellular phone in the program van to solicit money from local individuals who inquired about the program or to contact former benefactors or those who might contribute if only asked. One informant noted he never missed a pastor. Church groups, ministerial groups, and business organizations were all targets for fund-raising. The Exchange Club (Tacoma downtown business association) donated $10,000 to $20,000 (Milstead, 1993, p. 210). Some workers ask for personal checks from friends and acquaintances. One service worker made broad hints of donations to the interviewer.

Public funding for research is limited. Sources for private funding also were limited and were becoming more fragmented as more NEPs sought expansion of private funds. Research is needed to determine the effectiveness of the harm reduction model, the effects of multiple drug use over time, and policy aspects of drug services.

The last problem is a paradox. When needle exchanges are operating well (i.e., fewer needles are being found in neighborhoods, and addicts are becoming empowered and responsible), the "problem" loses some of its intensity and funding is cut. One administrator says that this attitude is extremely shortsighted on the part of politicians and may lead to a reversal of the gains of the programs.

Political Systems

Rotterdam. Historically, the Netherlands has been a consociational democracy (Lijphart, 1974). This typology is indicative of a fragmented political culture based on deep cleavages among religions within the country, especially between Catholics and Calvinists (Reformed and Dutch Reformed). Political parties and health care services are structured along these major religious divisions. As late as the 1890s, the Dutch government frequently delegated activities to municipalities, which often did not have adequate funds. As a result, citizens and groups were obligated to fill in. This was true especially in health care. Religious groups founded charity institutions and paid for them through church collections. As a result, health care was organized as a private initiative. Competition among religious communities often produced fragmented and incomplete health care services. Citizens complained, and in 1919 the Dutch government passed the Health Act, which established the Health Council, an advisory body to the central authority. Over the years there has been some softening of the boundaries among the religious groups and structures. Today, while the divisions still exist, there is less sectarian antagonism among the younger citizens and a more pervasive attitude throughout the country of political tolerance and compromise.

New York City. One of the most significant government events came in the form of a court decision relevant to the NEP in New York City. Nearly all respondents spoke of the 1991 arrests of eight people for possessing needles at the exchange program; some informants had been defendants. All of those arrested were acquitted of criminal charges. Manhattan Criminal Court Judge Laura Drager considered testimony from many individuals and organizations. Activists solicited testimony from local drug users whose personal stories were compelling in their intensity and their pleas for help to seek treatment and prevent HIV transmission. Manhattan Borough President Ruth Messinger confessed to being against the program originally but admitted she had changed her opinion after having gone personally to an exchange site. Researchers in the field of drugs and HIV/AIDS marshaled their political forces and educated the court on the incidence, prevalence, and transmission of the virus. Interviewees noted that a report from the National Commission on AIDS linked needle exchange and AIDS and was strongly supportive of needle exchange (National Commission on AIDS, 1991).

In a landmark decision on June 25, 1991, Manhattan Criminal Court Judge Drager ruled that the defendants' possession of needles was a "medical necessity" that was intended to prevent a greater societal harm, AIDS ("Judge

Acquits," 1991; "Manhattan Criminal Court," 1991). She held that the AIDS epidemic is a "grave medical emergency" that justifies illegal conduct. She distinguished between death by dirty needles versus drug addiction by clean needles and determined that in this age of the AIDS crisis "the defendants' actions sought to avoid the greater harm" (Decision and Order, 1991). The finding of the court did not provide legal action to allow exchange programs. However, after much political activism, a waiver was granted by the state health commissioner for the two programs in the Bronx and Harlem, effective June 1, 1992.

Tacoma.   The history of most respondants in Tacoma includes social and political action. Several talked about having marched together in civil rights actions in the South in the 1960s and having worked together for local political issues. The inbred quality of the policy community in Tacoma was reflected in the language they used. Many informants used the same phrases and terms, such as "bridge to treatment" and drug "users" rather than "addicts" (a term several stated is pejorative and outdated) (Milstead, 1993, p. 148). Another noted that "people know each other, they get their arms around each other" and talk together. Kingdon (1995) notes that familiarity can spawn stability and a common outlook, but even he did not describe as tight a network as observed in Tacoma.

The mood in Tacoma did not involve antagonism about political issues but about a legal one. Concern continued that the needle exchange was patently illegal. Respondents spoke of considering ways to get the issue before the court without making it a criminal case as in New York City. Purchase and his friends reasoned that they might have a clearer decision if the case were heard in civil court where the issue would not be criminalized. After much thought, they convinced the health department to ask the attorney general for Washington State for an opinion on the legality of NEPs. The 1989 response was that the programs were illegal, based on the drug paraphernalia law. The city of Tacoma then agreed to withhold its part of the funding designated for the needle exchange from a joint city-county budget until the legality of the program was established. This allowed the health department to sue to recover the funds. By organizing the political forces in this way, the case would be heard in a civil, not a criminal, court where criminality would not be at issue. Many respondents commented on the courage of the director of the health department in permitting this idea to go forward.

The judge ruled that although it is illegal to distribute needles and syringes without a prescription, health department workers were exempt because, as municipal officers, they were carrying out their legal duty to prevent the spread of disease (Shatzkin, 1990b). The exemption allowed the local health officer broad powers to take extraordinary measures to stop an epidemic. Most respondents confided that the term "officer" had been thought of in the past as the police. It was a matter of reframing the definition to accommodate the health officer.

Although the paraphernalia act was a general statute, the judgment noted that the AIDS act that had been passed by the Washington legislature and signed by the governor was a more specific statute regarding IV needles and HIV control. In the latter law, regional directors of AIDS services networks were required to develop strategies to reduce HIV transmission to high-risk groups "possibly including needle sterilization" and authorizing "appropriate materials." These sections of the law were interpreted as indications that the legislature considered that transmission of HIV through unsterile needles could be addressed by trading them for sterile ones (i.e., in effect, sterilizing them) in an exchange program.

The third component of the judgment noted that Washington Governor Gardner vetoed a portion of a 1989 drug act that would have banned NEPs. The veto stated that NEPs offer a way to limit the spread of the virus and, as a governor acts as part of the legislature when he vetoes bills, he was speaking for the legislative intent.

Organized political forces were seen at an intense level in this scenario. Experts in public health, law enforcement, AIDS prevention, drug treatment, and research worked together as a body to prepare and present a united appeal to the court. Their innovation of the "friendly" lawsuit between the city and county to force the issue and to place it in civil court so as not to confound the question with issues of morality was an indicator of an educated, creative group who operated comfortably with ideas and second-order change. The incentives of personal interests and values within the policy stream combined with organized forces in the political stream and were viewed as promoting the public good. The supportive members believed in the "rightness" of NEPs and their ability to reduce the transmission of HIV/AIDS, and they convinced the board of health, citizens, and the court of the merit.

Health Systems

Health Care Delivery   The Rotterdam policy community centers on the Ministry of Welfare, Health, and Cultural Affairs, which has responsibility for health policy. Health care essentially is publicly funded and privately administered. With few exceptions, everyone who lives in the Netherlands is covered by health insurance (Brasker, 1989). The National Health Service Law was enacted in 1966 and is known as the Health Insurance Act. This law regulates compulsory insurance for employees who earn an annual base salary. Those who earn more than the base salary must purchase their own insurance from a plethora of private insurance companies, the largest of which is Silver Cross, a sister organization to Blue Cross in the United States. Since 1989, all employees have contributed a percentage of their salaries toward the national health insurance plan. A basic package of health care consists of a choice of family physician, certain specialists, dental care, medicines, and hospital nursing care (*Fact Sheet*, 1989). The Exceptional Medical Expenses Act of 1968 (AWBZ) is a scheme for insuring everyone for long-term medical conditions (*Fact Sheet*, 1989). The Sickness Benefits Act provides unemployment benefits to those who cannot work due to sickness, disability, or accident (Buning and Verheijen, 1990). Complementary health care services, such as manual therapy, naturopathy, acupuncture, and paranormal medicine, are accepted as positive approaches. Government grants are awarded for research to document the effectiveness of these modes of treatment.

Health care consists of curative care (a two-tier system of family physician and hospital specialist) and preventive care. Hospitals mostly are proprietary organizations that are administered with public funds in a competitive market atmosphere. Regional planning by means of boards and councils regulates the types of services offered. Generalist physicians (family physicians) are paid by the government. They may enroll 3,000 families and are paid for the number of enrollees, not the number of services or visits provided, a system known in the United States as *capitation*. This has the effect of encouraging efficient medicine and of discouraging frequent office visits. Physician specialists are employees of hospitals and must be referred by generalists.

In the 1980s, the central government of the Netherlands, in a move toward decentralization, decided to concentrate drug assistance in four cities: Amsterdam, Rotterdam, The Hague, and Utrecht (*Odyssee Information*, 1992). The cities are autonomous entities; that is, they make their own policies and plan their own programs independently. The four cities set up committees with representation from other smaller cities and towns within their pre-scribed geographic areas. The committees develop local policy, plan specific programs, and draft budgets that are approved by central government.

Fourteen percent of Rotterdam's residents are immigrants, predominantly from Surinam, Turkey, Morocco, and the Antilles. Many of them are Moslem, a religion that has a strong taboo against injecting foreign substances into the body, including drugs and tattoos. Due to cultural practice, those immigrants with drug problems tend to smoke rather than inject. However, interviewees stated that migrants from northern France and Belgium have easy access to pills in their countries and bring them to Holland to sell so that they can buy heroin to take back to their countries for resale or use.

The scope of the drug and AIDS problems in Rotterdam is in proportion to that of the whole country. The Netherlands has a population of 15 million. There are approximately 20,000 hard drug users, and the number has stabilized. Rotter-dam has a population of nearly 600,000 with 3,000 users, most of whom are mul-tidrug users. According to several respondents, a recent report of drug use in four countries (United Kingdom, Germany, Sweden, and the Netherlands) docu-ments that 0.13 percent of the population in each of the four countries are users. These figures were cited by many informants to dispute the common misconcep-tion that drug use in the Netherlands is higher than anywhere in Europe.

In Rotterdam, unlike Tacoma or New York City, the site of the drug prob-lem is not on the street as much as in houses. Groups may "shoot up" together as a type of ritual behavior. This is done in "shooting galleries" (rooms or buildings appropriated for this activity) or at home. Because of this, street models for needle exchange are not popular. Most programs are within com-munity health organizations.

Implementation Problems

Problems often occur as implementation proceeds (Yanow, 1987). Common problematic themes include lack of money for basic services, too few treatment slots for too many clients, and not enough money for research. Rotterdam has particular problems with decentralization of government, but government fragmentation also is seen in New York between city and state provision of services. A move toward community-based organizations and a mix of public and private funding for neighborhood services is noted in all three sites.

Problems relating specifically to needle-exchange programs include the need for smaller sharps boxes, a need for protection from weather at street sites, and expanded service options. Tacoma informants noted a problem with court judgments that are restrictive to drug users. Both New York City and Tacoma noted some continued police harassment. Members of the New York City program fear losing the personal relationships they have established with clients, a value held by workers in all of the NEPs.

One problem that highlights the moral and ethical strength of the originators of the New York City NEP centered around the appropriate disposal of medical waste; that is, contaminated needles and syringes. The workers were cognizant of the hazardous material they were collecting. Federal regulations require that dirty needles and syringes cannot be thrown in general trash. Workers originally collected dirty needles and put them in large jugs that were meant to be used for commercial bottled drinking water in office buildings. The jugs then were stored under the bed of one of the workers. When gallons and gallons of dirty needles filled the room and colleagues were afraid of being arrested with the hundreds of needles, the group looked for a safe place to dispose of this hazardous waste. They agreed to take them to the Manhattan Department of Health, where they dumped them surreptitiously and ran. They were in a double bind because they knew they were breaking a state drug paraphernalia law. However, a positive effect of this near-disaster was that the group's camaraderie was strengthened when they told the researcher their stories of hardship and risk. They acknowledged a certain "bonding" and reflected a sense of pride, amazement, and laughter as they recounted their tales.

In Tacoma, Purchase made arrangements with the health department for safe disposal of contaminated needles, a process that was controlled strictly through guidelines established by the federal Occupational Safety and Health Administration. Medical waste cannot be dropped into public containers and cannot be added to general trash. Puncture-resistant containers must be used to prevent needles from sticking through and inadvertently puncturing and contaminating the disposer. Temperature range must be controlled if the waste is incinerated, and air pollution standards are specified for exhaust. The health department quickly began providing safe containers for use.

Even though there is much support for the program in many areas, the courts inadvertently pose a problem. One worker talked about SOAPs and SODAs, acronyms for Stay Out of the Area of Prostitutes and Stay Out of Drug

Areas. If a client is charged with a drug offense or prostitution, a judge may order a SOAP or SODA in lieu of a jail sentence. It serves as a formal, legal warning. If the person is caught later in either area by the police, a jail sentence will be imposed immediately. The NEP is set in an area where drugs are bought and sold. There is an assumption that people who are at the exchange are using drugs. The exchange, therefore, serves as a focus for locating or identifying drug users, which certainly is not a goal.

Several Rotterdam service providers and policy makers stated angrily that a major problem in drug treatment is the industry itself. Treatment programs are revenue centers because of the money they generate from insurance companies. Most treatment programs are methadone programs that require a 6-week hospitalization, which is paid for by insurance. In addition, the programs require abstinence from all drugs. Treatment centers face a big loss of revenue if needle exchanges flourish and addicts continue to use IV drugs.

Conclusion

A model for analyzing nursing and health policy has been presented. The model is comprehensive and can serve as a framework for conceptualizing and implementing the process of inquiry into policy issues between and among countries. Advanced practice nurses are encouraged to cultivate an expansive intellect and consider all local health and nursing interests in the context of a global perspective. APNs should use the model, evaluate the components, and validate the model's utility or improve it.

There is a dearth of policy research on nursing at the international level, and little comparative research has been done by nurses. The policy field is appropriate for APNs who have integrated the multiple roles of the professional nurse into their practices. Nurses have an obligation to extend scientific inquiry beyond national borders and can serve as role models for those who are beginning an interest in a broader arena. Nurses are mentors and experts who are accountable to clients and consumers of health care, to nurse colleagues for authoring (Kennedy and Charles, 1997), and to other health professionals and policy makers for leadership in providing intelligent, insightful health care. The potential for contributing to knowledge of health, nursing, and public policy is unlimited.

Discussion Points

1. State three reasons for conducting a comparative study of health problems.
2. Describe the type of government and general governmental structure in two countries in which you note a serious health problem. Identify where you could obtain resources about each country. At what level would your action be most beneficial?
3. Compare the values of family, language, and food in two countries. What are the implications of your analysis in planning for health care in each country?
4. How might not including minorities in a country bias or skew a research study?

5. What resources does a researcher use in a country in which he or she does not know the language? What are the advantages and disadvantages of conducting a study under these circumstances?
6. In studying two countries with differing economic systems, what common indicators may be used to reduce variance?
7. In studying two countries with differing political systems, what common indicators may be used to reduce variance?
8. What indicators are useful in comparing two different health care systems?

References

Aides to William J. Bennett, head of the Bush Administration's anti-drug program, protest health and human services department plan to support needle exchange. (1989). *New York Times*, 10 March, pp. 1–14.

Almond, G. A. and Powell, Jr., G. B. (1992). *Comparative Politics Today: A World View* (5th ed.). New York: HarperCollins Publishers.

Bardach, E. (1977). *The Implementation Game: What Happens After a Bill Becomes a Law*. Cambridge, MA: MIT Press.

Bowen, E. (1982). The Pressman-Wildavsky paradox: Four addenda on why models based on probability theory can predict implementation success and suggest useful tactical advice for implementers. *Journal of Public Policy* 2(1), 22.

Brasker, H. M. (1989). *Health Insurance in the Netherlands*. Rijswijk: Ministry of Welfare, Health & Cultural Affairs.

Buning, A. de C. and Verheijen, L. (1990). *The Netherlands in Brief*. The Hague: Foreign Information Service, Ministry of Foreign Affairs.

Campinha-Bacote, J. (2002). The process of cultural competence in the delivery of health care services: A model of care. *Journal of Transcultural Nursing 13*(3), 181–184.

Cantori, L. J. (Ed.). (1974). *Comparative Political Systems*. Boston: Holbrook Press.

Cuomo administration reportedly decides. (1988). *New York Times*, 31 January, p. 1.

Decision and order, *People of the State of New York v. Bordowitz et al.* Docket No. 90N0248423, June 25, 1991.

Dexter, L. A. (1970). *Elite and Specialized Interviewing*. Evanston, IL: Northwestern University Press.

Dogan, M. and Pelassy, D. (1984). *How to Compare Nations*. Chatham, NJ: Chatham House Publishers, Inc.

Dr. Louis Sullivan, Secretary of HHS, endorses needle exchange program. (1989). *New York Times*, 9 March, p. 9.

Durant, R. F. and Diehl, P. F. (1989). Agendas, alternatives, and public policy: Lessons from the U.S. foreign policy arena. *Journal of Public Policy 9*(2), 179, 205.

Elmore, R. F. (1979–1980). Backward mapping: Implementation research and policy decisions. *Political Science Quarterly 94*(4), 601.

Elovich, R. and Sorge, R. (1991). Toward a community-based needle exchange for New York City. *AIDS & Public Policy Journal 6*(4), 165, 172.

Evans, H. Needle exchange program is still mostly in vain. (1988a). *New York Daily News*, 28 December, p. A–1.

Evans, H. New assault on AIDS. (1988b). *New York Daily News,* 6 November, pp. F–13, 14.

Fact Sheet on the Netherlands. (1989). Rijswijk: Ministry of Welfare, Health and Cultural Affairs.

Fact Sheet: Tacoma-Pierce County, Washington State. (1992). Tacoma, WA: Tacoma-Pierce County Chamber of Commerce.

Ginzburg, H. M. (1989). Needle exchange programs: A medical or a policy dilemma? *American Journal of Public Health 79*(10), 1350, 1351.

Goldman, J. J. Twin epidemics in NY linked by addict's needle. (1987). *Los Angeles Times,* 16 February, p. B–12.

Gonzalez, D. (1992). Where children live in fear: Life in Red Hook, Brooklyn. *The New York Times,* 20 December, p. 16.

Goulet, C., Polomeno, V., Laizner, A. M., Marcil, I., and Lang, A. (2003). Translation and validation of a French version of Brown's Support Behaviors Inventory in Perinatal Health. *Western Journal of Nursing Research 25*(5), 561–582.

Grund, J. C., Kaplan, C. D., and Adriaans, N. F.P. (1991). Needle sharing in the Netherlands: An ethnographic analysis. *American Journal of Public Health 8*(12), 1602–1607.

Heidenheimer, A. J., Heclo, H., and Adams, C. T. (1983). *Comparative Public Policy* (2nd ed.). New York: St. Martin's Press.

Huntington, S. (1968). *Political Order in Changing Societies.* New Haven, CT: Yale University Press.

Inciardi, J. A. (1990). AIDS, a strange disease of uncertain origins. *American Behavioral Scientist 33*(4), 97–407.

Joseph, S. C. and Des Jarlais, D. C. (1989). *AIDS Updates 2*(5), 1, 8.

Judge acquits 4. (1991). *New York Times,* 8 November, p. 7.

Kennedy, E. and Charles, S. C. (1997). *Authority.* New York: Simon & Schuster.

King, W. Making a point. (1988). *Seattle Times,* 10 August, p. F–8.

Kingdon, J. W. (1995). *Agendas, Alternatives, and Public Policies* (2nd ed.). Boston: Little, Brown and Company.

Leininger, M. M. (Ed.). (1991). *Culture Care Diversity & Universality: A Theory of Nursing.* New York: National League for Nursing Press.

Lerner, A. W. and Wanat, J. (1983). Fuzziness and bureaucracy. *Public Administration Review,* November–December, pp. 500, 509.

Lijphart, A. (1974). The comparative method and methodological developments. In L. Cantori (Ed.). *Comparative Political Systems.* Boston: Holbrook Press.

Lipsky, M. (1980). *Street-Level Bureaucracy.* New York: Russel Sage Foundation.

Manhattan Criminal Court Judge Laura E. Drager. (1991). *New York Times,* 26 June, p. 1.

Maples, P. Needle exchange gains backing in AIDS fight. (1991). *Dallas Morning News,* 18 August, p. E–13.

Mazmanian, D. A. and Sabatier, P. A. (1983). *Implementation and Public Policy.* Dallas, TX: Scott, Foresman & Company.

McLuhan, M. and Fiore, Q. (1968). *War and Peace in the Global Village.* New York: McGraw-Hill.

Mechanic, D. (1990). Improving health status through health policy: An agenda for nursing leaders. In *Nursing Leadership: Global Strategies*, C. M. Fagin (Ed.). New York: National League for Nursing, pp. 181–188.

Milstead, J. A. (1997). A social mandate: APN leadership for the whole policy process. *Advanced Practice Nursing Quarterly 3*(3), 1, 8.

Milstead, J. A. (1993). The advancement of policy implementation theory: An analysis of three needle exchange programs (Doctoral dissertation). University of Georgia, Athens.

Mohr, L. B. (1980). *Impact Analysis for Program Evaluation*. Chicago: The Dorsey Press.

National Commission on AIDS. (1991, July). Report: The twin epidemics of substance use and HIV. Washington, DC: U.S. Government Printing Office.

Nicholson, J. Rangel blasts city's needle program. (1988). *New York Post*, 9 November, p. G–1.

Needle swap program gaining favor. (1991). *New York Times*, 30 October, p. 16.

New York State AIDS official Dr. Don C. Des Jarlais. (1988). *New York Times*, 6 June, p. 3.

New York State Assembly's Republican minority. (1988). *New York Times*, 18 February, p. 1.

New York State Health Commissioner Dr. David Axelrod says. (1988). *New York Times*, 15 March, p. 5.

Odyssee Information: Drugs and Relief Operations in Rotterdam. (1992). Amsterdam: ROTOR Offsetdruk BV.

Pressman, J. and Wildavsky, A. B. (1973). *Implementation: How Great Expectations in Washington are Dashed in Oakland; Or, Why It's Amazing That Federal Programs Work at all*. Berkeley: University of California Press.

Private Drug Abuse Agency. (1988). *New York Times*, 8 January, p. 1.

Pye, L. and Verba, S. (Eds.). (1965). *Political Culture and Political Development*. Princeton, NJ: Princeton University Press.

Quade, E. S. (1982). *Analysis for Public Decision* (2nd ed.). New York: North Holland.

Rose, R. (1991). What is lesson-drawing? *Journal of Public Policy 11*(1), 3–30.

Rosenwald, L. Tacoma man supplies syringes free of charge to drug abusers. (1989). *The Spokesman-Review* [Spokane, WA], 1 January. Accessed NewsBank, Health, 1989, fiche 1, grid C11.

Ross, C. A. (2002). Building bridges to promote globalization in nursing: The development of a Hermanamiento. *Journal of Transcultural Nursing 11*(1), 64–67.

Rossi, P. H. and Freeman, H. E. (1995). *Evaluation a Systematic Approach* (5th ed.). Beverly Hills, CA: Sage Publications.

Schneider, A. and Ingram, H. (1990). Behavioral assumptions of policy tools. *Journal of Politics 52*(2), 510–529.

Shatzkin, K. A coming of age for needle exchange. (1990a). *Seattle* [WA] *Times*, 12 October. Accessed NewsBank, Health, 1990, fiche 111, grid A9.

Shatzkin, K. Tacoma needle exchanges ruled legal. (1990b). *Seattle* [WA] *Times*, 17 February, pp. A1, A5.

Tacoma supports needle exchange to combat AIDS. (1989). *Seattle* [WA] *Independent*, 5 January, p. 1.

Thomas, S. B. and Quinn, S. C. (1991). The Tuskegee syphilis study, 1932 to 1972: Implications for HIV education and AIDS risk reduction education programs in the black community. *American Journal of Public Health 8*(11), 1498–1505.

Van Meter, D. S. and Van Horn, C. (1975). The policy implementation process: A conceptual framework. *Administration and Society 6*(2), 455–468.

Villarruel, A. M., Gallegos, E. C., Cherry, C. J., and Refugio de Duran, M. (2003). La uniendo de fronteras: Collaboration to develop HIV prevention strategies for Mexican and Latino youth. *Journal of Transcultural Nursing 14*(3), 193–206.

Watzlawick, R., Weakland, C. E., and Fisch, R. (1974). *Change.* New York: WW Norton Co.

Yanow, D. (1987). Criticism: What implementation research has not taught us. *Policy Studies Review 7*(2), 103.

Zonana, V. F. An activist group for the '80s aims to shame people into action. (1989). *The Los Angeles Times,* 4 April. Accessed NewsBank, Health, 1989, fiche 42, grid G1-2.

Index